BEYOND MYALGIC EN
CHRONIC FATIGUE SYNDROME

Redefining an Illness

Committee on the Diagnostic Criteria for
Myalgic Encephalomyelitis/Chronic Fatigue Syndrome

Board on the Health of Select Populations

INSTITUTE OF MEDICINE
OF THE NATIONAL ACADEMIES

THE NATIONAL ACADEMIES PRESS
Washington, D.C.
www.nap.edu

THE NATIONAL ACADEMIES PRESS 500 Fifth Street, NW Washington, DC 20001

NOTICE: The project that is the subject of this report was approved by the Governing Board of the National Research Council, whose members are drawn from the councils of the National Academy of Sciences, the National Academy of Engineering, and the Institute of Medicine. The members of the committee responsible for the report were chosen for their special competences and with regard for appropriate balance.

This study was supported by Contract No. HHSN263201200074I between the National Academy of Sciences and the National Institutes of Health. Any opinions, findings, conclusions, or recommendations expressed in this publication are those of the author(s) and do not necessarily reflect the views of the organizations or agencies that provided support for the project.

International Standard Book Number-13:   978-0-309-31689-7
International Standard Book Number-10:   0-309-31689-8
Library of Congress Control Number: 2015934699

Additional copies of this report are available for sale from the National Academies Press, 500 Fifth Street, NW, Keck 360, Washington, DC 20001; (800) 624-6242 or (202) 334-3313; http://www.nap.edu.

For more information about the Institute of Medicine, visit the IOM home page at: **www.iom.edu.**

The serpent has been a symbol of long life, healing, and knowledge among almost all cultures and religions since the beginning of recorded history. The serpent adopted as a logotype by the Institute of Medicine is a relief carving from ancient Greece, now held by the Staatliche Museen in Berlin.

Cover design by LeAnn Locher, LeAnn Locher & Associates.

Suggested citation: IOM (Institute of Medicine). 2015. *Beyond myalgic encephalomyelitis/chronic fatigue syndrome: Redefining an illness.* Washington, DC: The National Academies Press.

"Knowing is not enough; we must apply.
Willing is not enough; we must do."
—Goethe

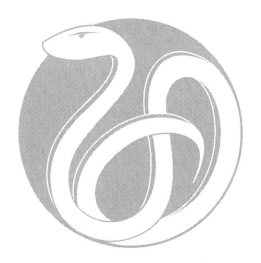

INSTITUTE OF MEDICINE
OF THE NATIONAL ACADEMIES

Advising the Nation. Improving Health.

THE NATIONAL ACADEMIES
Advisers to the Nation on Science, Engineering, and Medicine

The **National Academy of Sciences** is a private, nonprofit, self-perpetuating society of distinguished scholars engaged in scientific and engineering research, dedicated to the furtherance of science and technology and to their use for the general welfare. Upon the authority of the charter granted to it by the Congress in 1863, the Academy has a mandate that requires it to advise the federal government on scientific and technical matters. Dr. Ralph J. Cicerone is president of the National Academy of Sciences.

The **National Academy of Engineering** was established in 1964, under the charter of the National Academy of Sciences, as a parallel organization of outstanding engineers. It is autonomous in its administration and in the selection of its members, sharing with the National Academy of Sciences the responsibility for advising the federal government. The National Academy of Engineering also sponsors engineering programs aimed at meeting national needs, encourages education and research, and recognizes the superior achievements of engineers. Dr. C. D. Mote, Jr., is president of the National Academy of Engineering.

The **Institute of Medicine** was established in 1970 by the National Academy of Sciences to secure the services of eminent members of appropriate professions in the examination of policy matters pertaining to the health of the public. The Institute acts under the responsibility given to the National Academy of Sciences by its congressional charter to be an adviser to the federal government and, upon its own initiative, to identify issues of medical care, research, and education. Dr. Victor J. Dzau is president of the Institute of Medicine.

The **National Research Council** was organized by the National Academy of Sciences in 1916 to associate the broad community of science and technology with the Academy's purposes of furthering knowledge and advising the federal government. Functioning in accordance with general policies determined by the Academy, the Council has become the principal operating agency of both the National Academy of Sciences and the National Academy of Engineering in providing services to the government, the public, and the scientific and engineering communities. The Council is administered jointly by both Academies and the Institute of Medicine. Dr. Ralph J. Cicerone and Dr. C. D. Mote, Jr., are chair and vice chair, respectively, of the National Research Council.

www.national-academies.org

Reviewers

This report has been reviewed in draft form by individuals chosen for their diverse perspectives and technical expertise, in accordance with procedures approved by the National Research Council's Report Review Committee. The purpose of this independent review is to provide candid and critical comments that will assist the institution in making its published report as sound as possible and to ensure that the report meets institutional standards for objectivity, evidence, and responsiveness to the study charge. The review comments and draft manuscript remain confidential to protect the integrity of the deliberative process. We wish to thank the following individuals for their review of this report:

Italo Biaggioni, Vanderbilt University
Susan Cockshell, University of Adelaide
Stephen Gluckman, University of Pennsylvania
Maureen R. Hanson, Cornell University
Ben Katz, Ann and Robert H. Lurie Children's Hospital of Chicago
Charles Lapp, Hunter-Hopkins Center, P.A.
Michael L. LeFevre, University of Missouri School of Medicine
Susan Levine, Medical Office of Susan M. Levine
Jose Montoya, Stanford University Medical Center
Daniel Peterson, Sierra Internal Medicine
Michael I. Posner, University of Oregon
Katherine Rowe, Royal Children's Hospital
Christopher Snell, University of the Pacific

Rudd Vermeulen, CFS/ME Medical Centre
Yasuyoshi Watanabe, RIKEN Center for Life Science Technologies

Although the reviewers listed above provided many constructive comments and suggestions, they were not asked to endorse the report's conclusions or recommendations, nor did they see the final draft of the report before its release. The review of this report was overseen by **David Challoner,** University of Florida, and **Georges Benjamin,** American Public Health Association. Appointed by the Institute of Medicine, they were responsible for making certain that an independent examination of this report was carried out in accordance with institutional procedures and that all review comments were carefully considered. Responsibility for the final content of this report rests entirely with the authoring committee and the institution.

Contents

Boxes, Figures, and Tables

BOXES

FIGURES

xiii

TABLES

Preface

This study was sponsored by the U.S. Department of Health and Human Services Office on Women's Health, the National Institutes of Health, the Centers for Disease Control and Prevention (CDC), the Food and Drug Administration, the Agency for Healthcare Research and Quality, and the Social Security Administration, and conducted by a committee convened by the Institute of Medicine (IOM). The committee was asked to define diagnostic criteria for myalgic encephalomyelitis/chronic fatigue syndrome, to propose a process for reevaluation of these criteria in the future, and to consider whether a new name for this disease is warranted. The committee carefully reviewed the peer-reviewed literature on the multifaceted manifestations of this disease, and taking into account the clearly expressed views of hundreds of patients and their advocates, developed evidence-informed diagnostic criteria for this complex, multisystem, frequently undiagnosed, and often life-altering condition. The committee was able to redefine the diagnostic criteria for this disease so that they are easy to understand and apply and capture the essence of the disease's unique symptomatology. The committee recommends an evidence-based, disinterested procedure by which these criteria can be refined in the future on the basis of new research.

Listening to the comments and testimony provided for this study, as well as examining advocacy websites and the *Voice of the Patient* report, the committee determined that the name "chronic fatigue syndrome" has done a disservice to many patients and that the name "myalgic encephalomyelitis" does not accurately describe the major features of the disease. In their place, the committee proposes "systemic exertion intolerance disease" as a name that better captures the full scope of this disorder.

The committee owes a debt of gratitude to all of those who volunteered their time and shared their expertise by presenting at its public meetings, including Dr. Sara Eggers, Dr. Leonard A. Jason, Dr. Akifumi Kishi, Dr. Gudrun Lange, Dr. Nancy Lee, Dr. Susan Maier, and Dr. Elizabeth Unger. The committee also thanks all the patient advocates who spoke during its public sessions, including Lori Chapo-Kroger, Carol Head, Gabby Klein, Joseph Landson, Pat LaRosa, Denise Lopez-Majano, Robert Miller, Charmian Proskauer, Jennie Spotila, and Annette Whittemore. Collectively, the wide variety of viewpoints expressed by these speakers provided valuable insight into the complexity of the disease and helped the committee develop its approach to and thought process regarding its statement of task.

The committee wishes to express its sincere appreciation to National Academies Research Center staff Daniel Bearss and Rebecca Morgan for their support with the comprehensive literature review conducted for this study. The evidence reviewed was enriched by research materials shared by agencies and organizations such as the CDC Multi-Site Clinical Study of CFS, Chronic Fatigue Initiative, Massachusetts CFIDS/ME & FM Association, PANDORA Org, Phoenix Rising, Solve ME/CFS Initiative, and by researchers and advocates, including Dr. Byron Hyde, Dr. Leonard Jason, Dr. Lisa Petrison, Dr. Suzanne Vernon, Mary Dimmock, Denise Lopez-Majano, Courtney Miller, and Jennie Spotila. The committee is extremely grateful for these contributions.

The committee also is grateful to the study consultants: Rona Briere for copyediting the report; René Gonin for his support in interpreting the methodology of relevant literature; LeAnn Locher for designing the cover of the report; and Troy Petenbrink, who provided his expertise in health communications to help the committee develop a dissemination plan for the recommendations in this report.

The committee could not have done its work without the extraordinary efforts of the staff of the IOM, including Carmen Mundaca-Shah, study director; Kate Meck, associate program officer; Jonathan Schmelzer, research associate; and Adriana Moya and Sulvia Doja, senior program assistants. Their work was invaluable.

Finally, the committee would like to offer its profound thanks to the many patients and advocates who offered their knowledge, experiences, and feedback to inform its work throughout the study process. The success of this project is directly related to the support and assistance received from those passionate about this topic. The committee's goal in addressing this task was to ensure that these patients receive the diagnoses and treatment they require and deserve. It is to them and to their return to health that this work is dedicated.

Ellen Wright Clayton, *Chair*
Committee on the Diagnostic Criteria for
Myalgic Encephalomyelitis/Chronic Fatigue Syndrome

Acronyms and Abbreviations

5-HT	5 hydroxytryptamine
5-HTT	serotonin transporter
17-OHP	17-hydroxyprogesterone
A4	androstenedione
AAMC	Association of American Medical Colleges
ACR	American College of Rheumatology
ACTH	adrenocorticotropin hormone
ADH	antidiuretic hormone
AHRQ	Agency for Healthcare Research and Quality
AIDS	acquired immune deficiency syndrome
ANA	antinuclear antibody
ANT	Attention Network Test
ASP	Autonomic Symptom Profile
AVP	arginine vasopressin
B.	Borrelia
BMI	body mass index
BPI	Brief Pain Inventory
bpm	beats per minute
CANTAB	Cambridge Neuropsychological Test Automated Battery
CART	classification and regression tree
CBT	cognitive-behavioral therapy
CCC	Canadian Consensus Criteria

CDC	Centers for Disease Control and Prevention
CFIDS	chronic fatigue and immune dysfunction syndrome
CFS	chronic fatigue syndrome
CFSAC	Chronic Fatigue Syndrome Advisory Committee
CHF	congestive heart failure
CHQ	Child Health Questionnaire
CMV	cytomegalovirus
COMPASS	Composite Autonomic Symptom Score
CPAP	continuous positive airway pressure
CPET	cardiopulmonary exercise test
CRH	corticotropin-releasing hormone
CVDB	Chronic Viral Diseases Branch
DHEA	dehydroepiandrosterone
DPHQ	DePaul Pediatric Health Questionnaire
dsDNA	double-stranded deoxyribonucleic acid
DSM	*Diagnostic and Statistical Manual of Mental Disorders*
EBV	Epstein-Barr virus
EDS	Ehlers-Danlos syndrome
EEG	electroencephalogram
ELISA	enzyme-linked immunosorbent assay
FDA	Food and Drug Administration
FDI	Functional Disability Inventory
FIQ	Fibromyalgia Impact Questionnaire
FIQR	Revised Fibromyalgia Impact Questionnaire
FM	fibromyalgia
fMRI	functional magnetic resonance imaging
FMS	fibromyalgia syndrome
GAO	Government Accountability Office[1]
HC	healthy control
HD	hemodialysis
HepC	chronic hepatitis C
HHS	Department of Health and Human Services
HHV	human herpes virus
HIV	human immunodeficiency virus
HPA	hypothalamic-pituitary-adrenal (axis)
HRQOL	health-related quality of life

---

[1]Known as General Accounting Office until 2004.

HTLV	human T-cell lymphotropic virus
IACFS/ME	International Association for Chronic Fatigue Syndrome/ Myalgic Encephalomyelitis
IADL	instrumental activity of daily living
IBS	irritable bowel syndrome
ICD-10	*International Classification of Diseases* (Tenth Revision)
IDEA	Individuals with Disabilities Education Act
IFA	immunofluorescence assay
IGF-1	insulin-like growth factor 1
IGFBP-1	insulin-like growth factor-binding protein 1
IgG	immunoglobulin G
IgM	immunoglobulin M
IL	interleukin
IOM	Institute of Medicine
IVIG	intravenous immunoglobulin
JAK-STAT	Janus kinase/signal transducer and activator of transcription
LBNP	lower-body negative pressure
LDST	low-dose synacthen test
MCS	multiple chemical sensitivity
MD	major depression
MDI	medically determinable impairment
ME	myalgic encephalomyelitis
ME-ICC	International Consensus Criteria for ME
MOS	Medical Outcomes Study
MPS	myofascial pain syndrome
MRI	magnetic resonance imaging
MRS	magnetic resonance spectroscopy
MS	multiple sclerosis
MSD	musculoskeletal disease
MSIDS	multi-systemic infectious disease syndrome
MSLT	multiple sleep latency test
NICE	British National Institute for Health and Clinical Excellence
NIH	National Institutes of Health
NK	natural killer
NKCS	nature killer cells syndrome
NMH	neurally mediated hypotension

NREM   non-rapid eye movement
NYHA   New York Heart Association Functional Classification

ODP   Office of Disease Prevention
OFFER   Organization for Fatigue & Fibromyalgia Education &
                Research
OGS   Orthostatic Grading Scale
OH   orthostatic hypotension
OHQ   Orthostatic Hypotension Questionnaire
ORWH   Office of Research on Women's Health
OWH   Office on Women's Health

P2P   Pathways to Prevention
PANDORA   Patient Alliance for Neuro-endocrine-immune Disorders
                Organization for Research and Advocacy
PASAT   Paced Auditory Serial Addition Test
PBL   peripheral blood lymphocyte
PBMC   peripheral blood mononuclear cell
PCOCA   Patient-Centered Outreach and Communication Activity
PCP   primary care provider
PCR   polymerase chain reaction
Peds QL   Pediatrics Quality of Life Inventory
PEM   post-exertional malaise
PENE   post-exertional neuroimmune exhaustion
PET   positron emission tomography
POTS   postural orthostatic tachycardia syndrome
PPS   post-polio syndrome
PROMIS   Patient-Reported Outcomes Measurement Information
                System
PSG   polysomnography
PSQI   Pittsburgh Sleep Quality Index
PTSD   posttraumatic stress disorder

QOL   quality of life
QUADAS   Quality Assessment of Diagnostic Accuracy Studies (tool)

RA   rheumatoid arthritis
REM   rapid eye movement
RNA   ribonucleic acid
RP   role-physical

SAHS   sleep apnea/hypopnea syndrome
SDB   sleep disordered breathing

SEID	systemic exertion intolerance disease
SF-36	Short Form 36-Item Questionnaire
SI	Symptom Inventory
SIP-ab	Sickness Impact Profile-alertness behavior
SSA	Social Security Administration
SSc	scleroderma/systemic sclerosis
SWS	slow wave sleep
TMJ	temporomandibular joint syndrome
TNF	tumor necrosis factor
TPRI	total peripheral resistance index
TSH	thyroid-stimulating hormone
VAS	visual analog scale
VCA	viral capsid antigen
VT	vitality (subscale of the MOS SF-36)
WMS-R	Wechsler Memory Scale-Revised
WSAS	Work and Social Adjustment Scale

Summary

Myalgic encephalomyelitis (ME) and chronic fatigue syndrome (CFS) are serious, debilitating conditions that impose a burden of illness on millions of people in the United States and around the world. Somewhere between 836,000 and 2.5 million Americans are estimated to have these disorders (Jason et al., 1999, 2006b). The cause of ME/CFS remains unknown, although in many cases, symptoms may have been triggered by an infection or other prodromal event, such as "immunization, anesthetics, physical trauma, exposure to environmental pollutants, chemicals and heavy metals, and rarely blood transfusions" (Carruthers and van de Sande, 2005, p. 1). Over a period of decades, clinicians and researchers developed separate case definitions and diagnostic criteria for ME and CFS, although the terms denote conditions with similar symptoms. The literature analysis conducted in support of this study took into consideration the variability in the definitions used in the studies reviewed. For the purposes of this report, the umbrella term "ME/CFS" is used to refer to both conditions.

Diagnosing ME/CFS in the clinical setting remains a challenge. Patients often struggle with their illness for years before receiving a diagnosis, and an estimated 84 to 91 percent of patients affected by ME/CFS are not yet diagnosed (Jason et al., 2006b; Solomon and Reeves, 2004). In multiple surveys, 67 to 77 percent of patients have reported that it took longer than 1 year to get a diagnosis, and about 29 percent have reported that it took longer than 5 years (CFIDS Association of America, 2014; ProHealth, 2008). Seeking and receiving a diagnosis can be a frustrating process for several reasons, including skepticism of health care providers about the serious nature of ME/CFS and the misconception that it is a psychogenic illness or even a figment of the patient's imagination. Less than one-third of medical schools include ME/CFS-specific information in the curriculum (Peterson et al., 2013), and only 40 percent of medical textbooks include information on the disorder (Jason et al., 2010). ME/CFS often is seen as a diagnosis of exclusion, which also can lead to delays in diagnosis or to misdiagnosis of a psychological problem (Bayliss et al., 2014; Fossey et al., 2004; Jason and Richman, 2008). Once diagnosed, patients frequently complain that their health care providers do not know how to deliver appropriate care for their condition, and often subject them to treatment strategies that exacerbate their symptoms.

ME/CFS can cause significant impairment and disability that have negative economic consequences at both the individual and the societal level. At least one-quarter of ME/CFS patients are house- or bedbound at some point in their lives (Marshall et al., 2011; NIH, 2011; Shepherd and Chaudhuri, 2001). The direct and indirect economic costs of ME/CFS to society have been estimated at $17 to $24 billion annually (Jason et al., 2008), $9.1 billion of which has been attributed to lost household and labor force productivity (Reynolds et al., 2004). High medical costs combined with reduced earning capacity often have devastating effects on patients' financial status.

Literature on mortality associated with ME/CFS is sparse. One study found that cancer, heart disease, and suicide are the most common causes of death among those diagnosed with ME/CFS, and people with ME/CFS die from these causes at younger ages than others in the general population. However, the authors note that these results cannot be generalized to the overall population of ME/CFS patients because of the methodological limitations of the study (Jason et al., 2006a).

CONTEXT FOR THIS STUDY

This study was sponsored by the Office on Women's Health within the Department of Health and Human Services (HHS), the National Institutes of Health (NIH), the Centers for Disease Control and Prevention (CDC), the Food and Drug Administration, the Agency for Healthcare Research and Quality, and the Social Security Administration. The study was commissioned in response to a recommendation from HHS's Chronic Fatigue Syndrome Advisory Committee (CFSAC), which comprises 11 voting members, including the chair, who provide advice and recommendations to the Secretary of HHS on issues related to ME/CFS. In 2012, the CFSAC recommended that HHS "promptly convene . . . at least one stakeholders' (ME/CFS experts, patients, advocates) workshop in consultation with CFSAC members to reach a consensus for a case definition useful for research, diagnosis and treatment of ME/CFS beginning with the 2003

Canadian Consensus Definition for discussion purposes."[1] Given the well-established and well-regarded consensus process used by the Institute of Medicine (IOM), HHS contracted with the IOM in September 2013 to conduct this study.

In the weeks that followed, many advocates were greatly disappointed that HHS did not follow the CFSAC's specific recommendation. Patients, advocates, researchers, and clinicians expressed strong opposition to the study, arguing that the IOM lacks the expertise to develop clinical case definitions and that the inclusion of non-ME/CFS experts in this process would move the science backward. An open letter was sent to the Secretary of HHS, signed by 38 U.S.-based biomedical researchers and clinicians, declaring that consensus had been reached on the use of the Canadian clinical case definition (often called the Canadian Consensus Criteria [CCC]) for diagnosis of ME/CFS, and requesting that the IOM study be canceled and the funds used to support further ME/CFS research instead (An Open Letter, 2013).

CHARGE TO THE COMMITTEE

To conduct this study, the IOM convened the Committee on the Diagnostic Criteria for Myalgic Encephalomyelitis/Chronic Fatigue Syndrome. The HHS sponsors charged the committee with evaluating the current criteria for diagnosis of ME/CFS and recommending clinical diagnostic criteria that would address the needs of health care providers, patients, and their caregivers. Specifically, the committee was asked to

- conduct a study to identify the evidence for various clinical diagnostic criteria for ME/CFS using a process with input from stakeholders, including practicing clinicians and patients;
- develop evidence-based clinical diagnostic criteria for ME/CFS for use by clinicians, using a consensus-building methodology;
- recommend whether new terminology for ME/CFS should be adopted; and
- develop an outreach strategy for disseminating the new criteria nationwide to health professionals.

The committee was also asked to distinguish among disease subgroups, develop a plan for updating the new criteria, and make recommendations for the plan's implementation. The statement of task requested that the committee's recommendations consider unique diagnostic issues facing people

---

[1] CFSAC recommendations can be accessed at http://www.hhs.gov/advcomcfs/recommendations/10032012.html (accessed January 13, 2015).

with ME/CFS, related specifically to gender and particular subgroups with substantial disability and extending across the life span. The committee was not asked to investigate the etiology, pathophysiology, pathogenesis, or treatment of ME/CFS. The complete statement of task is provided in Chapter 1.

THE COMMITTEE'S APPROACH

The Committee on the Diagnostic Criteria for Myalgic Encephalo-myelitis/Chronic Fatigue Syndrome comprised 15 members with expertise in clinical care for ME/CFS, pediatrics, infectious disease, epidemiology, immunology, rheumatology, behavioral health, pain, sleep, primary care, genetics, exercise physiology, neurology/neuropathology, clinical case definitions, and consensus processes. In addition to their scientific expertise, two committee members are or have been patients, and one is a family member/caregiver of a patient with ME/CFS.

The committee engaged in a number of activities to inform its work:

- The committee heard testimony, primarily from patients and advocates, on two occasions. The agendas for these sessions are provided in Appendix A.
- The committee carefully considered hundreds of public comments submitted through its public portal for this study.[2]
- The committee heard testimony from selected experts in this field (see Appendix A).
- The committee conducted a comprehensive literature review. The review included a search of eight databases for all articles published since 1950 related to ME, CFS, ME/CFS, and other terms used to describe this disorder (criteria for the literature search are presented in Chapter 1). Additional citations and grey literature (i.e., non-commercially published) were identified by the IOM staff, committee members, and the public and from references in pertinent articles. After a preliminary review of the literature, the committee directed the IOM staff to divide the articles into topics most central to its work: eight symptoms or symptom categories (for children/adolescents and adults) and three additional topics. For some of these topics, the committee reviewed abstracts of all of the relevant literature. For other topics, the committee developed specific questions with inclusion/exclusion criteria, which the IOM staff used to exclude irrelevant abstracts. In all cases, research groups of two

---

[2] Public testimony and other materials submitted to the committee are available by request through the National Academies' Public Access Records Office.

to five committee members assigned to each topic reviewed the abstracts to determine which articles were pertinent to the committee's charge. These groups then read the full text of these articles, extracting their findings and using an adapted "GRADE grid" to record judgments as to whether there was sufficient evidence that certain symptoms and abnormalities define either ME/CFS or a particular subtype of the disorder (see Appendix B for the grid template) (Guyatt et al., 2008; Jaeschke et al., 2008).

- The committee received and considered preliminary findings from CDC's ongoing Multi-Site Clinical Assessment of CFS. The committee was unable, however, to obtain input from NIH's Evidence-based Methodology Workshop for ME/CFS until after this study was concluded.

- The committee consulted with a health communications specialist and a statistician to obtain additional expertise in addressing the statement of task.

In deliberating on its recommendations, the committee carefully considered the above sources of information. The collated judgments were used to facilitate discussion. Final recommendations regarding diagnostic criteria were made by consensus after deliberation by the committee as a whole.

OVERVIEW OF THE REPORT

Chapters 1 through 3 of this report summarize the history and background of ME/CFS and compare various existing definitions and terminology for the disorder proposed to date. They also address the extensive concerns that have been raised by patients and advocates regarding public perceptions of this disorder, in particular the term "chronic fatigue syndrome." Chapters 4 and 5 review the scientific evidence to identify which symptoms are necessary to diagnose this disease. Chapter 6 examines this evidence further with a particular focus on pediatrics. Chapter 7 presents the committee's recommendations, including new diagnostic criteria and a new name for ME/CFS, and operationalizes the new criteria. Finally, Chapter 8 details a dissemination strategy for the committee's recommendations.

RECOMMENDATIONS

The primary message of this report is that ME/CFS is a serious, chronic, complex, and systemic disease that frequently and dramatically limits the activities of affected patients. In its most severe form, this disease can consume the lives of those whom it afflicts. It is "real." It is not appropriate to dismiss these patients by saying, "I am chronically fatigued, too."

BOX S-1
Proposed Diagnostic Criteria for ME/CFS

Diagnosis requires that the patient have the following three symptoms:

1. A substantial reduction or impairment in the ability to engage in pre-illness levels of occupational, educational, social, or personal activities that persists for more than 6 months and is accompanied by fatigue, which is often profound, is of new or definite onset (not lifelong), is not the result of ongoing excessive exertion, and is not substantially alleviated by rest,
2. Post-exertional malaise,* and
3. Unrefreshing sleep*

At least one of the two following manifestations is also required:

1. Cognitive impairment* or
2. Orthostatic intolerance

---

* Frequency and severity of symptoms should be assessed. The diagnosis of ME/CFS should be questioned if patients do not have these symptoms at least half of the time with moderate, substantial, or severe intensity.

Based on a comprehensive review of the evidence and input from the patient, advocacy, and research communities, the committee decided that new diagnostic criteria (see Box S-1), which are more focused on the central symptoms of ME/CFS than many other definitions, are warranted for this disorder. These more focused diagnostic criteria will make it easier for clinicians to recognize and accurately diagnose these patients in a timelier manner. These new criteria led the committee to create the diagnostic algorithm shown in Figure S-1.

The committee weighed several factors in reaching consensus on these diagnostic criteria: (1) the frequency and severity with which these symptoms were experienced by patients, (2) the strength of the scientific literature, and (3) the availability of objective measures supporting the association of particular symptoms with the diagnosis. Patient reports and symptom surveys as well as scientific evidence consistently showed that impaired function, post-exertional malaise (an exacerbation of some or all of an individual's ME/CFS symptoms after physical or cognitive exertion, or orthostatic stress that leads to a reduction in functional ability), and unrefreshing sleep are characteristic symptoms almost universally present

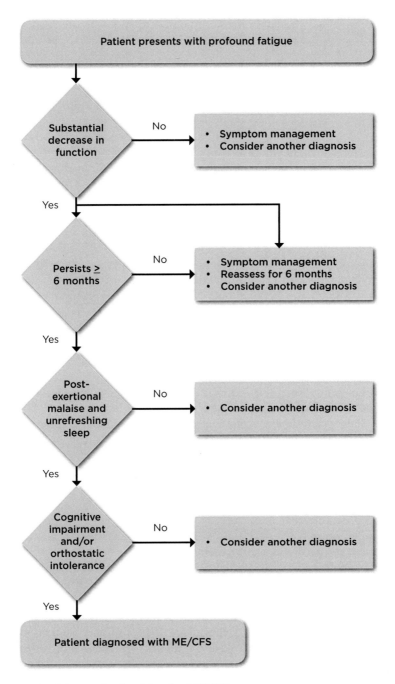

FIGURE S-1 Diagnostic algorithm for ME/CFS.

in ME/CFS; thus, the committee considered them to be core symptoms. The committee also found that cognitive impairment and orthostatic intolerance are frequently present in ME/CFS patients and have distinctive findings in these individuals that, particularly when viewed together with the core symptoms, distinguish ME/CFS from other fatiguing disorders. It is essential that clinicians assess the severity and duration of symptoms over an extended period of time because moderate or greater frequency and severity of symptoms are required to distinguish ME/CFS from other illnesses. Regarding the duration of the illness, the proposed criteria require 6 months to make a diagnosis in light of evidence that many other causes of similar fatigue do not last beyond 6 months (Jason et al., 2014; Nisenbaum et al., 1998).

The central point the committee wishes to emphasize is that ME/CFS is a diagnosis to be made. One of the committee's most important conclusions is that a thorough history, physical examination, and targeted work-up are necessary and often sufficient for diagnosis. The new criteria will allow a large percentage of undiagnosed patients to receive an accurate diagnosis and appropriate care. Patients who have not yet been symptomatic for 6 months should be followed over time to see whether they meet the criteria for ME/CFS at a later time. The committee emphasizes that although some patients previously diagnosed with ME/CFS may not meet the proposed criteria, clinicians should address their symptoms and concerns.

> **Recommendation 1: Physicians should diagnose myalgic encephalomyelitis/chronic fatigue syndrome if diagnostic criteria are met following an appropriate history, physical examination, and medical work-up. A new code should be assigned to this disorder in the *International Classification of Diseases*, Tenth Revision (ICD-10), that is not linked to "chronic fatigue" or "neurasthenia."**

To assist clinicians in making a diagnosis of ME/CFS, the committee developed a table that includes terms commonly used by patients to describe their symptoms; potential questions clinicians can use to elicit the presence of symptoms as well as their frequency and severity; in-office tests and observations that support the diagnosis; and more complex tests that may be helpful in cases of diagnostic uncertainty or long-term management (see Tables 7-1 and 7-2 in Chapter 7).

> **Recommendation 2: The Department of Health and Human Services should develop a toolkit appropriate for screening and diagnosing patients with myalgic encephalomyelitis/chronic fatigue syndrome in a wide array of clinical settings that commonly encounter these patients, including primary care practices, emergency departments, mental/behavioral health clinics, physical/occupational therapy units,**

and medical subspecialty services (e.g., rheumatology, infectious diseases, neurology).

CDC's *CFS Toolkit* (CDC, 2014) and the International Association for CFS/ME's *Primer for Clinical Practitioners* (IACFS/ME, 2014) may be potential places to start, but both need updating in a number of areas in light of the findings presented in this report. The development of clinical questionnaire or history tools that are valid across populations of patients and readily usable in the clinical environment should be an urgent priority. The DePaul Symptom Questionnaire, which has been used extensively in research (DePaul Research Team, 2010), as well as CDC's Symptom Inventory (Wagner et al., 2008), may provide a solid basis from which to begin developing questionnaires and interview guides that can be validated for clinical use.

It has become increasingly clear that many patients with ME/CFS have other disorders as well, some of which—including fibromyalgia, irritable bowel syndrome, metabolic syndrome, sleep disorders, and depression—may have symptoms that overlap with those of ME/CFS (Buchwald and Garrity, 1994; Johnson et al., 1996; Maloney et al., 2010). Some of these other disorders may develop in response to the burdens of this disorder. The committee decided against developing a comprehensive list of potential comorbid conditions, but it does point to conditions identified by the ME-International Consensus Criteria (Carruthers et al., 2011) and the CCC (Carruthers et al., 2003). The committee recognizes that diagnosis and treatment of comorbid conditions is necessary when caring for patients.

> Recommendation 3: A multidisciplinary group should reexamine the diagnostic criteria set forth in this report when firm evidence supports modification to improve the identification or care of affected individuals. Such a group should consider, in no more than 5 years, whether modification of the criteria is necessary. Funding for this update effort should be provided by nonconflicted sources, such as the Agency for Healthcare Research and Quality through its Evidence-based Practice Centers process, and foundations.

Although there was sufficient evidence with which to carry out the first steps of its task, the committee was struck by the relative paucity of research on ME/CFS conducted to date. Remarkably little research funding has been made available to study the etiology, pathophysiology, and effective treatment of this disease, especially given the number of people afflicted. Thus, the committee was unable to define subgroups of patients or even to clearly define the natural history of the disease. More research is essential.

Future diagnostic research will be most instructive when protocols include patients identified using the committee's proposed diagnostic criteria as well as patients with other complex fatiguing disorders. Almost all of the studies conducted to date have compared patients with ME/CFS with healthy controls rather than with patients with these other fatiguing disorders. As a result, there is a paucity of data to guide clinicians in distinguishing among these disorders, a gap that urgently needs to be filled.

Finding the cause of and cure for ME/CFS may require research that enlists large numbers of patients with this disorder from which important subsets can be identified in terms of disease symptomatology, responses to physical and cognitive stressors, brain imaging, the microbiome, virology, immune function, and gene expression. Integrative approaches using systems biology may be useful in unraveling illness triggers. Studies aimed at assessing the natural history of the disease and its temporal characteristics (onset, duration, severity, recovery, and functional deficits) are essential for a better understanding of ME/CFS.

It is encouraging to note that progress already is being made in understanding the etiology, natural history, pathophysiology, and effective treatment of ME/CFS using a variety of physiological and molecular methods. Several large cohort studies are now under way. The committee expects that this research will lead to findings that can be used to further refine the diagnosis of this disorder and the elaboration of clinically pertinent subtypes. As a result, the committee calls for a reevaluation of the evidence in no more than 5 years using the methods recommended in the IOM report *Clinical Practice Guidelines We Can Trust* (IOM, 2011).

The criteria proposed here will not improve the diagnosis and care of patients unless health care providers use them. The committee developed an outreach strategy for disseminating the clinical diagnostic criteria resulting from this study nationwide to health care professionals so that patients will receive this diagnosis in an accurate and timely manner. The committee believes that focusing dissemination efforts on reaching primary care and other providers who encounter these patients will increase awareness of and familiarity with the new criteria in a way that will be most beneficial to patients with ME/CFS.

Despite misconceptions about ME/CFS and other barriers to its accurate diagnosis among health care professionals, it is important that the dissemination of the new diagnostic criteria proposed in this report build on previous efforts that have helped increase awareness of ME/CFS among health professionals and the public. Key to this effort will be the continued positioning of ME/CFS as a legitimate disease that occurs in both children and adults and should be properly diagnosed and treated. As the dissemination strategy is implemented, it will also be important for HHS to include an evaluation component to monitor progress. The evaluation should encompass both quantitative and qualitative measures.

The committee devoted significant effort to the question of whether a new name for this disorder is warranted, heeding both the clear call by patients and advocates as well as the sponsors' request. The committee was swayed by the commonly expressed view of patients that the term "chronic fatigue syndrome" has led to misperceptions on the part of clinicians and the public. The committee deemed the term "myalgic encephalomyelitis," although commonly endorsed by patients and advocates, to be inappropriate because of the general lack of evidence of brain inflammation in ME/CFS patients, as well as the less prominent role of myalgia in these patients relative to more core symptoms. The committee was convinced of the value of creating a name that conveys the central elements of this disease, a practice for which there is much precedent in medicine for disorders whose etiology or pathophysiology is not yet well understood. After extensive consideration, and being mindful of the concerns expressed by patients and their advocates, the committee recommends that the disorder described in this report be named "systemic exertion intolerance disease" (SEID). "Systemic exertion intolerance" captures the fact that exertion of any sort—physical, cognitive, emotional—can adversely affect these patients in many organ systems and in many aspects of their lives. The committee intends for this name to convey the complexity and severity of this disorder.

> **Recommendation 4: The committee recommends that this disorder be renamed "systemic exertion intolerance disease" (SEID). SEID should replace myalgic encephalomyelitis/chronic fatigue syndrome for patients who meet the criteria set forth in this report.**

In conclusion, the committee hopes that the diagnostic criteria set forth in this report, based on a comprehensive review of the literature, will promote the prompt diagnosis of patients with this complex, multisystem, and often devastating disorder; enhance public understanding; and provide a firm foundation for future improvements in diagnosis and treatment.

REFERENCES

An Open Letter. 2013. *An open letter to the honorable Kathleen Sebelius, U.S. Secretary of Health and Human Services*, September 23, 2013. https://dl.dropboxusercontent. com/u/89158245/Case%20Definition%20Letter%20Sept%2023%202013.pdf (accessed January 12, 2015).

Bayliss, K., M. Goodall, A. Chisholm, B. Fordham, C. Chew-Graham, L. Riste, L. Fisher, K. Lovell, S. Peters, and A. Wearden. 2014. Overcoming the barriers to the diagnosis and management of chronic fatigue syndrome/ME in primary care: A meta synthesis of qualitative studies. *BMC Family Practice* 15(1):44.

Buchwald, D., and D. Garrity. 1994. Comparison of patients with chronic fatigue syndrome, fibromyalgia, and multiple chemical sensitivities. *Archives of Internal Medicine* 154(18):2049-2053.

Carruthers, B. M., and M. I. van de Sande. 2005. *Myalgic encephalomyelitis/chronic fatigue syndrome: A clinical case definition and guidelines for medical practitioners: An overview of the Canadian consensus document.* Vancouver, BC: Carruthers and van de Sande.

Carruthers, B. M., A. K. Jain, K. L. De Meirleir, D. L. Peterson, N. G. Klimas, A. M. Lerner, A. C. Bested, P. Flor-Henry, P. Joshi, A. C. P. Powles, J. A. Sherkey, and M. I. van de Sande. 2003. Myalgic encephalomyelitis/chronic fatigue syndrome: Clinical working case definition, diagnostic and treatment protocols (Canadian case definition). *Journal of Chronic Fatigue Syndrome* 11(1):7-115.

Carruthers, B. M., M. I. van de Sande, K. L. De Meirleir, N. G. Klimas, G. Broderick, T. Mitchell, D. Staines, A. C. P. Powles, N. Speight, R. Vallings, L. Bateman, B. Baumgarten-Austrheim, D. S. Bell, N. Carlo-Stella, J. Chia, A. Darragh, D. Jo, D. Lewis, A. R. Light, S. Marshall-Gradisbik, I. Mena, J. A. Mikovits, K. Miwa, M. Murovska, M. L. Pall, and S. Stevens. 2011. Myalgic encephalomyelitis: International consensus criteria. *Journal of Internal Medicine* 270(4):327-338.

CDC (Centers for Disease Control and Prevention). 2014. *CDC CFS toolkit.* http://www.cdc.gov/cfs/toolkit (accessed January 12, 2015).

CFIDS (Chronic Fatigue and Immune Dysfunction Syndrome) Association of America. 2014. *ME/CFS road to diagnosis survey.* Charlotte, NC: CFIDS Association of America.

DePaul Research Team. 2010. *DePaul Symptom Questionnaire.* http://condor.depaul.edu/ljason/cfs/measures.html (accessed August 20, 2014).

Fossey, M., E. Libman, S. Bailes, M. Baltzan, R. Schondorf, R. Amsel, and C. S. Fichten. 2004. Sleep quality and psychological adjustment in chronic fatigue syndrome. *Journal of Behavioral Medicine* 27(6):581-605.

Guyatt, G. H., A. D. Oxman, G. E. Vist, Y. Falck-Ytter, P. Alonso-Coello, and H. J. Schünemann. 2008. GRADE: An emerging consensus on rating quality of evidence and strength of recommendations. *British Medical Journal* 336.

IACFS/ME (International Association for Chronic Fatigue Syndrome/Myalgic Encephalomyelitis). 2014. *ME/CFS: Primer for clinical practitioners.* Chicago, IL: IACFS/ME.

IOM (Institute of Medicine). 2011. *Clinical practice guidelines we can trust.* Washington, DC: The National Academies Press.

Jaeschke, R., G. H. Guyatt, P. Dellinger, H. Schünemann, M. M. Levy, R. Kunz, S. Norris, and J. Bion. 2008. Use of GRADE grid to reach decisions on clinical practice guidelines when consensus is elusive. *British Medical Journal* 337:a744.

Jason, L. A., and J. A. Richman. 2008. How science can stigmatize: The case of chronic fatigue syndrome. *Journal of Chronic Fatigue Syndrome* 14(4):85-103.

Jason, L. A., J. A. Richman, A. W. Rademaker, K. M. Jordan, A. V. Plioplys, R. R. Taylor, W. McCready, C. F. Huang, and S. Plioplys. 1999. A community-based study of chronic fatigue syndrome. *Archives of Internal Medicine* 159(18):2129-2137.

Jason, L., K. Corradi, S. Gress, S. Williams, and S. Torres-Harding. 2006a. Causes of death among patients with chronic fatigue syndrome. *Health Care for Women International* 27(7):615-626.

Jason, L., S. Torres-Harding, and M. Njok. 2006b. The face of CFS in the U.S. *CFIDS Chronicle* 16-21. http://www.researchgate.net/profile/Leonard_Jason/publication/236995875_The_Face_of_CFS_in_the_U.S/links/00b7d51acf6823bccb000000.pdf (accessed March 3, 2015).

Jason, L. A., M. C. Benton, L. Valentine, A. Johnson, and S. Torres-Harding. 2008. The economic impact of ME/CFS: Individual and societal costs. *Dynamic Medicine* 7(6).

Jason, L. A., E. Paavola, N. Porter, and M. L. Morello. 2010. Frequency and content analysis of chronic fatigue syndrome in medical text books. *Australian Journal of Primary Health* 16(2):174-178.

Jason, L. A., B. Z. Katz, Y. Shiraishi, C. Mears, Y. Im, and R. R. Taylor. 2014. Predictors of post-infectious chronic fatigue syndrome in adolescents. *Health Psychology & Behavioural Medicine* 2(1):41-51.

Johnson, S. K., J. DeLuca, and B. H. Natelson. 1996. Depression in fatiguing illness: Comparing patients with chronic fatigue syndrome, multiple sclerosis and depression. *Journal of Affective Disorders* 39(1):21-30.

Maloney, E. M., R. S. Boneva, J. M. Lin, and W. C. Reeves. 2010. Chronic fatigue syndrome is associated with metabolic syndrome: Results from a case-control study in Georgia. *Metabolism: Clinical & Experimental* 59(9):1351-1357.

Marshall, R., L. Paul, and L. Wood. 2011. The search for pain relief in people with chronic fatigue syndrome: A descriptive study. *Physiotherapy Theory & Practice* 27(5):373-383.

NIH (National Institutes of Health). 2011. *State of the knowledge workshop. Myalgic encephalomyelitis/chronic fatigue syndrome (ME/CFS) research: Workshop report.* Bethesda, MD: Office of Research on Women's Health, NIH, U.S. Department of Health and Human Services.

Nisenbaum, R., M. Reyes, A. C. Mawle, and W. C. Reeves. 1998. Factor analysis of unexplained severe fatigue and interrelated symptoms: Overlap with criteria for chronic fatigue syndrome. *American Journal of Epidemiology* 148(1):72-77.

Peterson, T. M., T. W. Peterson, S. Emerson, E. Regalbuto, M. A. Evans, and L. A. Jason. 2013. Coverage of CFS within U.S. medical schools. *Universal Journal of Public Health* 1(4):177-179.

ProHealth. 2008. *A profile of ME/CFS patients: How many years and how many doctors?* http://www.prohealth.com/library/showarticle.cfm?libid=13672 (accessed August 13, 2014).

Reynolds, K. J., S. D. Vernon, E. Bouchery, and W. C. Reeves. 2004. The economic impact of chronic fatigue syndrome. *Cost Effectiveness and Resource Allocation* 2(4).

Shepherd, C., and A. Chaudhuri. 2001. *ME/CFS/PVFS: An exploration of the key clinical issues.* Buckingham, UK: The ME Association.

Solomon, L., and W. C. Reeves. 2004. Factors influencing the diagnosis of chronic fatigue syndrome. *Archives of Internal Medicine* 164(20):2241-2245.

Wagner, D., R. Nisenbaum, C. Heim, J. F. Jones, E. R. Unger, and W. C. Reeves. 2008. Psychometric properties of the CDC symptom inventory for assessment of chronic fatigue syndrome. In *Alterations in diurnal salivary cortisol rhythm in a population-based sample of cases with chronic fatigue syndrome (CFS)*, edited by U. M. Nater, L. S. Youngblood, J. F. Jones, E. R. Unger, A. H. Miller, W. C. Reeves, and C. Heim. *Psychosomatic Medicine* 70:298-305.

1

Introduction

Myalgic encephalomyelitis (ME) and chronic fatigue syndrome (CFS) are debilitating conditions that affect somewhere between 836,000 and 2.5 million Americans (Jason et al., 1999, 2006b). Despite having different definitions, ME and CFS often are used interchangeably to refer to an illness characterized by profound fatigue and autonomic and neurocognitive symptoms. Throughout this report, the umbrella term "ME/CFS" is used to refer to ME and CFS. However, the literature analysis conducted in support of this study took into consideration the variability among the definitions used in the studies reviewed.

The cause of ME/CFS remains unknown, although in many cases, symptoms may be triggered by an infection or other prodromal events such as "immunization, anesthetics, physical trauma, exposure to environmental pollutants, chemicals and heavy metals, and rarely blood transfusions" (Carruthers and van de Sande, 2005, p. 1). An estimated 84 to 91 percent of patients affected by the condition are not yet diagnosed (Jason et al., 2006b; Solomon and Reeves, 2004), and people with ME/CFS often struggle with their illness for years before receiving a diagnosis. In multiple surveys, 67 to 77 percent of patients reported that it took longer than 1 year to receive a diagnosis, and about 29 percent reported that it took longer than 5 years (CFIDS Association of America, 2014; ProHealth, 2008).

Seeking and receiving a diagnosis can be a frustrating process for patients with ME/CFS for several reasons, including a lack of understanding of diagnosis and treatment of the condition among health care providers and skepticism about whether it is in fact a true medical condition. Less than one-third of medical schools include ME/CFS-specific information in their curriculum (Peterson et al., 2013), and only 40 percent of medical textbooks include information on the condition (Jason et al., 2010). Some studies on awareness of ME/CFS have found high awareness among health care providers, but many providers believe it is a psychiatric/psychological illness or at least has a psychiatric/psychological component (Brimmer et al., 2010; Jason and Richman, 2008; Unger, 2011). ME/CFS often is seen as a diagnosis of exclusion, which also can lead to delays in diagnosis or misdiagnosis of a psychological problem (Bayliss et al., 2014; Fossey et al., 2004). Once diagnosed, moreover, many people with ME/CFS report being subject to hostile attitudes from their health care providers (Anderson and Ferrans, 1997; David et al., 1991), as well as to treatment strategies that exacerbate their symptoms (Twemlow et al., 1997).

ME/CFS can cause significant impairment and disability that have negative economic consequences at the individual and societal levels. At least one-quarter of ME/CFS patients are house- or bedbound at some point in their lives (Marshall et al., 2011; NIH, 2011; Shepherd and Chaudhuri, 2001). The direct and indirect economic costs of ME/CFS to society are estimated to be between $17 and $24 billion annually (Jason et al., 2008), $9.1 billion of which can be attributed to lost household and labor force productivity (Reynolds et al., 2004). Together, high medical costs and reduced earning capacity often have devastating effects on patients' financial situations (Reynolds et al., 2004).

Literature on mortality associated with ME/CFS is sparse. One study found that cancer, heart disease, and suicide are the most common causes of death among those diagnosed with ME/CFS, and people with ME/CFS die from these causes at younger ages than others in the general population. However, the authors note that these results cannot be generalized to the overall population of ME/CFS patients because of the methodological limitations of the study (Jason et al., 2006a).

This report, based on a study conducted by a committee convened by the Institute of Medicine (IOM), documents the evidence base for ME/CFS. The committee also proposes clear and concise diagnostic criteria designed to improve the ability of health care providers to diagnose this disorder.

CHARGE TO THE COMMITTEE

The Committee on the Diagnostic Criteria for Myalgic Encephalomyelitis/Chronic Fatigue Syndrome was charged by the Department of Health and Human Services (HHS) sponsors with evaluating the current criteria for diagnosis of ME/CFS and recommending clinical diagnostic criteria that would address the needs of health care providers, patients, and their caregivers. Specifically, the committee was asked to

- conduct a study to identify the evidence for various clinical diagnostic criteria for ME/CFS using a process with input from stakeholders, including practicing clinicians and patients;
- develop evidence-based clinical diagnostic criteria for ME/CFS for use by clinicians, using a consensus-building methodology;
- recommend whether new terminology for ME/CFS should be adopted; and
- develop an outreach strategy for disseminating the new criteria nationwide to health professionals.

The committee was also asked to distinguish among disease subgroups, develop a plan for updating the new criteria, and make recommendations for the plan's implementation. The statement of task requested that the committee's recommendations consider unique diagnostic issues facing people with ME/CFS, related specifically to gender and particular subgroups with substantial disability and extending across the life span. The committee was not asked to investigate the etiology, pathophysiology, pathogenesis, or treatment of ME/CFS. The complete statement of task is provided in Box 1-1.

The committee comprised 15 members with expertise in clinical care for ME/CFS, pediatrics, infectious disease, epidemiology, immunology, rheumatology, behavioral health, pain, sleep, primary care, genetics, exercise physiology, neurology/neuropathology, and clinical case definitions. In addition to their scientific expertise, two committee members are or have been patients, and one is a family member/caregiver of a patient with ME/CFS.

CONTEXT FOR THIS STUDY

This study was sponsored by the Office on Women's Health within HHS, the National Institutes of Health (NIH), the Centers for Disease Control and Prevention (CDC), the Food and Drug Administration, the Agency for Healthcare Research and Quality, and the Social Security Administration. The study was commissioned in response to a recommendation from HHS's Chronic Fatigue Syndrome Advisory Committee (CFSAC), which comprises 11 voting members, including the chair, who provide advice and recommendations to the Secretary of HHS on issues related to ME/CFS. Of the 11 members, 7 are required to be scientists with demonstrated expertise in ME/CFS biomedical research, and 4 should have expertise in health care delivery, private health care services or insurers, or voluntary organizations

BOX 1-1
Institute of Medicine Study on Diagnostic Criteria for ME/CFS:
Statement of Task

An Institute of Medicine (IOM) committee will comprehensively evaluate the current criteria for the diagnosis of Myalgic Encephalomyelitis/Chronic Fatigue Syndrome (ME/CFS). The committee will consider the various existing definitions and recommend clinical diagnostic criteria for the disorder to address the needs of health providers, patients and their caregivers.

The committee will also distinguish between disease subgroups, develop a plan for updating the new criteria, and make recommendations for its implementation. Any recommendations made by the committee will consider unique diagnostic issues facing people with ME/CFS, specifically related to: gender, across the life span, and specific subgroups with substantial disability.

Specifically the IOM will:

- Conduct a study to identify the evidence for various diagnostic clinical criteria of ME/CFS using a process with stakeholder input, including practicing clinicians and patients;
- Develop evidence-based clinical diagnostic criteria for ME/CFS for use by clinicians, using a consensus-building methodology;
- Recommend whether new terminology for ME/CFS should be adopted; and
- Develop an outreach strategy to disseminate the definition nationwide to health professionals.

Over the 18 months, the committee will consider four topic areas and produce a consensus report with recommendations. The recommendations will have a domestic focus; however, major international issues may be identified. As the committee reviews the literature, efforts that have already been completed on this topic area will be considered, including the 2003 ME/CFS Canadian Consensus Criteria, the 2007 British National Institute for Health and Clinical Excellence (NICE) Clinical Guidelines for CFS/ME, the 2010 Revised Canadian Consensus Criteria, the 2011 ME International Consensus Criteria, and data from the ongoing CDC Multi-Site Clinical Study of CFS. In an effort to minimize overlap and maximize synergy, the committee will seek input from the NIH Evidence-based Methodology Workshop for ME/CFS.

working with ME/CFS patients.[1] In 2012, the CFSAC recommended that HHS "promptly convene . . . at least one stakeholders' (ME/CFS experts, patients, advocates) workshop in consultation with the CFSAC members to reach a consensus for a case definition useful for research, diagnosis

---

[1] The HHS website can be accessed at http://www.hhs.gov/advcomcfs/charter/index.html (accessed January 13, 2015).

and treatment of ME/CFS beginning with the 2003 Canadian Consensus Definition for discussion purposes."[2] Given the well-established and well-regarded consensus process used by the IOM, HHS contracted with the IOM in September 2013 to conduct this study.

In the weeks that followed, many advocates were greatly disappointed that HHS did not follow the CFSAC recommendation as it was intended. Patients, advocates, researchers, and clinicians expressed strong opposition to the study, arguing that the IOM lacks the expertise to develop clinical case definitions and that the inclusion of non-ME/CFS experts in this process would move the science backward. An open letter was sent to the Secretary of HHS, signed by 38 U.S.-based biomedical researchers and clinicians, declaring that consensus had been reached on the use of the Canadian clinical case definition (often called the Canadian Consensus Criteria [CCC]) for diagnosis of ME/CFS, and requesting that the IOM study be canceled and the funds used to support further ME/CFS research instead (see Chapter 3 for a discussion of current diagnostic criteria) (An Open Letter, 2013).

THE COMMITTEE'S APPROACH

The committee held five meetings and two public sessions during the course of its work (see Appendix A for the agendas for the public sessions). Throughout the study, many people with ME/CFS and their family members and friends, as well as the study sponsors and other organizations and individuals, provided valuable input to the committee about their concerns, burdens, hopes, and challenges. Some quotes throughout the report highlight perspectives shared during the public sessions and in emails to the committee. In addition to its meetings and public sessions, the committee sought information from relevant concurrent research efforts and undertook a comprehensive review of the scientific literature and other available evidence on ME/CFS. The committee consulted with a health communications specialist and a statistician to obtain additional expertise in addressing its statement of task. The committee's approach to this study is described in more detail below.

Public Sessions and Public Comments

In the two public sessions, the committee heard testimony from patients, their family members, advocates, and researchers in the field. The

---

[2] CFSAC recommendations can be accessed at http://www.hhs.gov/advcomcfs/recommendations/10032012.html (accessed January 13, 2015).

committee also reviewed and carefully considered hundreds of comments received from the public.[3]

Input from Other Groups

As requested in its statement of task, the committee sought data from the ongoing CDC Multi-Site Clinical Study of CFS. The CDC study has collected standardized data on major illness domains of CFS from patients in seven practices around the country (Unger, 2013). Dr. Elizabeth Unger, principal investigator of the CDC study, presented the study's preliminary results at the committee's first public session. Throughout the study, the committee communicated questions and data requests to CDC through the IOM staff. Dr. Unger and her team provided analyses requested by the committee.[4] The committee recognizes that these findings are preliminary and have not been independently verified, and thus should be interpreted with caution. These data are appropriately cited throughout this report.

The study's statement of task also directed the committee to seek input from NIH's Evidence-based Methodology Workshop for ME/CFS, a process now referred to as Pathways to Prevention (P2P). The NIH P2P workshop was originally intended to complement the present study by developing a re-search case definition for ME/CFS (CFSAC, 2012). However, in remarks on behalf of the P2P workshop process at the committee's first public session, Susan Maier, Deputy Director for NIH's Office of Research on Women's Health, stated that the goal of the P2P workshop was not to develop a re-search case definition but to suggest a research agenda for ME/CFS based on an unbiased review of the evidence. She also expressed a desire to work with this committee throughout the P2P process. However, the planning group for the P2P workshop declined to share any data with the committee.

Literature Review

Throughout the study, the IOM staff maintained an EndNote library to organize the committee's research. The foundation for this library was a broad search of eight databases for all articles related to ME, CFS, ME/CFS, and other terms used to describe this disorder (such as post-viral fatigue syndrome) published since 1950. This search was run regularly to identify peer-reviewed articles published through May 30, 2014. Additional citations and grey literature (i.e., non-commercially published) were identified by the IOM staff,

---

[3] Public testimony and other materials submitted to the committee are available upon request from the National Academies' Public Access Records Office.
[4] Ibid.

committee members, and the public and from references in pertinent articles. See Figure 1-1 for additional information on the initial search results.

The committee was charged with reviewing the evidence for various diagnostic clinical criteria for ME/CFS. Existing diagnostic criteria refer to a minimum of nine distinct symptoms, so the evidence for clinical criteria spans a wide range of disciplines. After a preliminary review of the literature, the committee directed the IOM staff to divide the articles into topics most central to its work: eight symptoms or symptom categories (for children/adolescents and adults) and three additional topics. For some of these topics, the committee reviewed all of the relevant literature, while for others, the

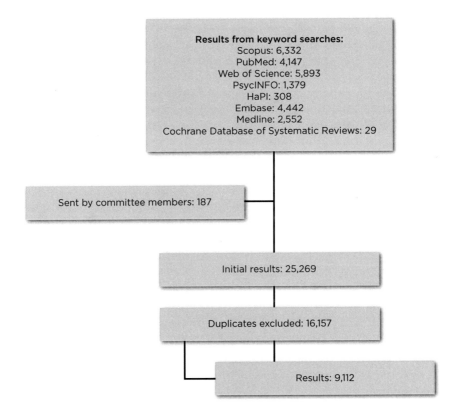

FIGURE 1-1 Initial results (as of January 2014) of the committee's broad literature search.
NOTE: Through May 2014 the committee received regular updates on this search strategy. The committee also received additional literature from members of the public and identified further resources throughout the study.

committee conducted targeted literature searches. All of the topic areas are listed below; those in italics were identified for targeted searches.

- Symptoms or symptom categories
  - *Autonomic manifestations*
  - Fatigue
  - Immune manifestations
  - *Neurocognitive manifestations*
  - Neuroendocrine manifestations
  - Pain
  - *PEM (post-exertional malaise)*
  - *Sleep*
- Additional topics
  - Disability and impairment
  - Infections and ME/CFS
  - *Symptom constructs and clusters*

For the topics identified for targeted searches, the committee and the IOM staff worked together to identify priority research questions and to develop targeted search strategies for gathering literature relevant to answering these questions. The targeted searches were run in the same eight databases as the general search and also included articles published from 1950 through May 30, 2014. The IOM staff evaluated the results of each targeted search according to predefined inclusion and exclusion criteria, and they provided a list of abstracts to research groups of two to five committee members assigned to each topic. The research groups reviewed the abstracts and identified articles appropriate for full-text review. Articles addressing diagnosis (e.g., a particular biomarker) and prognosis (e.g., the relationship between a feature and an outcome) and those defining manifestations of ME/CFS subgroups (cluster of symptoms and signs) were selected. The overall intent was to identify information on symptoms and objectively measurable signs (such as laboratory and imaging abnormalities) that are associated with ME/CFS and could be useful in defining ME/CFS or discriminating it—or subgroups—from other conditions. The results of the targeted searches are presented in Tables 1-1 and 1-2.

The research groups read the full-text articles and extracted information into spreadsheets, including information about study populations, sample sizes, methods, findings, and conclusions. The data extraction spreadsheets also included items adapted from Quality Assessment of Diagnostic Accuracy Studies (QUADAS) criteria (Whiting et al., 2003) and Hoy and colleagues (2012) to help assess study quality. The research groups presented summaries of the literature and assessments of its quality to the entire committee.

TABLE 1-1 Targeted Search Results: Adults

Topic	Search Results	Fulfilled Criteria	Deemed Relevant
Autonomic manifestations	785	89	86
Neurocognitive manifestations*	685	71	67
Post-exertional malaise (PEM)	354	77	70
Sleep	354	87	78
Symptom clusters	120	35	18

NOTES: Search results = number of references returned from the targeted search after removing duplicates. Fulfilled criteria = number of references that fulfilled inclusion criteria for the targeted search after a review of abstracts. Deemed relevant = number of references that were determined to be relevant to the topic questions and reviewed in full.

   * Because of the large number of results, the committee reviewed only papers published during the past 10 years with the understanding that older research is considered and cited in the introduction and discussion sections of more recent literature.

TABLE 1-2 Targeted Search Results: Pediatrics

Topic	Search Results	Fulfilled Criteria	Deemed Relevant
Autonomic manifestations	172	27	22
Neurocognitive manifestations	144	13	12
Post-exertional malaise (PEM)	43	8	7
Sleep	68	10	8

NOTES: Search results = number of references returned from the targeted search after removing duplicates. Fulfilled criteria = number of references that fulfilled inclusion criteria for the targeted search after a review of abstracts. Deemed relevant = number of references that were determined to be relevant to the topic questions and reviewed in full.

Committee's Deliberation and Consensus Process

The committee carefully considered the testimony and public comments received and the results of the literature review as it deliberated on its recommendations concerning (1) symptoms and abnormalities that must be present to make the diagnosis of ME/CFS, (2) symptoms and abnormalities that can support the diagnosis but are not required in all cases, and (3) exclusionary and comorbid conditions. The committee adapted a "GRADE grid" to record individual judgments as to whether there is sufficient evidence that certain symptoms and abnormalities define either ME/CFS or a particular subtype of ME/CFS (see Appendix B for the grid template) (Guyatt et al., 2008; Jaeschke et al., 2008). The collated judgments were used to facilitate further discussion, which led to consensus among the committee members on final recommendations regarding diagnostic criteria. The committee then considered the recommended criteria and revisited the public comments to inform its decision making on whether a different name or set of names might be appropriate for ME/CFS.

Consultants

To fulfill its statement of task with respect to developing an outreach strategy for disseminating the diagnostic criteria for ME/CFS, the committee consulted with a communication specialist with expertise in dissemination for health care professionals. The committee worked with the consultant to explain the needs and priorities for and the audiences to be reached with this strategy. After an initial meeting, the consultant worked with a group of three committee members to develop the strategy, which was discussed during the last committee meeting. The final outreach strategy presented in this report incorporates the committee's review and feedback.

The committee also consulted with a statistician who reviewed and summarized 18 papers that use statistical methods to analyze symptom data from ME/CFS patients. The committee discussed the information provided by this consultant to determine whether the data presented in these papers could be used to identify subgroups of patients with ME/CFS.

OVERVIEW OF THE REPORT

The remainder of this report is organized as follows:

- **Chapter 2** provides additional background information on ME/CFS, including its history, its terminology, and its burden and impact.
- **Chapter 3** presents a comparison of five current sets of case definitions and diagnostic criteria, a discussion that supports the committee's proposal for new terminology for ME/CFS. This chapter also presents the committee's assessment of the literature on ME/CFS symptom constructs and clusters.
- **Chapter 4** reviews the evidence on the major symptoms of ME/CFS (fatigue, post-exertional malaise [PEM], sleep abnormalities, neurocognitive manifestations, and orthostatic intolerance and autonomic dysfunction).
- **Chapter 5** reviews the evidence on other symptoms and manifestations commonly presented in ME/CFS patients, such as pain, immune abnormalities, neuroendocrine abnormalities, and an association with infection.
- **Chapter 6** reviews the evidence on pediatric ME/CFS.

- **Chapter 7** presents the committee's recommendations for new diagnostic criteria and new terminology for ME/CFS and for updating of the new diagnostic criteria.
- **Chapter 8** presents the committee's plan for dissemination of the new criteria to health professionals nationwide.

REFERENCES

An Open Letter. 2013. *An open letter to the honorable Kathleen Sebelius, U.S. Secretary of Health and Human Services*, September 23, 2013. https://dl.dropboxusercontent.com/u/89158245/Case%20Definition%20Letter%20Sept%2023%202013.pdf (accessed January 12, 2015).

Anderson, J. S., and C. E. Ferrans. 1997. The quality of life of persons with chronic fatigue syndrome. *Journal of Nervous and Mental Disease* 185(6):359-367.

Bayliss, K., M. Goodall, A. Chisholm, B. Fordham, C. Chew-Graham, L. Riste, L. Fisher, K. Lovell, S. Peters, and A. Wearden. 2014. Overcoming the barriers to the diagnosis and management of chronic fatigue syndrome/ME in primary care: A meta synthesis of qualitative studies. *BMC Family Practice* 15(1):44.

Brimmer, D. J., F. Fridinger, J. M. Lin, and W. C. Reeves. 2010. U.S. healthcare providers' knowledge, attitudes, beliefs, and perceptions concerning chronic fatigue syndrome. *BMC Family Practice* 11:28.

Carruthers, B. M., and M. I. van de Sande. 2005. *Myalgic encephalomyelitis/chronic fatigue syndrome: A clinical case definition and guidelines for medical practitioners: An overview of the Canadian consensus document.* Vancouver, BC: Carruthers and van de Sande.

CFIDS (Chronic Fatigue and Immune Dysfunction Syndrome) Association of America. 2014. *ME/CFS road to diagnosis survey.* Charlotte, NC: CFIDS Association of America.

CFSAC (Chronic Fatigue Syndrome Advisory Committee). 2012. *The twenty-second meeting of the Chronic Fatigue Syndrome Advisory Committee*, October 3, 2012. Washington, DC: U.S. Department of Health and Human Services.

David, A. S., S. Wessely, and A. J. Pelosi. 1991. Chronic fatigue syndrome: Signs of a new approach. *British Journal of Hospital Medicine* 45(3):158-163.

Fossey, M., E. Libman, S. Bailes, M. Baltzan, R. Schondorf, R. Amsel, and C. S. Fichten. 2004. Sleep quality and psychological adjustment in chronic fatigue syndrome. *Journal of Behavioral Medicine* 27(6):581-605.

Guyatt, G. H., A. D. Oxman, G. E. Vist, Y. Falck-Ytter, P. Alonso-Coello, and H. J. Schünemann. 2008. GRADE: An emerging consensus on rating quality of evidence and strength of recommendations. *British Medical Journal* 336(7650):924-926.

Hoy, D., P. Brooks, A. Woolf, F. Blyth, L. March, C. Bain, P. Baker, E. Smith, and R. Buchbinder. 2012. Assessing risk of bias in prevalence studies: Modification of an existing tool and evidence of interrater agreement. *Journal of Clinical Epidemiology* 65(9):934-939.

Jaeschke, R., G. H. Guyatt, P. Dellinger, H. Schünemann, M. M. Levy, R. Kunz, S. Norris, and J. Bion. 2008. Use of GRADE grid to reach decisions on clinical practice guidelines when consensus is elusive. *British Medical Journal* 337:a744.

Jason, L. A., and J. A. Richman. 2008. How science can stigmatize: The case of chronic fatigue syndrome. *Journal of Chronic Fatigue Syndrome* 14(4):85-103.

Jason, L. A., J. A. Richman, A. W. Rademaker, K. M. Jordan, A. V. Plioplys, R. R. Taylor, W. McCready, C. F. Huang, and S. Plioplys. 1999. A community-based study of chronic fatigue syndrome. *Archives of Internal Medicine* 159(18):2129-2137.

Jason, L., K. Corradi, S. Gress, S. Williams, and S. Torres-Harding. 2006a. Causes of death among patients with chronic fatigue syndrome. *Health Care for Women International* 27(7):615-626.

Jason, L., S. Torres-Harding, and M. Njok. 2006b. The face of CFS in the U.S. *CFIDS Chronicle* 16-21. http://www.researchgate.net/profile/Leonard_Jason/publication/236995875_The_Face_of_CFS_in_the_U.S/links/00b7d51acf6823bccb000000.pdf (accessed March 3, 2015).

Jason, L. A., M. C. Benton, L. Valentine, A. Johnson, and S. Torres-Harding. 2008. The economic impact of ME/CFS: Individual and societal costs. *Dynamic Medicine* 7(6).

Jason, L. A., E. Paavola, N. Porter, and M. L. Morello. 2010. Frequency and content analysis of chronic fatigue syndrome in medical text books. *Australian Journal of Primary Health* 16(2):174-178.

Marshall, R., L. Paul, and L. Wood. 2011. The search for pain relief in people with chronic fatigue syndrome: A descriptive study. *Physiotherapy Theory & Practice* 27(5):373-383.

NIH (National Institutes of Health). 2011. *State of the knowledge workshop. Myalgic encephalomyelitis/chronic fatigue syndrome (ME/CFS) research: Workshop report.* Bethesda, MD: Office of Research on Women's Health, NIH, U.S. Department of Health and Human Services.

Peterson, T. M., T. W. Peterson, S. Emerson, E. Regalbuto, M. A. Evans, and L. A. Jason. 2013. Coverage of CFS within U.S. medical schools. *Universal Journal of Public Health* 1(4):177-179.

ProHealth. 2008. *A profile ME/CFS patients: How many years and how many doctors?* http://www.prohealth.com/library/showarticle.cfm?libid=13672 (accessed August 13, 2014).

Reynolds, K. J., S. D. Vernon, E. Bouchery, and W. C. Reeves. 2004. The economic impact of chronic fatigue syndrome. *Cost Effectiveness and Resource Allocation* 2(4).

Shepherd, C., and A. Chaudhuri. 2001. *ME/CFS/PVFS: An exploration of the key clinical issues.* Buckingham, UK: The ME Association.

Solomon, L., and W. C. Reeves. 2004. Factors influencing the diagnosis of chronic fatigue syndrome. *Archives of Internal Medicine* 164(20):2241-2245.

Twemlow, S. W., S. L. Bradshaw, Jr., L. Coyne, and B. H. Lerma. 1997. Patterns of utilization of medical care and perceptions of the relationship between doctor and patient with chronic illness including chronic fatigue syndrome. *Psychological Reports* 80(2):643-658.

Unger, A. 2011. CFS knowledge and illness management behavior among U.S. healthcare providers and the public. Paper read at IACFS/ME Biennial International Conference Ottawa, Ontario, Canada.

Unger, E. 2013. Measures of CFS in a multi-site clinical study. Paper read at FDA Scientific Drug Development Workshop, April 26, 2013, Washington, DC.

Whiting, P., A. W. Rutjes, J. B. Reitsma, P. M. Bossuy, and J. Kleijnen. 2003. The development of QUADAS: A tool for the quality assessment of studies of diagnostic accuracy included in systematic reviews. *BMC Medical Research Methodology* 3(25):1-13.

2

Background

As background for the remainder of the report, this chapter presents a brief history of ME/CFS, a discussion of the terminology used for this illness, and a summary of the burden it imposes in the United States.

HISTORY OF ME/CFS

As noted in Chapter 1, "ME/CFS" is an umbrella term that includes myalgic encephalomyelitis (ME) and chronic fatigue syndrome (CFS). For decades, clinicians and researchers developed separate case definitions and diagnostic criteria for ME (Carruthers et al., 2011; Hyde, 2007; Ramsay, 1988a) and CFS (Fukuda et al., 1994; Holmes et al., 1988; Kitani et al., 1992; Reeves et al., 2005; Sharpe, 1991), although the terms describe conditions with similar symptoms and unknown etiology. In the World Health Organization's *International Classification of Diseases,* Tenth Revision, which will be implemented in October 2015, both ME and CFS are coded identically and classified as disorders of the nervous system (ICD G93.3). However "fatigue syndrome," which clinicians may view as synonymous with CFS, is classified under mental and behavioral disorders (ICD F48.0).[1]

More recent efforts to develop diagnostic criteria for this condition(s) have used the term "ME/CFS" or "CFS/ME" (Carruthers and van de Sande,

---

[1] The World Health Organization's *International Classification of Diseases*, Tenth Revision, can be accessed at http://apps.who.int/classifications/icd10/browse/2015/en (accessed February 13, 2015).

2005; Carruthers et al., 2003; Government of South Australia et al., 2004; Jason et al., 2006b, 2010; NICE, 2007). However, there is still disagreement as to whether ME and CFS are separate conditions or are similar enough to belong under an umbrella term such as ME/CFS (Jason et al., 2014).

Myalgic Encephalomyelitis

Beginning in 1934, a series of outbreaks of a previously unknown illness were recorded around the world (Acheson, 1959; Parish, 1978, 1980). The illness was initially confused with poliomyelitis, but it was eventually differentiated and became known as "epidemic neuromyasthenia" (Parish, 1978). The term "benign myalgic encephalomyelitis" was first used in the 1950s to describe a similar outbreak at the Royal Free Hospital in London (Wojcik et al., 2011). The details of each outbreak vary, but in general, patients experienced a variety of symptoms, including malaise, tender lymph nodes, sore throat, pain, and signs of encephalomyelitis (Lancet, 1955). Although the cause of the condition could not be determined, it appeared to be infectious, and the term "benign myalgic encephalomyelitis" eventually was chosen to reflect "the absent mortality, the severe muscular pains, the evidence of parenchymal damage to the nervous system, and the presumed inflammatory nature of the disorder" (Acheson, 1959, p. 593). The syndrome usually appeared in epidemics, but some sporadic cases were identified as well (Price, 1961).

In 1970, two psychiatrists in the United Kingdom reviewed the reports of 15 outbreaks of benign myalgic encephalomyelitis and concluded that these outbreaks "were psychosocial phenomena caused by one of two mechanisms, either mass hysteria on the part of the patients or altered medical perception of the community" (McEvedy and Beard, 1970, p. 11). They based their conclusions on the higher prevalence of the disease in females and the lack of physical signs in these patients. The researchers also recommended that the disease be renamed "myalgia nervosa." Although these findings were strongly refuted by Dr. Melvin Ramsay, the proposed psychological etiology created great controversy and convinced health professionals that this was a plausible explanation for the condition (Speight, 2013).

Over time, Dr. Ramsay's work demonstrated that, although this disease rarely resulted in mortality, it was often severely disabling, and as a result, the prefix "benign" was dropped (Ramsay, 1988a; Ramsay et al., 1977; Wojcik et al., 2011). In 1986, Dr. Ramsay published the first diagnostic criteria for ME, a condition characterized by a unique form of muscle fatigability whereby, even after a minor degree of physical effort, 3 or more days elapse before full muscle power is restored; extraordinary variability or fluctuation of symptoms even in the course of one day; and an alarming chronicity (Ramsay, 1986).

Despite Dr. Ramsay's work and a U.K. independent report recognizing that ME is not a psychological entity (CFS/ME Working Group, 2002), the health care community generally still doubts the existence or seriousness of this disease. This perception may partly explain the relatively limited research efforts to study ME in fields other than psychiatry and psychology.

Chronic Fatigue Syndrome

In the mid-1980s, two large outbreaks of an illness in Nevada and New York resembling mononucleosis attracted national attention. The illness was characterized by "chronic or recurrent debilitating fatigue and various combinations of other symptoms, including sore throat, lymph node pain and tenderness, headache, myalgia, and arthralgias" (Holmes et al., 1988, p. 387). The illness was initially linked to Epstein-Barr virus and became known as "chronic Epstein-Barr virus syndrome" (Holmes et al., 1988). In 1987, the Centers for Disease Control and Prevention (CDC) convened a working group to reach consensus on the clinical features of the illness. This group recognized that CFS was not new and had been known by many different names throughout history, "each reflecting a particular concept of the syndrome's etiology and epidemiology" (Straus, 1991, p. S2). Many of these names were gradually rejected as new research ruled out various causes of the illness, including Epstein-Barr virus. Therefore, the CDC group chose "chronic fatigue syndrome" as a more neutral and inclusive name, noting that "myalgic encephalomyelitis" was the name most accepted in other parts of the world (Holmes et al., 1988). The first definition of CFS was published in 1988, and although the cause of the illness remains unknown, there have been several attempts to update this definition (Fukuda et al., 1994). Chapter 3 provides more information on some of the most recent case definitions and diagnostic criteria.

TERMINOLOGY

Although a variety of names have been proposed for this illness, the most commonly used today are "chronic fatigue syndrome," "myalgic encephalomyelitis,"[2] and the umbrella term "ME/CFS." Reaching consensus on a name for this illness is particularly challenging in part because its etiology and pathology remain unknown (CFS/ME Working Group, 2002).

---

[2] The most commonly used term around the world is "myalgic encephalomyelitis," although a U.S. consensus group endorsed "encephalopathy" instead. The committee uses the former term throughout this report.

For years, patients, clinicians, and researchers have debated changing the name of the illness.

The term "chronic fatigue syndrome" has been the object of particular criticism from patients, as reflected in hundreds of comments the committee received from the public, both in person and electronically, during the course of this study (FDA, 2013).[3] Surveys conducted by ME/CFS advocacy organizations have found that 85 to 92 percent of respondents want that name to be changed (Jason et al., 2004). Their most common complaints are that this name is stigmatizing and trivializing, causing people not to take the disorder seriously (Jason and Richman, 2008). Patients and advocates told the committee that the name "chronic fatigue syndrome" leads others, including clinicians, to think that patients are malingering and to ask whether the illness is "real." Patients reported that many clinicians are dismissive, making such comments as "I feel tired all the time, too."[4] Many respondents objected specifically to the use of "fatigue" in the name because they do not believe fatigue to be the defining characteristic of this illness.[5] For example, the following comment was submitted to the committee:

> I believe that the words "Chronic Fatigue" are the kiss of death. Who in this over-wrought, stress-driven society isn't "fatigued" a good deal of the time? What people don't get is that this fatigue for people like me keeps me in bed for days at a time and prevents me from doing everyday errands and even simple house tasks on some days.[6]

In addition to difficult interactions with health care providers, patients have reported several other ways in which the stigmatization of ME/CFS affects them, including financial instability (such as job loss or demotion), social disengagement, and feeling the need to hide their symptoms in front of others (Assefi et al., 2003; Dickson et al., 2007; Green et al., 1999).

Comments submitted to the committee also noted that other illnesses, such as Parkinson's disease, are not named after their symptoms.[7] Patients often pointed out that ME/CFS, which includes symptoms in multiple systems that occur for an extended period of time, involves much more than fatigue, a level of complexity and impact not conveyed by the term "chronic fatigue syndrome." The term "chronic fatigue syndrome" also may be difficult to understand in populations where English is not the primary language (Bayliss et al., 2014). Many patients prefer "myalgic encephalomyelitis," a term first used in 1956, because they believe it better reflects the medical

---

[3] Personal communication; public comments submitted to the IOM Committee on the Diagnostic Criteria for Myalgic Encephalomyelitis/Chronic Fatigue Syndrome for meeting 3, 2014.
[4] Ibid.
[5] Ibid.
[6] Ibid.
[7] Ibid.

nature of the illness (Jason et al., 2004; Ramsay, 1988b). However, there are patients and researchers who maintain that ME and CFS are two different illnesses and oppose simply changing the name of CFS to ME (Twisk, 2014).[8]

Partly in response to the concerns that have been expressed about CFS and to a lesser extent ME, particularly by patients, the committee was asked to recommend whether new terminology for ME/CFS should be adopted, a request that is addressed in Chapter 7. As noted in Chapter 1, the committee uses the umbrella term "ME/CFS" to refer to ME and CFS throughout this report.

BURDEN OF ME/CFS

> My personal experience of having ME/CFS feels like permanently having the flu, a hangover, and jet lag while being continually electrocuted (which means that pain plays at least as much of a role in my condition as fatigue).[9]

As noted in Chapter 1, ME/CFS affects between 836,000 and 2.5 million people in the United States (Jason et al., 1999, 2006a; Reynolds et al., 2004). It affects more women than men, and although many seeking care for ME/CFS are Caucasian, the illness may be more common in minority groups (Jason et al., 1999, 2009, 2011; Reyes et al., 2003). The average age of onset is 33, although ME/CFS may begin as early as age 10 and as late as age 77 (NIH, 2011). Symptoms can persist for years, and most patients never regain their premorbid level of health or functioning (Nisenbaum et al., 2000; Reyes et al., 2003; Reynolds et al., 2004). The duration of ME/CFS and the potentially debilitating consequences of symptoms can be an enormous burden for patients, their caregivers, the health care system, and society.

Disability and Impairment

Several ME/CFS symptoms—including fatigue, cognitive dysfunction, pain, sleep disturbance, post-exertional malaise, and secondary depression or anxiety—may contribute to impairment or disability (Andersen et al., 2004; Tiersky et al., 2001). Patients with ME/CFS have been found to be more functionally impaired than those with other disabling illnesses, including type 2 diabetes mellitus, congestive heart failure, hypertension, depression, multiple sclerosis, and end-stage renal disease (Jason and Richman,

---

[8] Ibid.
[9] Ibid.

2008; Twisk, 2014). Symptoms can be severe enough to preclude patients from completing everyday tasks, and 25-29 percent of patients report being house- or bedbound by their symptoms. Many patients feel unable to meet their family responsibilities and report having to reduce their social activities (NIH, 2011). However, these data include only patients who were counted in clinics or research studies and may underrepresent the extent of the problem by excluding those who are undiagnosed or unable to access health care (Wiborg et al., 2010). More information on disability in ME/CFS can be found in Appendix C.

Health Care Costs and Utilization

Patients with ME/CFS spend considerably more on health care than the general medical patient population (Twemlow et al., 1997). They also see more physicians and visit their health care providers more often relative to the general medical patient population (Thanawala and Taylor, 2007; Twemlow et al., 1997). Many patients report barriers to accessing health care as well, including the nature of their illness and financial considerations (Lin et al., 2009; Thanawala and Taylor, 2007).

Household Income

ME/CFS symptoms often are so debilitating that patients are unable to work or attend school full-time (Crawley et al., 2011; Solomon et al., 2003; Taylor and Kielhofner, 2005; Twemlow et al., 1997). A review of 15 studies conducted between 1966 and 2004 showed that unemployment rates among those with the disorder ranged from 35 to 69 percent in 13 of these studies (Taylor and Kielhofner, 2005). ME/CFS was found to account for $8,554 in lost household earnings, 19 percent of which was attributable to lower educational attainment (Lin et al., 2011). Another study, conducted among ME/CFS patients in Kansas, found that ME/CFS resulted in reduced household and labor force productivity that caused individual income losses of approximately $20,000 annually (Taylor and Kielhofner, 2005). Reductions in employment and productivity per hour resulted in a 37 percent reduction in household productivity and a 54 percent reduction in labor force productivity (Reynolds et al., 2004).

Economic Costs

As noted, ME/CFS often lasts for many years, and beyond lost income, inflicts substantial economic costs at both the individual and the societal level. In one study, annual direct medical costs per ME/CFS patient ranged from $2,342 in a community-based sample (previously undiagnosed) to

$8,675 in a tertiary sample (already diagnosed) (Jason et al., 2008). Another study found that individuals with ME/CFS incurred $3,286 in annual direct medical costs (Lin et al., 2011). The direct and indirect economic costs of ME/CFS to society are estimated to be approximately over $18 to $24 billion annually (Jason et al., 2008).

REFERENCES

Acheson, E. D. 1959. The clinical syndrome variously called benign myalgic encephalomyelitis, Iceland disease and epidemic neuromyasthenia. *American Journal of Medicine* 26(4):569-595.

Andersen, M. M., H. Permin, and F. Albrecht. 2004. Illness and disability in Danish chronic fatigue syndrome patients at diagnosis and 5-year follow-up. *Journal of Psychosomatic Research* 56(2):217-229.

Assefi, N. P., T. V. Coy, D. Uslan, W. R. Smith, and D. Buchwald. 2003. Financial, occupational, and personal consequences of disability in patients with chronic fatigue syndrome and fibromyalgia compared to other fatiguing conditions. *Journal of Rheumatology* 30(4):804-808.

Bayliss, K., L. Riste, L. Fisher, A. Wearden, S. Peters, K. Lovell, and C. Chew-Graham. 2014. Diagnosis and management of chronic fatigue syndrome/myalgic encephalitis in black and minority ethnic people: A qualitative study. *Primary Health Care Research & Development* 15(2):143-152.

Carruthers, B., and M. I. van de Sande. 2005. *Myalgic encephalomyelitis/chronic fatigue syndrome: A clinical case definition and guidelines for medical practitioners: An overview of the Canadian consensus document.* Vancouver, BC: Carruthers and van de Sande.

Carruthers, B. M., A. K. Jain, K. L. De Meirleir, D. L. Peterson, N. G. Klimas, A. M. Lemer, A. C. Bested, P. Flor-Henry, P. Joshi, A. C. P. Powles, J. A. Sherkey, and M. I. van de Sande. 2003. Myalgic encephalomyelitis/chronic fatigue syndrome: Clinical working case definition, diagnostic and treatment protocols (Canadian case definition). *Journal of Chronic Fatigue Syndrome* 11(1):7-115.

Carruthers, B. M., M. I. van de Sande, K. L. De Meirleir, N. G. Klimas, G. Broderick, T. Mitchell, D. Staines, A. C. P. Powles, N. Speight, R. Vallings, L. Bateman, B. Baumgarten-Austrheim, D. S. Bell, N. Carlo-Stella, J. Chia, A. Darragh, D. Jo, D. Lewis, A. R. Light, S. Marshall-Gradisbik, I. Mena, J. A. Mikovits, K. Miwa, M. Murovska, M. L. Pall, and S. Stevens. 2011. Myalgic encephalomyelitis: International consensus criteria. *Journal of Internal Medicine* 270(4):327-338.

CFS/ME (Chronic Fatigue Syndrome/Myalgic Encephalomyelitis) Working Group. 2002. *Report to the chief medical officer of an independent working group.* http://www.erythos.com/gibsonenquiry/Docs/CMOreport.pdf (accessed January 12, 2015).

Crawley, E. M., A. M. Emond, and J. A. C. Sterne. 2011. Unidentified chronic fatigue syndrome/myalgic encephalomyelitis (CFS/ME) is a major cause of school absence: Surveillance outcomes from school-based clinics. *BMJ Open* 1(2).

Dickson, A., C. Knussen, and P. Flowers. 2007. Stigma and the delegitimation experience: An interpretative phenomenological analysis of people living with chronic fatigue syndrome. *Psychology & Health* 22(7):851-867.

FDA (Food and Drug Administration). 2013. *The voice of the patient: Chronic fatigue syndrome and myalgic encephalomyelitis.* Bethesda, MD: Center for Drug Evaluation and Research (CDER), FDA.

Fukuda, K., S. E. Straus, I. Hickie, M. C. Sharpe, J. G. Dobbins, A. Komaroff, A. Schluederberg, J. F. Jones, A. R. Lloyd, S. Wessely, N. M. Gantz, G. P. Holmes, D. Buchwald, S. Abbey, J. Rest, J. A. Levy, H. Jolson, D. L. Peterson, J. Vercoulen, U. Tirelli, B. Evengård, B. H. Natelson, L. Steele, M. Reyes, and W. C. Reeves. 1994. The chronic fatigue syndrome: A comprehensive approach to its definition and study. *Annals of Internal Medicine* 121(12):953-959.

Government of South Australia, Human Services, The University of Adelaide, Adelaide Western Division of General Practice, and MEICFS Society (SA), Inc. 2004. *ME/CFS guidelines myalgic encephalopathy (ME)/chronic fatigue syndrome (CFS): Management guidelines for general practitioners: A guideline for the diagnosis and management of ME/CFS in the community and primary care setting.* http://www.investinme.org/Documents/PDFdocuments/c6a_mecfsguidelines.pdf (accessed January 12, 2015).

Green, J., J. Romei, and B. H. Natelson. 1999. Stigma and chronic fatigue syndrome. *Journal of Chronic Fatigue Syndrome* 5(2):63-95.

Holmes, G. P., J. E. Kaplan, N. M. Gantz, A. L. Komaroff, L. B. Schonberger, S. E. Straus, J. F. Jones, R. E. Dubois, C. Cunningham-Rundles, S. Pahwa, G. Tosato, L. S. Zegans, D. T. Purtilo, N. Brown, R. T. Schooley, and I. Brus. 1988. Chronic fatigue syndrome: A working case definition. *Annals of Internal Medicine* 108(3):387-389.

Hyde, B. M. 2007. *The nightingale, mylagic encephalomyelitis (ME) definition.* Ottawa, Canada: Nightingale Research Foundation.

Jason, L. A., and J. A. Richman. 2008. How science can stigmatize: The case of chronic fatigue syndrome. *Journal of Chronic Fatigue Syndrome* 14(4):85-103.

Jason, L. A., J. A. Richman, A. W. Rademaker, K. M. Jordan, A. V. Plioplys, R. R. Taylor, W. McCready, C. F. Huang, and S. Plioplys. 1999. A community-based study of chronic fatigue syndrome. *Archives of Internal Medicine* 159(18):2129-2137.

Jason, L., C. Holbert, S. Torres-Harding, and R. Taylor. 2004. Stigma and the term chronic fatigue syndrome. *Journal of Disability Policy Studies* 14(4):222-228.

Jason, L., S. Torres-Harding, and M. Njok. 2006a. The face of CFS in the U.S. *CFIDS Chronicle* 16-21. http://www.researchgate.net/profile/Leonard_Jason/publication/236995875_The_Face_of_CFS_in_the_U.S/links/00b7d51acf6823bccb000000.pdf (accessed March 3, 2015).

Jason, L. A., D. S. Bell, K. Rowe, E. L. S. Van Hoof, K. Jordan, C. Lapp, A. Gurwitt, T. Miike, S. Torres-Harding, and K. De Meirleir. 2006b. A pediatric case definition for myalgic encephalomyelitis and chronic fatigue syndrome. *Journal of Chronic Fatigue Syndrome* 13(2-3):1-44.

Jason, L. A., M. C. Benton, L. Valentine, A. Johnson, and S. Torres-Harding. 2008. The economic impact of ME/CFS: Individual and societal costs. *Dynamic Medicine* 7(6).

Jason, L. A., N. Porter, M. Brown, V. Anderson, A. Brown, J. Hunnell, and A. Lerch. 2009. CFS: A review of epidemiology and natural history studies. *Bulletin of the IACFS/ME* 17(3):88-106.

Jason, L. A., M. Evans, N. Porter, M. Brown, A. Brown, J. Hunnell, V. Anderson, A. Lerch, K. De Meirleir, and F. Friedberg. 2010. The development of a revised Canadian myalgic encephalomyelitis chronic fatigue syndrome case definition. *American Journal of Biochemistry and Biotechnology* 6:120-135.

Jason, L. A., N. Porter, J. Hunnell, A. Rademaker, and J. A. Richman. 2011. CFS prevalence and risk factors over time. *Journal of Health Psychology* 16(3):445-456.

Jason, L. A., M. Sunnquist, A. Brown, M. Evans, and J. L. Newton. 2014. Are myalgic encephalomyelitis and chronic fatigue syndrome different illnesses? A preliminary analysis. *Journal of Health Psychology* [Epub ahead of print].

Kitani, T., H. Kuratsune, and K. Yamaguchi. 1992. Diagnostic criteria for chronic fatigue syndrome by the CFS study group in Japan. *Nippon Rinsho. Japanese Journal of Clinical Medicine* 50(11):2600-2605.

Lancet. 1955. Public health: Outbreak at the royal free. *Lancet* 266(6885):351-352.

Lin, J. M. S., D. J. Brimmer, R. S. Boneva, J. F. Jones, and W. C. Reeves. 2009. Barriers to healthcare utilization in fatiguing illness: A population-based study in georgia. *BMC Health Services Research* 9.

Lin, J. M. S., S. C. Resch, D. J. Brimmer, A. Johnson, S. Kennedy, N. Burstein, and C. J. Simon. 2011. The economic impact of chronic fatigue syndrome in Georgia: Direct and indirect costs. *Cost Effectiveness and Resource Allocation* 9(1).

McEvedy, C. P., and A. W. Beard. 1970. Concept of benign myalgic encephalomyelitis. *British Medical Journal* 1(5687):11-15.

NICE (National Institute for Health and Clinical Excellence). 2007. *Chronic fatigue syndrome/ myalgic encephalomyelitis (or encephalopathy): Diagnosis and management of CFS/ME in adults and children.* London, UK: NICE.

NIH (National Institutes of Health). 2011. *State of the knowledge workshop. Myalgic encephalomyelitis/chronic fatigue syndrome (ME/CFS) research: Workshop report.* Bethesda, MD: Office of Research on Women's Health, NIH, U.S. Department of Health and Human Services.

Nisenbaum, R., A. Jones, J. Jones, and W. Reeves. 2000. Longitudinal analysis of symptoms reported by patients with chronic fatigue syndrome. *Annals of Epidemiology* 10(7):458.

Parish, J. G. 1978. Early outbreaks of "epidemic neuromyasthenia." *Postgraduate Medical Journal* 54(637):711-717.

Parish, J. G. 1980. *The American term "epidemic neuromyasthenia" refers to a condition similar to "ME." Icelandic disease is the original name for the illness.* http://www. meresearch.org.uk/wp-content/uploads/2012/11/ResearchPublications1934-1980.pdf (accessed January 12, 2015).

Price, J. L. 1961. Myalgic encephalomyelitis. *Lancet* 1(7180):737-738.

Ramsay, A. M. 1986. The definitive description of ME. http://www.meactionuk.org.uk/ramsey. html (accessed June 25, 2014).

Ramsay, A. M. 1988a. Myalgic encephalomyelitis, or what? *Lancet* 2(8602):100.

Ramsay, A. M. 1988b. *Myalgic encephalomyelitis and postviral fatigue states: The saga of royal free disease,* 2nd ed. London, UK: Gower Publishing Corporation.

Ramsay, A. M., E. G. Dowsett, J. V. Dadswell, W. H. Lyle, and J. G. Parish. 1977. Icelandic disease (benign myalgic encephalomyelitis or royal free disease). *British Medical Journal* 1(6072):1350.

Reeves, W. C., D. Wagner, R. Nisenbaum, J. F. Jones, B. Gurbaxani, L. Solomon, D. A. Papanicolaou, E. R. Unger, S. D. Vernon, and C. Heim. 2005. Chronic fatigue syndrome—a clinically empirical approach to its definition and study. *BMC Medicine* 3:19.

Reyes, M., R. Nisenbaum, D. C. Hoaglin, E. R. Unger, C. Emmons, B. Randall, J. A. Stewart, S. Abbey, J. F. Jones, N. Gantz, S. Minden, and W. C. Reeves. 2003. Prevalence and incidence of chronic fatigue syndrome in Wichita, Kansas. *Archives of Internal Medicine* 163(13):1530-1536.

Reynolds, K. J., S. D. Vernon, E. Bouchery, and W. C. Reeves. 2004. The economic impact of chronic fatigue syndrome. *Cost Effectiveness and Resource Allocation* 2(4).

Sharpe, M. C. 1991. A report-chronic fatigue syndrome: Guidelines for research. *Journal of the Royal Society of Medicine* 84(2):118-121.

Solomon, L., R. Nisenbaum, M. Reyes, D. A. Papanicolaou, and W. C. Reeves. 2003. Functional status of persons with chronic fatigue syndrome in the Wichita, Kansas, population. *Health and Quality of Life Outcomes* 1.

Speight, N. 2013. Myalgic encephalomyelitis/chronic fatigue syndrome: Review of history, clinical features, and controversies. *Saudi Journal of Medicine & Medical Sciences* 1(1):11-13.

Straus, S. E. 1991. History of chronic fatigue syndrome. *Reviews of Infectious Diseases* 13(Suppl. 1):S2-S7.

Taylor, R. R., and G. W. Kielhofner. 2005. Work-related impairment and employment-focused rehabilitation options for individuals with chronic fatigue syndrome: A review. *Journal of Mental Health* 14(3):253-267.

Thanawala, S., and R. R. Taylor. 2007. Service utilization, barriers to service access, and coping in adults with chronic fatigue syndrome. *Journal of Chronic Fatigue Syndrome* 14(1):5-21.

Tiersky, L. A., J. DeLuca, N. Hill, S. K. Dhar, S. K. Johnson, G. Lange, G. Rappolt, and B. H. Natelson. 2001. Longitudinal assessment of neuropsychological functioning, psychiatric status, functional disability and employment status in chronic fatigue syndrome. *Applied Neuropsychology* 8(1):41-50.

Twemlow, S. W., S. L. Bradshaw, Jr., L. Coyne, and B. H. Lerma. 1997. Patterns of utilization of medical care and perceptions of the relationship between doctor and patient with chronic illness including chronic fatigue syndrome. *Psychological Reports* 80(2):643-658.

Twisk, F. N. 2014. The status of and future research into myalgic encephalomyelitis and chronic fatigue syndrome: The need of accurate diagnosis, objective assessment, and acknowledging biological and clinical subgroups. *Frontiers in Physiology* 5:109.

Wiborg, J. F., S. van der Werf, J. B. Prins, and G. Bleijenberg. 2010. Being homebound with chronic fatigue syndrome: A multidimensional comparison with outpatients. *Psychiatry Research* 177(1-2):246-249.

Wojcik, W., D. Armstrong, and R. Kanaan. 2011. Chronic fatigue syndrome: Labels, meanings and consequences. *Journal of Psychosomatic Research* 70(6):500-504.

3

Current Case Definitions and Diagnostic Criteria, Terminology, and Symptom Constructs and Clusters

A central element of the committee's charge was to "consider the various existing definitions [for ME/CFS] and recommend clinical diagnostic criteria for the disorder to address the needs of health providers, patients and their caregivers." At least 20 sets of case definitions or diagnostic criteria currently exist for ME/CFS (Brurberg et al., 2014), yet as noted in Chapter 1, many ME/CFS patients struggle for years before being diagnosed. In one survey, more than 70 percent of ME/CFS patients reported seeing four or more doctors before receiving a diagnosis (CFIDS Association of America, 2014). During the committee's first meeting, Dr. Nancy Lee spoke on behalf of the study sponsors, acknowledging "the considerable need for faster and more accurate diagnoses for patients" and expressing her hope that this committee would "provide guidance to the broader medical community on how to identify and diagnose ME/CFS in the clinical setting."[1] To set the stage for the chapters of this report that offer this guidance, this chapter provides some background information on case definitions and diagnostic criteria for ME/CFS, a brief review of some of the existing case definitions and diagnostic criteria, a discussion of the terminology used to refer to this illness, and a review of the literature on symptom constructs and clusters.

---

[1] A video of Dr. Lee's remarks can be accessed at http://iom.edu/Activities/Disease/DiagnosisMyalgicEncephalomyelitisChronicFatigueSyndrome/2014-JAN-27/Videos/Session%20Background/3-Lee-Video.aspx (accessed January 13, 2015).

CASE DEFINITIONS AND DIAGNOSTIC CRITERIA

Clinicians use diagnoses to manage illness, provide appropriate treatment, and predict prognosis. Diagnostic criteria provide guidance to clinicians on the specific signs, symptoms, or test results that indicate the presence of an illness, and classifying patients into diagnostic categories facilitates communication among clinicians and researchers (Coggon et al., 2005; Jason et al., 2006). Case definitions are a specific type of diagnostic criteria used to define an illness and are generally used for disease surveillance or investigations of infectious disease outbreaks (CDC, 2013). They are used to identify patients with a specific illness and are essential for disease-related research (Christley et al., 2011). Case definitions work well for illnesses for which the underlying pathology is understood and can be observed; establishing the presence of disease-specific pathology through examination or testing provides a gold standard for diagnosis of a particular disease, and potential case definitions can be compared against this standard. Case definitions often are assessed in terms of sensitivity, or the ability to identify patients with an illness correctly, and specificity, or the ability to exclude patients that do not have the illness. The appropriate balance of sensitivity and specificity varies depending on the purpose of a case definition (Coggon et al., 2005).

When the underlying pathology of an illness is unknown, as with ME/CFS, there is no gold standard against which to assess the sensitivity or specificity of a case definition. In these circumstances, diagnostic criteria may be more useful for "classifying people for the ultimate purpose of preventing or managing illness." Then, the accuracy or precision of diagnostic criteria and case definitions may be assessed in terms of how well they "distinguish groups of people whose illnesses share the same causes or determinants of outcome (including response to treatment)" (Coggon et al., 2005, p. 950). There are many examples of diagnostic criteria for illnesses without a clearly observable pathology, such as the Jones criteria for acute rheumatic fever. No symptom, sign, or test can be used to diagnose acute rheumatic fever; the Jones criteria divide clinical and laboratory findings into major and minor manifestations. A diagnosis of acute rheumatic fever is indicated if a patient has evidence of a preceding group A streptococcal infection and either two major and one minor manifestations or one major and two minor manifestations (Dajani et al., 1992). Another example is the *Diagnostic and Statistical Manual of Mental Disorders* (DSM), which provides diagnostic criteria for mental disorders (such as autism and posttraumatic stress disorder) that are "concise, explicit, and intended to facilitate an objective assessment of symptom presentations in a variety of clinical settings" (APA, 2013, p. xli).

Existing Diagnostic Criteria for ME, CFS, and ME/CFS

Because the pathology of ME/CFS remains unknown and there is no diagnostic test for the disorder, most of the existing diagnostic criteria for ME/CFS were developed through the consensus of experts. This approach is not unusual for an illness without a gold standard for diagnosis; consensus-based diagnostic criteria have been developed, for example, for the functional gastrointestinal disorders and gastro-esophageal reflux disease (Drossman, 2006; Jason et al., 1999; Vakil et al., 2006). However, consensus reached by one group of experts is unlikely to represent all of the various perspectives within a field (Coggon et al., 2005; Morris and Maes, 2013; van der Meer and Lloyd, 2012). Further, diagnostic criteria developed by consensus of a group are likely to reflect the biases of the individuals within that group (Morris and Maes, 2013; van der Meer and Lloyd, 2012). This committee acknowledges that it faced the same limitations in fulfilling its charge to develop diagnostic criteria for ME/CFS using a consensus-based methodology; further discussion of this issue can be found in Chapter 7.

For this study, the committee was specifically asked to review the 2003 Canadian clinical case definition for ME/CFS (often called the Canadian Consensus Criteria [CCC]), the 2007 Clinical Guidelines for CFS/ME of the British National Institute for Health and Clinical Excellence (NICE), the 2010 revised Canadian Consensus Criteria for ME/CFS (Revised CCC), and the 2011 International Consensus Criteria for ME (ME-ICC). The committee also reviewed the case definition for CFS developed by Fukuda and colleagues (1994) (the Fukuda definition) because it has been used extensively to define research populations and is commonly used in clinical practice, as well as the case definitions developed for use in the pediatric population (Carruthers et al., 2003, 2011; Jason et al., 2006; Royal College, 2004). With the exception of the pediatric case definitions, which are discussed later in the chapter, the essential elements of these case definitions and diagnostic criteria, extracted from their original papers, are summarized in Table 3-1.

Fukuda Case Definition for CFS (1994)

In 1994, Fukuda and colleagues published a case definition for CFS and idiopathic chronic fatigue that was intended to guide research in adult populations (CDC, 2012). The Fukuda definition defines chronic fatigue as "self-reported persistent or relapsing fatigue lasting 6 or more consecutive months" and requires a clinical evaluation to identify or rule out medical or psychological conditions that could explain the chronic fatigue's presence. A diagnosis of CFS requires the absence of exclusionary conditions, severe chronic fatigue, and at least four of eight minor symptoms.

TABLE 3-1 Elements of Selected Case Definitions and Diagnostic Criteria for ME/CFS

	Fukuda Case Definition for CFS (1994)	Canadian Consensus Criteria for ME/CFS (2003)
Terminology	CFS	ME/CFS
Method of Development	Consensus process involving an international collaborative group of leading CFS researchers and clinicians (including input from patient group representatives).	Expert Medical Consensus Panel that comprehensively reviewed and analyzed CFS research evidence; grouped symptoms together that share a common region of pathogenesis.

NICE Clinical Guidelines for CFS/ME (2007)	Revised Canadian Consensus Criteria for ME/CFS (2010)	International Consensus Criteria for ME (2011)
CFS/ME	ME/CFS	ME
The guideline was developed by the National Collaborating Centre for Primary Care, which worked with a group of health care professionals, patients, and caregivers, and technical staff who reviewed the evidence and drafted the recommendations. The recommendations were finalized after public consultation.	Authors reviewed previous definitions and literature available; tried to limit the types of symptoms within each of the Canadian Consensus Criteria categories to allow investigators to more reliably categorize patients.	The expertise and experience of the Panel members as well as PubMed and other medical sources were utilized in a progression of suggestions/drafts/reviews/revisions. The authors achieved 100 percent consensus through a Delphi-type process. The Canadian Consensus Criteria were used as a starting point, but significant changes were made.

continued

TABLE 3-1 Continued

	Fukuda Case Definition for CFS (1994)	Canadian Consensus Criteria for ME/CFS (2003)
Required Symptom(s)	• Prolonged or chronic fatigue that persists or relapses for ≥ 6 months. • Four or more of the following concurrently present for ≥ 6 months: – impaired memory or concentration – sore throat – tender cervical or axillary lymph nodes – muscle pain – multi-joint pain – new headaches – unrefreshing sleep – post-exertion malaise	• Fatigue • Post-exertional malaise and/or fatigue • Sleep dysfunction • Pain • Two or more neurological/cognitive manifestations • At least one symptom from two of the following categories: – autonomic – neuroendocrine – immune • Illness lasting ≥ 6 months

NICE Clinical Guidelines for CFS/ME (2007)	Revised Canadian Consensus Criteria for ME/CFS (2010)	International Consensus Criteria for ME (2011)
• Fatigue (characterized by post-exertional malaise and/or fatigue) • One or more of the following: – difficulty with sleeping – muscle and/or joint pain – headaches – painful lymph nodes without pathological enlargement – sore throat – cognitive dysfunction – physical or mental exertion makes symptoms worse – general malaise or flu-like symptoms – dizziness and/or nausea – palpitations in the absence of identified cardiac pathology • Persistence of symptoms ≥ 4 months for adults and ≥ 3 months in children or young people	• Fatigue • Post-exertional malaise and/or post-exertional fatigue • Unrefreshing sleep or disturbance of sleep quantity or rhythm disturbance • Pain (or discomfort) that is often widespread and migratory in nature • Two or more neurological/cognitive manifestations • At least one symptom from two of the three categories: – autonomic manifestations – neuroendocrine manifestations – immune manifestations • Persistent or recurring symptoms for ≥ 6 months but not lifelong	• Post-exertional neuroimmune exhaustion (PENE) • At least one symptom from three of the following four neurological impairment categories: – neurocognitive impairments – pain – sleep disturbance – neurosensory, perceptual, and motor disturbances • Immune, gastrointestinal, and genitourinary impairments. At least one symptom from three of the following five categories: – flu-like symptoms – susceptibility to viral infections with prolonged recovery periods – gastrointestinal tract – genitourinary – sensitivities to food, medications, odors, or chemicals • At least one symptom from energy production/transportation impairments: – cardiovascular – respiratory – loss of thermostatic stability – intolerance of extremes of temperature

continued

TABLE 3-1 Continued

	Fukuda Case Definition for CFS (1994)	Canadian Consensus Criteria for ME/CFS (2003)

Exclusionary Conditions	• Any active medical condition that may explain the presence of chronic fatigue, such as
	  – untreated hypothyroidism, sleep apnea, and narcolepsy
	  – iatrogenic conditions, such as side effects of medication.
	• Any previously diagnosed medical condition whose resolution has not been documented beyond reasonable clinical doubt and whose continued activity may explain the chronic fatiguing illness. Such conditions may include
	  – previously treated malignancies
	  – unresolved cases of hepatitis B or C virus infection.
	• Any past or current diagnosis of:
	  – major depressive disorder with psychotic or melancholic features
	  – bipolar affective disorders
	  – schizophrenia of any subtype
	  – delusional disorders of any subtype
	  – dementias of any subtype
	  – anorexia nervosa
	  – bulimia nervosa.
	• Alcohol or other substance abuse within 2 years before the onset of the chronic fatigue and at any time afterward.
	• Severe obesity as defined by a body mass index (BMI) [body mass index = weight in kilograms/(height in meters)^2] equal to or greater than 45.
		Active disease processes that explain most of the major symptoms, including
		• Addison's disease
		• Cushing's syndrome
		• hypothyroidism
		• hyperthyroidism
		• iron deficiency, other treatable forms of anemia
		• iron overload syndrome
		• diabetes mellitus
		• cancer
		
		Also exclude:
		• treatable sleep disorders such as upper airway resistance syndrome and obstructive or central sleep apnea
		• rheumatological disorders such as rheumatoid arthritis, lupus, polymyositis, and polymyalgia rheumatica
		• immune disorders such as AIDS
		• neurological disorders such as multiple sclerosis (MS), Parkinsonism, myasthenia gravis, and B$_{12}$ deficiency
		• infectious diseases such as tuberculosis, chronic hepatitis, Lyme disease, etc.
		• primary psychiatric disorders and substance abuse

NICE Clinical Guidelines for CFS/ME (2007)	Revised Canadian Consensus Criteria for ME/CFS (2010)	International Consensus Criteria for ME (2011)

No list provided	Any active medical condition that may explain the presence of chronic fatigue, such as
	
	• untreated hypothyroidism
	• sleep apnea
	• narcolepsy
	• malignancies
	• leukemia
	• unresolved hepatitis
	• multiple sclerosis
	• juvenile rheumatoid arthritis
	• lupus erythematosus
	• HIV/AIDS
	• severe obesity (BMI greater than 40; but if weight gain follows onset of ME/CFS, the patient could meet the clinical criteria)
	• celiac disease
	• Lyme disease
	
	Also exclude active psychiatric conditions that may explain the presence of chronic fatigue, such as
	
	• schizophrenia or psychotic disorders
	• bipolar disorder
	• active alcohol or substance abuse—except as below:
	  – alcohol or substance abuse that has been successfully treated and resolved should not be considered exclusionary.
	• active anorexia nervosa or bulimia nervosa—except as below:
	  – eating disorders that have been treated and resolved should not be considered exclusionary.
	• depressive disorders with melancholic or psychotic features
		As in all diagnoses, exclusion of alternate explanatory diagnoses is achieved by the patient's history, physical examination, and laboratory/biomarker testing as indicated. It is possible to have more than one disease but it is important that each one is identified and treated. Primary psychiatric disorders, somatoform disorder, and substance abuse are excluded.

continued

TABLE 3-1 Continued

	Fukuda Case Definition for CFS (1994)	Canadian Consensus Criteria for ME/CFS (2003)
Comorbidities (not necessarily exclusionary)	The following conditions do not exclude a patient from the diagnosis of unexplained chronic fatigue.	Fibromyalgia syndrome (FMS), myofascial pain syndrome (MPS), temporomandibular joint syndrome (TMJ), irritable bowel syndrome (IBS), interstitial cystitis, irritable bladder syndrome, Raynaud's phenomenon, prolapsed mitral valve, depression, migraine, allergies, multiple chemical sensitivity (MCS), Hashimoto's thyroiditis, sicca syndrome, etc.

Under the Fukuda column, the following detailed list appears:

• Any condition defined primarily by symptoms that cannot be confirmed by diagnostic laboratory tests, including
  – fibromyalgia
  – anxiety disorders
  – somatoform disorders
  – nonpsychotic or nonmelancholic depression
  – neurasthenia
  – multiple chemical sensitivity disorder.
• Any condition under specific treatment sufficient to alleviate all symptoms related to that condition and for which the adequacy of treatment has been documented. Such conditions include
  – hypothyroidism for which the adequacy of replacement hormone has been verified by normal thyroid-stimulating hormone levels or
  – asthma in which the adequacy of treatment has been determined by pulmonary function and other testing.
• Any condition, such as Lyme disease or syphilis, that was treated with definitive therapy before development of chronic symptomatic sequelae.
• Any isolated and unexplained physical examination finding or laboratory or imaging test abnormality that is insufficient to strongly suggest the existence of an exclusionary condition. Such conditions include an elevated antinuclear antibody titer that is inadequate to strongly support a diagnosis of a discrete connective tissue disorder without other laboratory or clinical evidence.

NICE Clinical Guidelines for CFS/ME (2007)	Revised Canadian Consensus Criteria for ME/CFS (2010)	International Consensus Criteria for ME (2011)

No list provided	May have presence of concomitant disorders that do not adequately explain fatigue and are, therefore, not necessarily exclusionary.
	
	• Psychiatric diagnoses, such as
	  – anxiety disorders
	  – somatoform disorders
	  – depressive disorders
	• Other conditions defined primarily by symptoms that cannot be confirmed by diagnostic laboratory tests, such as
	  – multiple food and/or chemical sensitivity
	  – fibromyalgia
	• Any condition under specific treatment sufficient to alleviate all symptoms related to that condition and for which the adequacy of treatment has been documented.
	• Any condition that was treated with definitive therapy before development of chronic symptomatic sequelae.
	• Any isolated and unexplained physical examination, laboratory, or imaging test abnormality that is insufficient to strongly suggest the existence of an exclusionary condition.
		Fibromyalgia, MPS, TMJ, IBS, interstitial cystitis, Raynaud's phenomenon, prolapsed mitral valve, migraines, allergies, MCSs, Hashimoto's thyroiditis, sicca syndrome, reactive depression. Migraine and irritable bowel syndrome may precede ME but then become associated with it. Fibromyalgia overlaps.

SOURCES: Information excerpted from Carruthers et al., 2003, 2011; CDC, 2012; Fukuda et al., 1994; Jason et al., 2010; NICE, 2007; and Reeves et al., 2003.

The Fukuda definition does not require what some consider core symptoms of ME/CFS, such as post-exertional malaise (PEM) and neurocognitive symptoms. The definition has been criticized for being overly inclusive, particularly of patients whose symptoms may be caused by a psychiatric disorder. Because many of the minor symptoms overlap with the symptoms of major depression, patients with major depression may be misclassified by the Fukuda definition (Jason et al., 1999, 2010). Some criteria for fatigue severity and minor symptoms are listed in Table 3-1, but many have argued that the Fukuda definition fails to sufficiently operationalize the major and minor symptoms, leading to variations in the way these symptoms are interpreted (Jason et al., 1999; Reeves et al., 2003). Further, a major limitation of the Fukuda definition is that its criteria are polythetic, which inevitably leads to great heterogeneity among the group of patients diagnosed according to these criteria. For instance, two patients could have very little symptom overlap yet both be diagnosed with CFS.

The Fukuda definition indicates that patients who fail to meet its criteria for fatigue severity and at least four minor symptoms should be diagnosed with idiopathic chronic fatigue. The research guidelines recommend subgrouping cases of CFS or idiopathic chronic fatigue by the presence or absence of comorbid conditions, level of fatigue, duration of fatigue, and level of physical function (Fukuda et al., 1994). Despite the challenges noted above, the Fukuda case definition is the most widely used definition in ME/CFS research, and it is also used for clinical evaluation of patients (Brurberg et al., 2014; CDC, 2012).

Canadian Consensus Criteria for ME/CFS (2003)

Carruthers and colleagues (2003) published the CCC as a clinical working case definition to assist physicians and other clinicians in making a diagnosis of ME/CFS. Because fatigue can be present in many other illnesses, the CCC requires for a diagnosis of ME/CFS the presence of four cardinal symptoms—fatigue, PEM, sleep dysfunction, and pain—as well as minor symptoms grouped by region of pathogenesis (see Table 3-1). Thus, for a diagnosis of ME/CFS, the CCC requires that symptoms be present from the following six symptom categories for 6 months or longer:

- fatigue, including substantial reduction in activity level;
- PEM and/or post-exertional fatigue;
- sleep dysfunction;
- pain;
- neurologic/cognitive manifestations; and
- autonomic, neuroendocrine, or immune manifestations.

The authors intentionally included more symptoms than had been specified in previous diagnostic criteria to help clinicians identify patients with unique combinations of symptoms, and a symptom merely must be present to count toward a diagnosis.

NICE Clinical Guidelines for CFS/ME (2007)

In 2007, NICE published clinical guidelines for the diagnosis and management of ME/CFS, referred to as CFS/ME (NICE, 2007). The NICE criteria for diagnosis require the presence of fatigue and at least one other symptom, and these symptoms must have persisted for at least 4 months (see Table 3-1 for more information). Although the NICE criteria require fewer total symptoms relative to other diagnostic criteria for ME/CFS, the guidelines note that PEM or post-exertional fatigue, cognitive difficulties, sleep disturbance, and chronic pain are key features of the illness and that a diagnosis of ME/CFS should be reconsidered if none of these symptoms are present. As with other criteria, the NICE guidelines recommend that alternative diagnoses be ruled out before a diagnosis of ME/CFS is given. These guidelines also provide a list of "red flags" and potential comorbidities that should be investigated.

Revised Canadian Clinical Case Definition for ME/CFS (2010)

In 2010, Jason and colleagues revised the CCC and provided explicit rules for applying this case definition, including a questionnaire for assessing symptoms. The Revised CCC was intended to better operationalize the CCC. The authors provided operational definitions for several key symptoms to improve diagnostic reliability and use of the CCC in research studies (Jason et al., 2010, 2013b). For a diagnosis of ME/CFS, the Revised CCC requires the presence of symptoms from the same six categories (with some wording differences) as those of the original CCC (Jason et al., 2010).

The Revised CCC recommends the use of a structured questionnaire (the DePaul Symptom Questionnaire) (DePaul Research Team, 2010) to gather standardized information on symptoms as well as the use of the scales of the Short Form 36-Item Questionnaire (SF-36) of the Medical Outcomes Study to assess whether a patient has a substantial reduction in functioning (McHorney et al., 1993). A symptom must be present with moderate severity about half of the time to meet criteria for a symptom category, and a patient must score below a certain maximum score on at least two of the three scales of the SF-36 to meet criteria for a substantial reduction in functioning.

International Consensus Criteria for ME (2011)

Carruthers and colleagues (2011) published the ME-ICC for both clinical and research use. The authors started with the CCC and made extensive changes. Referring to "recent research and clinical experience that strongly point to widespread inflammation and multi-systemic neuropathology," the authors chose to use the term "ME" instead of "CFS" or "ME/CFS" (Carruthers et al., 2011, p. 327). This decision has been challenged by other researchers in the field who oppose the use of the term, asserting that there is no convincing evidence of inflammation in ME/CFS (van der Meer and Lloyd, 2012).

The ME-ICC no longer requires a 6-month waiting period before a diagnosis is made and includes operational notes for each of the symptom criteria. To be diagnosed, a patient must experience post-exertional neuroimmune exhaustion—the authors' term for PEM—as well as symptoms from three symptom categories:

- neurological impairments (which encompass neurocognitive impairments; pain; sleep disturbance; and neurosensory, perceptual, and motor disturbances);
- immune, gastrointestinal, and genitourinary impairments; and
- energy production/transportation impairments.

To receive a diagnosis of ME, a patient must have symptoms that result in a substantial reduction in activity compared with premorbid activity levels. A 50 percent reduction in pre-illness activity level is considered only a "mild" reduction. The ME-ICC does not provide guidelines on the severity or frequency of symptoms that must be present for a diagnosis (Jason et al., 2013b). It does not suggest the use of a standardized questionnaire for clinical diagnosis but recommends that all patients in research studies complete the International Symptom Scale to increase the reliability of data collection.

Comparison of Existing Diagnostic Criteria

The diagnostic criteria described above have similarities and differences. The Revised CCC and the ME-ICC share the most similarities with the CCC, but that is to be expected given that both used the CCC as a starting point. All of the criteria require that other explanations for a patient's symptoms be ruled out before a diagnosis of ME/CFS can be made, although the list of exclusionary conditions differs across the criteria. While all of the criteria make clear that they are describing and defining the same illness, some vary in the terminology used to refer to the illness or to specific symptoms. The following subsections compare some of the major components of the various diagnostic criteria and summarize the literature comparing the groups of patients identified by these criteria.

Required and Additional Symptoms

The existing diagnostic criteria focus on similar sets of symptoms, but they differ markedly in the number of symptoms required and how those symptoms are defined. The Fukuda definition and the NICE guidelines are perhaps the most straightforward. Both require persistent fatigue of new or definite onset; the NICE criteria require 1 additional symptom from a list of 10 minor symptoms, and the Fukuda definition requires 4 additional symptoms from a list of 8 minor symptoms. The CCC, Revised CCC, and ME-ICC require PEM (referred to in the ME-ICC as post-exertional neuroimmune exhaustion), while PEM is one of the minor symptoms in the Fukuda definition and listed as a feature of the fatigue required in the NICE guidelines. In addition to fatigue and PEM, pain and sleep disturbance are required symptoms for a diagnosis using the CCC and Revised CCC.

The CCC, Revised CCC, and ME-ICC divide additional symptoms into symptom categories. The CCC and Revised CCC require at least two neurological/cognitive manifestations and some combination of autonomic, neuroendocrine, and immune manifestations. The ME-ICC lists many of the same additional symptoms but categorizes them differently (see Table 3-1).

It is important to note that when diagnostic criteria require any symptom on a list to classify a patient as having a disease, they risk including groups of patients that do not suffer from the same disease. For instance, the CCC provides a list of several neurological impairments. If one of these symptoms is present, the patient is considered to have fulfilled the neurological impairment requirement. For example, reduced working memory and ataxia would both indicate neurocognitive impairment, but patients presenting with memory impairment might suffer from a different entity than patients with ataxia.

Comparison of Groups Selected by Various Diagnostic Criteria

Many patients with ME/CFS meet more than one set of diagnostic criteria given the overlap of symptoms among criteria. Several studies have compared the groups of patients selected using different ME/CFS criteria and found that the various criteria select groups of patients with differences in symptomatology and impairment (Jason et al., 2013b). Most of these studies have compared patients fulfilling the Fukuda definition with patients fulfilling another of the sets of ME/CFS criteria described above.

In general, the Fukuda definition identifies a larger, more heterogeneous group of patients compared with the other criteria (Jason et al., 2012a). The symptoms in the Fukuda definition can be present in other illnesses, and if exclusionary conditions are unknown or unaccounted for, patients with lupus or multiple sclerosis may be incorrectly diagnosed (Jason et al., 1997; King, 2003). Most patients that fulfill the CCC will also fulfill the Fukuda definition; not all patients fulfilling the Fukuda definition will also fulfill the CCC (Nacul et al., 2011; Pheby et al., 2011). Patients fulfilling the CCC have a higher prevalence and severity of symptoms than those fulfilling the Fukuda definition (Nacul et al., 2011). The CCC also has been shown to select patients with more functional impairment, fatigue, weakness, and neuropsychiatric and neurological symptoms relative to the Fukuda definition (Jason et al., 2004b; Morris and Maes, 2013; Watson et al., 2014). In addition, patients diagnosed with the CCC were found to have less psychiatric comorbidity than those diagnosed with the Fukuda definition (Jason et al., 2004b).

The CCC requires only the presence of a symptom to count toward a diagnosis, whereas the Revised CCC specifies that minimum levels of frequency and severity be present for a symptom to count toward a diagnosis. Fewer patients meet the criteria for ME/CFS under the Revised CCC than do so under the CCC or the Fukuda definition (Jason et al., 2012a). Up to 75 percent of patients fulfilling the Fukuda definition will also fulfill the CCC, suggesting that the CCC selects a subset of these patients (Jason et al., 2013a; Nacul et al., 2011). Patients fulfilling the Revised CCC have more severe functional impairment and physical and cognitive symptoms relative to those fulfilling the Fukuda definition. In contrast to the CCC, and perhaps as a result of requiring higher frequency and greater severity of symptoms, the Revised CCC identifies patients with significantly more psychiatric comorbidity compared with the Fukuda definition (Jason et al., 2012a).

The ME-ICC has been shown to select for a subset of patients that also meet the Fukuda definition. Patients that fulfill the ME-ICC have more severe functional impairment and more physical, mental, and cognitive problems than those that fulfill the Fukuda definition. There has been conflicting evidence on rates of psychiatric comorbidity in those fulfilling the ME-ICC compared with the Fukuda definition, which may be attributable to the different measures used in different studies (Brown et al., 2013b; Jason et al., 2014).

Challenges Created by Multiple Sets of Criteria

The way a definition is operationalized can dramatically affect the specificity of diagnostic criteria. Jason and colleagues (2013b) examined different thresholds for ME/CFS symptoms and found that merely requiring a symptom to be present without specifying a minimum level of frequency or severity resulted in more frequent misdiagnosis of healthy controls as having ME/CFS. Without a minimum threshold for assessing symptoms, 33.7 percent of healthy controls fulfilled the Fukuda definition, 20.7 percent fulfilled the CCC, and 14.6 percent fulfilled the ME-ICC. After applying minimum thresholds for frequency and severity (symptoms must be present at least half of the time with at least moderate severity), only 4.7 percent of healthy controls fulfilled the Fukuda definition, while 3.7 percent fulfilled both the CCC and ME-ICC. The operational ambiguity has important consequences for research in ME/CFS, as different studies operationalize the criteria in different ways, limiting comparisons across studies. Having different case definitions also has resulted in diagnostic unreliability and confusion for clinicians, patients, and their families.

In April 2014, the U.S. Social Security Administration—the government agency responsible for administering disability benefits—revised its guidelines for evaluating disability claims involving ME/CFS. The new ruling replaced previous guidelines, which were based on the Fukuda definition of CFS. The updated guidelines are based on adaptations of the Fukuda definition and some elements of the CCC and ME-ICC (Social Security Ruling, 2014). Although disability is a legal decision and not a medical diagnosis, the U.S. Social Security Administration's incorporation of more recent diagnostic criteria indicates the usefulness of these criteria for identifying ME/CFS. More information on disability related to ME/CFS can be found in Appendix C.

Validation of Diagnostic Criteria for ME/CFS

In a recent systematic review, Brurberg and colleagues (2014) identified 38 studies on comparison and evaluation of the existing diagnostic criteria for ME/CFS, which they considered "validation" studies. Their search strategy identified studies that either (1) independently applied multiple case definitions to the same population; or (2) sequentially applied multiple case definitions (with assumed increasing specificity) to the same population; or (3) indirectly compared prevalence estimates from multiple case definitions applied to different populations. All clinical and basic science studies were excluded. Most of these studies examined the Fukuda definition; there were a few validation studies for the CCC and ME-ICC and none for the NICE guidelines. Most of the studies had serious limitations, and there were no rigorous assessments of the reproducibility or feasibility of case definitions.

Pediatric Definitions

Although most of the diagnostic criteria described above were developed for adults, they have been used to diagnose children and adolescents in both clinical and research settings. ME/CFS usually is equally represented in younger male and female children, yet it occurs more frequently in female than in male adolescents (Royal College, 2004). Two case definitions have been developed specifically for children (one proposed by Jason and colleagues and one developed by the Royal College of Paediatrics), but the CCC, NICE guidelines, and ME-ICC include guidelines for diagnosing ME/CFS in children (Carruthers et al., 2003, 2011; Jason et al., 2006; NICE, 2007; Royal College, 2004). The concerns and limitations described above for the case definitions and diagnostic criteria for adults apply also to criteria used to diagnose children and adolescents.

Canadian Consensus Criteria for ME/CFS (2003)

Although there are no separate criteria for children in the CCC, these criteria note that children with ME/CFS usually have numerous symptoms, and "their hierarchy of symptom severity may vary from day to day" (Carruthers et al., 2003, p. 21). Children fulfilling the CCC may be diagnosed after the illness persists for 3 months (rather than the 6 months required for adults) (Carruthers et al., 2003).

Royal College of Paediatrics and Child Health Evidence-Based Guideline for the Management of CFS/ME in Children and Young People (2004) and NICE Guidelines (2007)

The Royal College of Paediatrics and Child Health proposed pediatric criteria for ME/CFS in 2004. The authors considered whether the shorter duration of 3 months for diagnosis rather than 6 months is appropriate in children. They concluded that, in the absence of compelling epidemiological data, the diagnosis of ME/CFS requires 6 months. They nonetheless suggest that pediatricians should be "prepared to make a positive diagnosis of CFS/ME when a child or young person has characteristic symptoms supported by normal results and when the symptoms are causing significant functional impairment. This diagnosis does not depend on a specific time frame, and a positive diagnosis of CFS/ME is not a prerequisite for the initiation of an appropriate management plan" (Royal College, 2004, p. 27). Nevertheless, the NICE guidelines, published in 2007, recommended a duration of symptoms of 3 months for children and young people (NICE, 2007).

International Association for CFS/ME Pediatric Case Definition (2006)

The International Association for CFS/ME's (IACFS/ME's) pediatric case definition, developed by Jason and colleagues (2006), incorporates elements of the Fukuda definition and the CCC and was intended to facilitate clinical and research diagnoses of ME/CFS in children and adolescents. Like the CCC, the pediatric definition requires 3 months of clinically evaluated, unexplained, persistent or relapsing chronic fatigue as well as cardinal symptoms of ME/CFS: PEM, unrefreshing sleep, pain, and neurocognitive manifestations. To fulfill the pediatric definition, a patient must also have some combination of autonomic, neuroendocrine, or immune manifestations. As noted in the CCC, the pediatric definition highlights "the individuality of symptom patterns and unpredictability of symptom severity among youngsters with ME/CFS" (Jason et al., 2006, p. 5). The pediatric definition also was intended to represent the importance of particular symptoms, including dizziness, decreased endurance with symptoms, pain, and flu-like symptoms.

The onset of ME/CFS symptoms in pediatric populations can be abrupt or insidious. This definition recommends that patients who have experienced symptoms for 1 to 2 months should be classified as "CFS-like." A small number of patients may present with no pain or sleep dysfunction or have only two to four of the cardinal ME/CFS symptoms described above. These individuals may be given a diagnosis of atypical pediatric ME/CFS (Jason et al., 2006). Subsequently, Jason and colleagues (2009) further subdivided these criteria into severe and moderate. As with the diagnostic criteria for adults, the pediatric definition includes a list of medical and psychiatric conditions that may also cause chronic fatigue and should be considered exclusionary.

International Consensus Criteria for Pediatric ME (2011)

The ME-ICC, as discussed above, was developed for both clinical and research use and includes considerations for diagnosing children and adolescents. The ME-ICC also emphasizes the fluctuation of symptoms and symptom severity in pediatric ME/CFS as well as the gradual onset of symptoms. In addition to PEM, the most prominent pediatric symptoms include headaches, neurocognitive impairments, and sleep disturbances. The ME-ICC also notes that pain in pediatric ME/CFS "may seem erratic and migrate quickly" and that "joint hypermobility is common" (Carruthers et al., 2011, p. 330).

Comparison of Pediatric Diagnostic Criteria

Differences among the diagnostic criteria for pediatric ME/CFS are similar to those among the adult criteria, but some aspects are consistent in most of the pediatric criteria. All the pediatric criteria except the Royal College of Paediatrics guideline recognize the more gradual or insidious onset of symptoms relative to adults, require that symptoms persist for a shorter period of time before diagnosis than in adults, and highlight the variability of symptoms and symptom severity in individual pediatric patients. They all note that ME/CFS symptoms often make it more difficult to do schoolwork, so children and adolescents with ME/CFS may be misclassified as having "school phobia."[2] All include information to help clinicians differentiate ME/CFS from school phobia (Carruthers et al., 2003, 2011; Jason et al., 2006). Although children with school phobia and ME/CFS may have similar complaints, symptoms of the former condition usually disappear when a child is allowed to stay home or on weekends or holidays (Jason et al., 2006). Moreover, children with school phobia continue to enjoy their hobbies and leisure activities, while children with ME/CFS are likely to abandon them to keep up in school and spend their out-of-school hours resting (Carruthers et al., 2011; Jason et al., 2006). School phobia is listed as a comorbidity in the IACFS/ME pediatric case definition, and "primary" school phobia is considered an exclusionary condition in the ME-ICC. Both of these criteria note that it is important to determine the timeline of symptoms, as school phobia may develop as a consequence of ME/CFS in situations where academic performance becomes difficult or bullying due to ME/CFS symptoms occurs (Carruthers et al., 2011; Jason et al., 2006). Jason and colleagues (2006) note that a comprehensive evaluation should be able to distinguish between the two conditions.

The use of different diagnostic criteria and case definitions has posed the same challenges for research into pediatric ME/CFS as it has for research with adults. The IACFS/ME pediatric case definition was developed years after similar criteria existed for adults, so it is not surprising that much of the research on pediatric populations has used the Fukuda definition (Jason et al., 2006). The use of different definitions to define research populations impedes the ability to compare results across studies.

Research Subgroups

The Fukuda definition identifies essential and optional variables for subgrouping patients in formal studies (research subgroups), yet many

---

[2] Japanese investigators have frequently used the term "school phobia" to refer to pediatric ME/CFS (Miike et al., 2004).

BOX 3-1
ME/CFS Research Subgroups

Clinical Stratification Variables

- Fulfillment of different case definitions or diagnostic criteria
- Illness onset: sudden or gradual
- Type, severity, or duration of symptoms
- Level of functional performance
- Gender
- Age
- Duration of illness
- Comorbid conditions
  - ME/CFS + fibromyalgia
  - ME/CFS + postural orthostatic tachycardia syndrome
  - ME/CFS + depression
  - ME/CFS + anxiety
- Pre-illness history and triggers

Biological Stratification Variables

- Exercise response
- Immunologic
- Infectious
- Endocrine
- Neurological
- Metabolic
- Genomic

SOURCES: Abbi and Natelson, 2013; Arroll and Senior, 2009; Aschbacher et al., 2012; Brenu et al., 2013; Brown et al., 2010, 2013a; Corradi et al., 2006; Fukuda et al., 1994; Janal et al., 2006; Jason et al., 2000, 2012b; Njoku et al., 2009; Reynolds et al., 2013; Twisk, 2014.

---

researchers have not examined subgroups of patients according to these guidelines. There are numerous ways to stratify patients with ME/CFS (see Box 3-1). Evidence specific to certain subgroups of ME/CFS is discussed in Chapters 4, 5, and 6.

TERMINOLOGY

In response to its directive to "recommend whether new terminology for ME/CFS should be adopted," the committee considered the variety of names that have been proposed for ME/CFS. Over the years, many patients and advocates have suggested a variety of other names they find more appropriate (Dimmock and Lazell-Fairman, 2014; Jason et al., 2001, 2004a).

BOX 3-2
Suggestions for a New Name Received from
Members of the Public

- Myalgic encephalomyelitis
- Myalgic encephalomyelitis/chronic fatigue syndrome (ME/CFS)
- Chronic fatigue and immune dysfunction syndrome (CFIDS)
- Activity-induced neuroimmune morbidity
- Autonomic nervous system dysfunction
- Autonomic nervous system immune mitochondrial dysfunction
- Body breakdown syndrome
- Brain dysfunction induced ME/CFS
- Brain stem infection
- Catastrophic multisystem dysfunction
- Chronic fatigue
- Chronic fatigue syndrome
- Chronic immune abnormality
- Chronic immune deficiency
- Chronic influenza syndrome
- Chronic myalgic encephalopathy syndrome
- Complex energy collapse syndrome
- Complex energy drain syndrome
- Cytokinitis
- Diffuse encephalomyelitic immune inflammatory syndrome
- Encephalomyelitic cytokine inflammatory cascade
- Encephalomyelitic cytokine syndrome
- Encephalomyelitic immune inflammatory cascade
- Encephalomyelitic immune syndrome
- Encephalomyelitis/chronic fatigue syndrome
- Energy collapse syndrome
- Epidemic neuro-myasthenia
- Immune dysfunction syndrome
- Immune neuroendocrine syndrome
- Immunity disease
- Mitochondrial dysfunction syndrome
- Mitochondrial failure syndrome

The committee asked members of the public to suggest a new name for the illness, and these suggestions can be found in Box 3-2. The most common suggestions were "myalgic encephalomyelitis," "myalgic encephalomyelitis/ chronic fatigue syndrome" (ME/CFS), and "chronic fatigue and immune dysfunction syndrome" (CFIDS). The most commonly used names include "chronic fatigue syndrome" and "myalgic encephalomyelitis," either of which may be used alone or in combination with others. Other names in-

- Mitochondrial immune dysfunction syndrome
- Multi-symptom cognitive and energy challenge
- Multi-system disease
- Multiple encephalomyelitis
- Multiple enervation disorder
- Multiple neuroimmune disorder
- Multi-systemic dysregulation
- Multi-systemic infectious disease syndrome (MSIDS)
- Myalgic encephalomyelitis fatigue syndrome
- Myalgic encephalomyopathy
- Nature killer cells syndrome (NKCS)
- Neural-endocrine exhaustive dysfunction
- Neurasthenia gravis
- Neuroendocrine immune collapse syndrome
- Neuroendocrine immune disease
- Neuroendocrine immune dysfunction
- Neuroendocrine immune dysfunction syndrome
- Neuroimmune disease
- Neuroimmune disorder
- Neuroimmune-endocrine muscular disease
- Neuroimmune inflammatory disease
- Neuroimmune microbe imbalance
- Neuroimmune spectrum disorder
- Neuro-myasthenia
- Nightingale's disease
- Peterson syndrome
- Peterson's disease
- Post-activity neuroimmune morbidity
- Post-polio syndrome (PPS)
- Ramsey's syndrome
- Severe systematic collapse
- Sophia Mirza disease
- Vagal gliosis
- Vagal neuropathy
- Anything but CFS

clude "benign myalgic encephalomyelitis," "post-viral fatigue syndrome," and "epidemic neuromyasthenia."

As discussed in Chapter 2, many patients and researchers are critical of the term "chronic fatigue syndrome," which is the name most commonly ascribed to this disease in the United States (but not in other parts of the world). Patients in particular find this term stigmatizing and trivializing, and there is evidence to support these perspectives. The way an illness is labeled affects the illness experience (Wojcik et al., 2011). Labels convey meanings that affect patients' perception of their illness as well as the reactions of others, including medical personnel, family members, and colleagues (Jason and Richman, 2008; Jason et al., 2002b; Wojcik et al., 2011). As noted in Chapter 2, patients have reported that many clinicians are dismissive, making such comments as "I am fatigued all the time, too." Perceptions of a patient by others are important because they have been shown to affect the course of a disorder and may be associated with different outcomes (Wojcik et al., 2011).

In addition to the personal experiences presented in Chapter 2, several investigators have examined the attitudes and beliefs elicited by different diagnostic labels for ME/CFS. Among medical students, the term "myalgic encephalomyelitis" was more likely to be classified as a disease than the term "chronic fatigue syndrome" (Erueti et al., 2012). Among medical trainees and college students, the term "myalgic encephalomyelitis" was "more likely to prompt beliefs in a physiological cause for the illness" than the term "chronic fatigue syndrome" (Jason et al., 2002b, 2004a, p. 223).

> **Conclusion:** *The committee agrees that the term "chronic fatigue syndrome" often results in stigmatization and trivialization and should no longer be used as the name of this illness.*

In considering which name would be most appropriate, the committee turned first to ME—"myalgic encephalomyelitis" or "encephalopathy." Historically, however, the diagnostic criteria for ME have required the presence of specific or different symptoms from those required by the diagnostic criteria for CFS; thus, a diagnosis of CFS is not equivalent to a diagnosis of ME. This term also fails to convey the full spectrum of this disorder. While the term "encephalopathy" suggests the presence of global brain dysfunction, a symptom supported by research, the term "encephalomyelitis" suggests brain inflammation, for which there is much less evidence at present. Similarly, the term "myalgia" refers to a symptom that is neither a distinguishing aspect of this illness nor a severe symptom in many patients with ME/CFS. The committee noted that many of the other proposed names focus on particular organ systems, while others suggest particular etiologies for this disorder, such as immune or infectious, which are not yet proven. The committee's recommendations for new terminology for ME/CFS are presented in Chapter 7.

SYMPTOM CONSTRUCTS AND CLUSTERS

Committee members read and reviewed selected articles with the following questions in mind: Is there a set of core symptom constructs that defines ME/CFS and distinguishes it from other disorders? Are there particular clusters or characteristics of symptoms that reliably identify subgroups of individuals with ME/CFS? (For more information on the methodology of the literature review, see Chapter 1.)

Many of the limitations of the evidence base on ME/CFS described elsewhere in this report apply to this literature (see Chapter 4). For example, studies used different measures to assess various symptoms. Some instruments measured the presence or absence of a symptom in a dichotomous manner; others categorized symptoms according to frequency or severity or both. Some studies evaluated a narrow or limited set of symptoms and failed to assess potentially relevant symptoms, such as PEM or flu-like complaints. The study investigators used a variety of analytic methods, including factor analysis, principal component analysis, cluster analysis, and classification and regression tree (CART). They rarely specified either the rationale for or the limitations of the method they chose. Small studies with few individuals sharing particular constellations of symptoms sometimes limited the ability to tease out distinct clusters or subgroups of ME/CFS patients.

Evidence

Key Symptom Constructs Identified by Factor Analyses

Several investigators used factor analysis to explore the relations or components of symptom constructs or to reduce large sets of symptom data to a few structural components. As these particular factor analyses did not differentiate among groups of people with and without illness, their findings cannot be used to create a discriminating case definition. In the absence of standard protocol, investigators assigned somewhat different names to groups of symptoms (e.g., "cognitive problems," "cognitive difficulties") and identified different numbers of factors (e.g., four to six) as important (Arroll and Senior, 2009; Jason et al., 2002a). They used different statistical approaches and made different decisions about how factors were "extracted" and "rotated."[3] Some used low threshold factor loading

---

[3] Factor extraction and rotation are essential steps in exploratory factor analysis. Extraction is performed to produce factor loadings with the hope of large loading on one factor and small loadings on other factors—this is known as "simple structure." There are several approaches to extraction, and principal axis factoring and maximum likelihood are considered the most appropriate methods for small sample sizes. Rotation then maximizes high loadings and minimizes low loadings to achieve the simplest structure. The two basic approaches to rotation are "orthogonal" and "oblique," with various algorithms to employ with each method. The former assumes no correlation between factors, and the latter assumes correlation (Kim and Mueller, 1978).

values, which resulted in retaining symptoms that contributed relatively little information. Only one study involved both an exploratory and a confirmatory analysis (Nisenbaum et al., 2004).

Most authors identify fatigue-type factors as an integral symptom construct of ME/CFS (Arroll and Senior, 2009; Jason and Taylor, 2002; Nisenbaum et al., 1998, 2004; Ray et al., 1992). In two studies, fatigue is considered part of a multidimensional construct encompassing fatigue, mood, and cognition (Nisenbaum et al., 1998, 2004), while in two other studies, fatigue is considered part of a bidimensional construct related to either rest or PEM (Arroll and Senior, 2009; Jason and Taylor, 2002). Several studies identify a "neurocognitive difficulty" factor that includes such symptoms as slowness of thought; mental fog; and problems with concentrating, memory, or understanding (Arroll and Senior, 2009; Hickie et al., 2009; Jason and Taylor, 2002; Ray et al., 1992). Some identify a "musculoskeletal" factor that includes such symptoms as muscle or joint aches and pains and weakness (Brimacombe et al., 2002; Hickie et al., 2009; Nisenbaum et al., 2004; Tseng and Natelson, 2004); a "viral flu-like" factor that includes such complaints as fever, sore throat, and tender lymph nodes (Brimacombe et al., 2002; Nisenbaum et al., 1998, 2004; Tseng and Natelson, 2004); an emotional distress or mood or anxiety disturbance factor (Arroll and Senior, 2009; Fostel et al., 2006; Hickie et al., 2009; Ray et al., 1992); a somatic factor that includes such gastrointestinal complaints as stomach pain or diarrhea (Arroll and Senior, 2009; Nisenbaum et al., 2004; Ray et al., 1992); and a sleep difficulties factor (Fostel et al., 2006; Hickie et al., 2009).

Symptom Constructs and Clusters That Distinguish ME/CFS Patients

Few studies examined whether particular symptom clusters or characteristics of symptom constructs (e.g., severity, frequency) differentiated individuals with ME/CFS from healthy individuals or individuals with fatigue due to conditions other than ME/CFS. One study involving 236 participants who had been diagnosed by physicians using either the Fukuda definition or the CCC and 86 healthy controls examined the frequency and severity of 54 symptoms reported on the DePaul Symptom Questionnaire (Jason et al., 2013b). Three symptom constructs (PEM, memory and concentration problems, unrefreshing sleep) were more prevalent among ME/CFS patients compared with other constructs (e.g., headaches, joint pain, muscle aches, sore throat, lymph node problems). Using a CART algorithm, the investigators found that three symptoms (fatigue or extreme tiredness, inability to focus on more than one item at a time, experiencing a dead or heavy feeling after starting to exercise) accurately classified 95.4 percent of the study participants as patients or healthy controls when a minimum frequency and severity score of 2 (symptom must be of at least moderate intensity and be present at least half of the time) was used for the symptoms.

A community-based study of 780 adults in Chicago who reported chronic fatigue symptoms subdivided the sample into individuals with (1) ME/CFS who had four or more symptoms of the Fukuda definition, (2) idiopathic chronic fatigue, or (3) fatigue explained by medical or psychiatric conditions (Jason et al., 2002a). Symptoms were assessed with the CFS Screening Questionnaire administered via telephone, and diagnoses were not verified by physician evaluation. Four factors—"lack of energy," "physical exertion," "cognitive functioning," and "fatigue and rest"—most accurately defined fatigue-related symptomatology in individuals with severe fatigue lasting 6 months or longer. The group with ME/CFS meeting the Fukuda definition consistently had more severe symptomatology for all four dimensions of fatigue compared with those in the idiopathic fatigue group. Another analysis of data from this study, limited to 166 individuals who were medically evaluated, identified three clusters of participants (Jason and Taylor, 2002). The cluster that contained the highest proportion of participants with ME/CFS was characterized by high post-exertional fatigue and fatigue not alleviated by rest.

A study conducted in Germany compared the presence or absence of 26 "unspecific" symptoms in outpatients with severe fatigue who had ME/CFS (n = 91), systemic lupus erythematosus (n = 41), or fibromyalgia (n = 58) (Linder et al., 2002). ME/CFS patients met the Fukuda definition for ME/CFS or for idiopathic chronic fatigue. Neither PEM nor post-exertional precipitation/exacerbation of symptoms was examined. Four analytic methods, including regression tree analysis and artificial neural network analysis, were used to generate classification criteria that would differentiate the patients with ME/CFS from those with lupus and fibromyalgia. Although the various analytic methods resulted in different optimum sets of classification criteria, symptoms that appeared to best differentiate ME/CFS patients from the other patients were "acute onset of fatigue" and "sore throat."

Hickie and colleagues (2009) analyzed heterogeneous data collected from 33 different studies in 21 countries. They found that patients diagnosed with ME/CFS, compared with people with chronic fatigue but no ME/CFS diagnosis, more commonly reported "musculoskeletal pain/fatigue" symptom factors (e.g., "pain in arms or legs") and "neurocognitive difficulties" (e.g., "poor concentration") and less commonly reported "sleep disturbance/fatigue" symptom factors (e.g., "waking up tired"). A study involving patients recruited both from tertiary clinics and through advertisements concluded that a broad diversity of ancillary symptoms distinguishes ME/CFS from other fatiguing syndromes and that exertional exhaustion helps separate ME/CFS and ME/CFS-like patients from healthy controls (Baraniuk et al., 2013).

Using data from a population-based telephone survey in San Francisco, Nisenbaum and colleagues (1998) attempted to identify the correlations between severe fatigue not explained by medical or psychiatric conditions and lasting either less than 6 months or 6 months or longer and 30 symptoms perceived to be "significant health problems" during the previous 4 weeks. A random sample of 1,078 adults with no fatigue and a total of 1,510 adults with unexplained severe fatigue were interviewed. Through common factor analysis, the authors identified three correlated factors ("fatigue-mood-cognition" symptoms, "flu-type" symptoms, and "visual impairment") that explained the correlations between fatigue lasting 6 months or longer and 14 interrelated symptoms. The authors could identify no factors that explained the correlations between fatigue lasting less than 6 months and other symptoms. They concluded that "these results provide empirical support for the interrelations among unexplained fatigue of ≥ 6 months' duration and symptoms included in the CFS case definition." They interpreted the study findings as suggesting that as unexplained fatigue continues (with 6 months being a possible threshold), other "natural" accompanying symptoms that may help define the presence of ME/CFS are likely to arise.

A second study by Nisenbaum and colleagues (2004) examined the presence or absence of 21 symptoms in 1,391 chronically fatigued patients, including 43 patients with diagnosed ME/CFS. Factor scores for three symptom areas (musculoskeletal, infection, and cognition-mood-sleep) were created, and cluster analysis was used to generate three groups of patients. Cluster 1 (n = 232) represented the healthiest patients and included very few patients with ME/CFS, while cluster 3 (n = 455) included most of the ME/CFS patients and patients who were most chronically unwell. Agreement between clusters and fatigue subgroups was poor. The authors concluded that ME/CFS may represent the severe end of a spectrum of "chronic unwellness syndrome" but that chronic unwellness per se is not sufficient to distinguish patients with ME/CFS from those with other fatigue states.

Symptom Constructs and Clusters That Identify Subgroups

A small study involving 114 participants meeting the Fukuda definition for ME/CFS who were recruited to participate in a trial used cluster analysis to identify three subgroups of patients: symptomatic and highly overextended individuals (n = 20), less symptomatic and moderately overextended individuals (n = 34), and symptomatic and mildly overextended individuals (n = 37) (Brown et al., 2013a). Overextension was measured by an "energy envelope quotient" calculated from self-rated measures of energy capacity and energy expended. The cluster of individuals who were symptomatic and mildly overextended had more pain than individuals in the other clusters. Another study involving the same patients found that patient fatigue patterns reported during a single day could be subtyped into the following three categories based on fatigue intensity and variability: group 1 had high fatigue intensity and low variability; group 2 "had moderate fatigue intensity and high variability, with fatigue intensity decreasing over time"; and group 3 "had moderate fatigue intensity and high variability, with fatigue intensity increasing over time" (Jason et al., 2012a, p. 4).

A study of 246 patients recruited from support groups who self-reported that they had been diagnosed with ME/CFS according to the Fukuda definition used cluster analysis to identify low, medium, and high symptomatology subgroups (Arroll and Senior, 2009). Individuals in the high symptomatology subgroup had high scores in all five factor domains (fibromyalgia syndrome [FMS]-like, depression/anxiety, fatigue/PEM, cognitive/neurological, irritable bowel syndrome [IBS]-like). Individuals in the low symptomatology subgroup had average scores in the depression/anxiety domain and low scores in all other domains.

Two studies explored gender differences in the expression of symptoms. One of these studies examined 121 patients meeting the Fukuda definition and found no gender differences in severity of fatigue or functional status; however, women were more likely than men to have flu-like symptoms and less likely to have comorbid depression (Tseng and Natelson, 2004). The second, larger study of 780 adults reporting chronic fatigue found that women experienced more difficulty with memory, concentration, and information processing than men (Jason et al., 2002a). This study also found that middle-aged and older individuals with chronic fatigue reported more difficulties with energy, tiredness, weakness, and fatigue and greater fatigue symptomatology following exertion relative to individuals younger than 40. Finally, individuals of low socioeconomic status reported more severe fatigue related to exertion compared with those of higher socioeconomic status.

One study examined differences in disease presentation in older and younger Fukuda-diagnosed ME/CFS patients (Lewis et al., 2013). The study matched 25 older patients (> 50) to 25 younger patients (16-29) on gender and length of history and found very different disease phenotypes between the two groups. Specifically, the older patients demonstrated greater fatigue, a higher rate of depression, greater autonomic dysfunction, lower baroflexic sensitivity, and more prolonged left ventricular ejection time. The findings of this study suggest a greater disease impact in older patients.

Summary

These studies provide insufficient evidence to conclude that a specific cluster of symptoms universally defines ME/CFS or that the presence of a particular cluster of symptoms reliably distinguishes among ME/CFS subgroups or distinguishes ME/CFS from other disorders. Individual symptom constructs that may help distinguish adults with ME/CFS from those with other conditions include intense fatigue or tiredness that is worsened by exertion and not alleviated by rest, neurocognitive difficulties characterized by slowness of thought or mental fog, and unrefreshing sleep. Severity scores for such constructs as fatigue appear to be higher in individuals with ME/CFS than in those without ME/CFS. Accordingly, it is important to consider symptom thresholds that take severity into account when operationalizing any diagnostic criteria for ME/CFS.

REFERENCES

Abbi, B., and B. H. Natelson. 2013. Is chronic fatigue syndrome the same illness as fibromyalgia: Evaluating the "single syndrome" hypothesis. *QJM: An International Journal of Medicine* 106(1):3-9.

APA (American Psychiatric Association). 2013. *Diagnostic and statistical manual of mental disorders*, 5th ed. Arlington, VA: APA.

Arroll, M. A., and V. Senior. 2009. Symptom typology and subgrouping. *Bulletin of the IACFS/ME* 17(2).

Aschbacher, K., E. K. Adam, L. J. Crofford, M. E. Kemeny, M. A. Demitrack, and A. Ben-Zvi. 2012. Linking disease symptoms and subtypes with personalized systems-based phenotypes: A proof of concept study. *Brain, Behavior, and Immunity* 26(7):1047-1056.

Baraniuk, J. N., O. Adewuyi, S. J. Merck, M. Ali, M. K. Ravindran, C. R. Timbol, R. Ray-Han, Y. Zheng, U. Le, R. Esteitie, and K. N. Petrie. 2013. A chronic fatigue syndrome (CFS) severity score based on case designation criteria. *American Journal of Translational Research* 5(1):53-68.

Brenu, E. W., S. Johnston, S. L. Hardcastle, T. K. Huth, K. Fuller, S. B. Ramos, D. R. Staines, and S. M. Marshall-Gradisnik. 2013. Immune abnormalities in patients meeting new diagnostic criteria for chronic fatigue syndrome/myalgic encephalomyelitis. *Molecular Biomarkers & Diagnosis* 4(3).

Brimacombe, M., D. Helmer, and B. H. Natelson. 2002. Clinical differences exist between patients fulfilling the 1988 and 1994 case definitions of chronic fatigue syndrome. *Journal of Clinical Psychology in Medical Settings* 9(4):309-314.

Brown, A. A., M. A. Evans, and L. A. Jason. 2013a. Examining the energy envelope and associated symptom patterns in chronic fatigue syndrome: Does coping matter? *Chronic Illness* 9(4):302-311.

Brown, A. A., L. A. Jason, M. A. Evans, and S. Flores. 2013b. Contrasting case definitions: The ME international consensus criteria vs. the Fukuda et al. CFS criteria. *North American Journal of Psychology* 15(1):103-120.

Brown, M. M., C. Kaplan, L. A. Jason, and C. B. Keys. 2010. Subgroups of chronic fatigue syndrome based on psychiatric disorder onset and current psychiatric status. *Health* 2(2):90-96.

Brurberg, K. G., M. S. Fonhus, L. Larun, and S. Flottorp. 2014. Case definitions for chronic fatigue syndrome/myalgic encephalomyelitis (CFS/ME): A systematic review. *BMJ Open* 4(2):1-12.

Carruthers, B. M., A. K. Jain, K. L. De Meirleir, D. L. Peterson, N. G. Klimas, A. M. Lemer, A. C. Bested, P. Flor-Henry, P. Joshi, A. C. P. Powles, J. A. Sherkey, and M. I. van de Sande. 2003. Myalgic encephalomyelitis/chronic fatigue syndrome: Clinical working case definition, diagnostic and treatment protocols (Canadian case definition). *Journal of Chronic Fatigue Syndrome* 11(1):7-115.

Carruthers, B. M., M. I. van de Sande, K. L. De Meirleir, N. G. Klimas, G. Broderick, T. Mitchell, D. Staines, A. C. P. Powles, N. Speight, R. Vallings, L. Bateman, B. Baumgarten-Austrheim, D. S. Bell, N. Carlo-Stella, J. Chia, A. Darragh, D. Jo, D. Lewis, A. R. Light, S. Marshall-Gradisbik, I. Mena, J. A. Mikovits, K. Miwa, M. Murovska, M. L. Pall, and S. Stevens. 2011. Myalgic encephalomyelitis: International consensus criteria. *Journal of Internal Medicine* 270(4):327-338.

CDC (Centers for Disease Control and Prevention). 2012. *Chronic fatigue syndrome: 1994 case definition.* http://www.cdc.gov/cfs/case-definition/1994.html (accessed December 16, 2013).

CDC. 2013. *National Notifiable Diseases Surveillance System (NNDSS): Case definitions.* http://wwwn.cdc.gov/nndss/script/casedefDefault.aspx (accessed July 4, 2014).

CFIDS (Chronic Fatigue and Immune Dysfunction Syndrome) Association of America. 2014. *ME/CFS road to diagnosis survey.* Charlotte, NC: CFIDS Association of America.

Christley, Y., T. Duffy, and C. R. Martin. 2011. Definitional criteria for chronic fatigue syndrome: A critical review. *Value in Health* 14(3):A31-A32.

Coggon, D., C. Martyn, K. T. Palmer, and B. Evanoff. 2005. Assessing case definitions in the absence of a diagnostic gold standard. *International Journal of Epidemiology* 34(4):949-952.

Corradi, K., L. A. Jason, and S. Torres-Harding. 2006. Exploratory subgrouping in CFS: Infectious, inflammatory, and other. *Advances in Psychology Research* 41:115-127.

Dajani, A. S., E. Ayoub, F. Z. Bierman, A. L. Bisno, F. W. Denny, D. T. Durack, P. Ferrieri, M. Freed, M. Gerber, E. L. Kaplan, A. W. Karchmer, M. Markowitz, S. H. Rahimtoola, S. T. Shulman, G. Stollerman, M. Takahashi, A. Taranta, K. A. Taubert, W. Wilson, and Endocarditis Special Writing Group of the Committee on Rheumatic Fever, and Kawasaki Disease of the Council on Cardiovascular Disease in the Young of the American Heart Association. 1992. Guidelines for the diagnosis of rheumatic fever. Jones criteria, 1992 update. *Journal of the American Medical Association* 268(15):2069-2073.

DePaul Research Team. 2010. *Depaul symptom questionnaire.* http://condor.depaul.edu/ljason/cfs/measures.html (accessed August 20, 2014).

Dimmock, M., and M. Lazell-Fairman. 2014. *Chronic fatigue syndrome: How to make a disease "evaporate."* https://dl.dropboxusercontent.com/u/89158245/CFS%20How%20to%20Make%20a%20Disease%20Evaporate%20May%202014.pdf (accessed January 12, 2015).

Drossman, D. A. 2006. The functional gastrointestinal disorders and the Rome III process. *Gastroenterology* 130(5):1377-1390.

Erueti, C., P. Glasziou, C. D. Mar, and M. L. van Driel. 2012. Do you think it's a disease?: A survey of medical students. *BMC Medical Education* 12:19.

Fostel, J., R. Boneva, and A. Lloyd. 2006. Exploration of the gene expression correlates of chronic unexplained fatigue using factor analysis. *Pharmacogenomics* 7(3):441-454.

Fukuda, K., S. E. Straus, I. Hickie, M. C. Sharpe, J. G. Dobbins, A. Komaroff, A. Schluederberg, J. F. Jones, A. R. Lloyd, S. Wessely, N. M. Gantz, G. P. Holmes, D. Buchwald, S. Abbey, J. Rest, J. A. Levy, H. Jolson, D. L. Peterson, J. Vercoulen, U. Tirelli, B. Evengård, B. H. Natelson, L. Steele, M. Reyes, and W. C. Reeves. 1994. The chronic fatigue syndrome: A comprehensive approach to its definition and study. *Annals of Internal Medicine* 121(12):953-959.

Hickie, I., T. Davenport, S. D. Vernon, R. Nisenbaum, W. C. Reeves, D. Hadzi-Pavlovic, A. Lloyd, and International Chronic Fatigue Syndrome Study Group. 2009. Are chronic fatigue and chronic fatigue syndrome valid clinical entities across countries and health-care settings? *Australian and New Zealand Journal of Psychiatry* 43:25-35.

Janal, M. N., D. S. Ciccone, and B. H. Natelson. 2006. Sub-typing CFS patients on the basis of "minor" symptoms. *Biological Psychology* 73(2):124-131.

Jason, L. A., and J. A. Richman. 2008. How science can stigmatize: The case of chronic fatigue syndrome. *Journal of Chronic Fatigue Syndrome* 14(4):85-103.

Jason, L. A., and R. R. Taylor. 2002. Applying cluster analysis to define a typology of chronic fatigue syndrome in a medically-evaluated, random community sample. *Psychology and Health* 17(3):323-337.

Jason, L. A., M. T. Ropacki, N. B. Santoro, J. A. Richman, W. Heatherly, R. Taylor, J. R. Ferrari, T. M. Haney-Davis, A. Rademaker, J. Dupuis, J. Golding, A. V. Plioplys, and S. Plioplys. 1997. A screening instrument for chronic fatigue syndrome: Reliability and validity. *Journal of Chronic Fatigue Syndrome* 3(1):39-59.

Jason, L. A., C. P. King, J. A. Richman, R. R. Taylor, S. R. Torres, and S. Song. 1999. U.S. case definition of chronic fatigue syndrome: Diagnostic and theoretical issues. *Journal of Chronic Fatigue Syndrome* 5(3-4):3-33.

Jason, L. A., R. R. Taylor, C. L. Kennedy, K. Jordan, S. Song, D. E. Johnson, and S. R. Torres. 2000. Chronic fatigue syndrome: Sociodemographic subtypes in a community-based sample. *Evaluation and the Health Professions* 23(3):243-263.

Jason, L. A., H. Eisele, and R. R. Taylor. 2001. Asessing attitudes toward new names for chronic fatigue syndrome. *Evaluation and the Health Professions* 24(4):424-435.

Jason, L. A., R. R. Taylor, C. L. Kennedy, K. Jordan, C. F. Huang, S. Torres-Harding, S. Song, and D. Johnson. 2002a. A factor analysis of chronic fatigue symptoms in a community-based sample. *Social Psychiatry & Psychiatric Epidemiology* 37(4):183-189.

Jason, L. A., R. R. Taylor, S. Plioplys, Z. Stepanek, and J. Shlaes. 2002b. Evaluating attributions for an illness based upon the name: Chronic fatigue syndrome, myalgic encephalopathy and Florence Nightingale disease. *American Journal of Community Psychology* 30(1):133-148.

Jason, L. A., C. Holbert, S. Torres-Harding, and R. Taylor. 2004a. Stigma and the term chronic fatigue syndrome. *Journal of Disability Policy Studies* 14(4):222-228.

Jason, L. A., S. R. Torres-Harding, A. Jurgens, and J. Helgerson. 2004b. Comparing the Fukuda et al. Criteria and the Canadian case definition for chronic fatigue syndrome. *Journal of Chronic Fatigue Syndrome* 12(1):37-52.

Jason, L. A., D. S. Bell, K. Rowe, E. L. S. Van Hoof, K. Jordan, C. Lapp, A. Gurwitt, T. Miike, S. Torres-Harding, and K. De Meirleir. 2006. A pediatric case definition for myalgic encephalomyelitis and chronic fatigue syndrome. *Journal of Chronic Fatigue Syndrome* 13(2-3):1-44.

Jason, L., N. Porter, E. Shelleby, L. Till, D. S. Bell, C. W. Lapp, K. Rowe, and K. De Meirleir. 2009. Severe versus moderate criteria for the new pediatric case definition for ME/CFS. *Child Psychiatry and Human Development* 40(4):609-620.

Jason, L. A., M. Evans, N. Porter, M. Brown, A. Brown, J. Hunnell, V. Anderson, A. Lerch, K. De Meirleir, and F. Friedberg. 2010. The development of a revised Canadian myalgic encephalomyelitis chronic fatigue syndrome case definition. *American Journal of Biochemistry and Biotechnology* 6(2):120-135.

Jason, L. A., A. Brown, E. Clyne, L. Bartgis, M. Evans, and M. Brown. 2012a. Contrasting case definitions for chronic fatigue syndrome, myalgic encephalomyelitis/chronic fatigue syndrome and myalgic encephalomyelitis. *Evaluation and the Health Professions* 35(3):280-304.

Jason, L. A., E. R. Unger, J. D. Dimitrakoff, A. P. Fagin, M. Houghton, D. B. Cook, G. D. Marshall, N. Klimas, and C. Snell. 2012b. Minimum data elements for research reports on CFS. *Brain, Behavior, and Immunity* 26(3):401-406.

Jason, L. A., A. Brown, M. Evans, M. Sunnquist, and J. L. Newton. 2013a. Contrasting chronic fatigue syndrome versus myalgic encephalomyelitis/chronic fatigue syndrome. *Fatigue* 1(3):168-183.

Jason, L. A., M. Sunnquist, A. Brown, M. Evans, S. Vernon, J. Furst, and V. Simonis. 2013b. Examining case definition criteria for chronic fatigue syndrome and myalgic encephalomyelitis. *Fatigue: Biomedicine, Health & Behavior* 2(1):40-56.

Jason, L. A., M. Sunnquist, A. Brown, M. Evans, and J. L. Newton. 2014. Are myalgic encephalomyelitis and chronic fatigue syndrome different illnesses? A preliminary analysis. *Journal of Health Psychology* [Epub ahead of print].

Kim, J. O., and C. W. Mueller. 1978. *Introduction to factor analysis: What it is and how to do it (quantitative application in the social sciences)*. Newbury Park, CA: SAGE.

King, C. P. 2003. The development of a diagnostic screening instrument for chronic fatigue syndrome. DePaul University, DePaul University Library, Chicago, IL.

Lewis, I., J. Pairman, G. Spickett, and J. L. Newton. 2013. Is chronic fatigue syndrome in older patients a different disease?—A clinical cohort study. *European Journal of Clinical Investigation* 43(3):302-308.

Linder, R., R. Dinser, M. Wagner, G. R. Krueger, and A. Hoffmann. 2002. Generation of classification criteria for chronic fatigue syndrome using an artificial neural network and traditional criteria set. *In Vivo* 16(1):37-43.

McHorney, C. A., J. E. Ware, Jr., and A. E. Raczek. 1993. The MOS 36-item Short-Form Health Survey (SF-36): II. Psychometric and clinical tests of validity in measuring physical and mental health constructs. *Medical Care* 31(3):247-263.

Miike, T., A. Tomoda, T. Jhodoi, N. Iwatani, and H. Mabe. 2004. Learning and memorization impairment in childhood chronic fatigue syndrome manifesting as school phobia in Japan. *Brain and Development* 26(7):442-447.

Morris, G., and M. Maes. 2013. Case definitions and diagnostic criteria for myalgic encephalomyelitis and chronic fatigue syndrome: From clinical-consensus to evidence-based case definitions. *Neuroendocrinology Letters* 34(3):185-199.

Nacul, L. C., E. M. Lacerda, D. Pheby, P. Campion, M. Molokhia, S. Fayyaz, J. C. Leite, F. Poland, A. Howe, and M. L. Drachler. 2011. Prevalence of myalgic encephalomyelitis/chronic fatigue syndrome (ME/CFS) in three regions of England: A repeated cross-sectional study in primary care. *BMC Medicine* 9:91.

NICE (National Institute for Health and Clinical Excellence). 2007. *Chronic fatigue syndrome/myalgic encephalomyelitis (or encephalopathy): Diagnosis and management of CFS/ME in adults and children*. London, UK: NICE.

Nisenbaum, R., M. Reyes, A. C. Mawle, and W. C. Reeves. 1998. Factor analysis of unexplained severe fatigue and interrelated symptoms: Overlap with criteria for chronic fatigue syndrome. *American Journal of Epidemiology* 148(1):72-77.

Nisenbaum, R., M. Reyes, E. R. Unger, and W. C. Reeves. 2004. Factor analysis of symptoms among subjects with unexplained chronic fatigue: What can we learn about chronic fatigue syndrome? *Journal of Psychosomatic Research* 56(2):171-178.

Njoku, M. G. C., L. A. Jason, N. Porter, and M. Brown. 2009. ME/CFS health outcomes: The interaction of mode of illness onset and psychiatric comorbidity. *International Journal of Human and Social Science* 4:420-425.

Pheby, D., E. Lacerda, L. Nacul, M. D. L. Drachler, P. Campion, A. Howe, F. Poland, M. Curran, V. Featherstone, S. Fayyaz, D. Sakellariou, and J. C. D. C. Leite. 2011. A disease register for ME/CFS: Report of a pilot study. *BMC Research Notes* 4.

Ray, C., W. R. Weir, S. Cullen, and S. Phillips. 1992. Illness perception and symptom components in chronic fatigue syndrome. *Journal of Psychosomatic Research* 36(3):243-256.

Reeves, W. C., A. Lloyd, S. D. Vernon, N. Klimas, L. A. Jason, G. Bleijenberg, B. Evengård, P. D. White, R. Nisenbaum, E. R. Unger, and Group International Chronic Fatigue Syndrome Study. 2003. Identification of ambiguities in the 1994 chronic fatigue syndrome research case definition and recommendations for resolution. *BMC Health Services Research* 3(1):25.

Reynolds, G. K., D. P. Lewis, A. M. Richardson, and B. A. Lidbury. 2013. Comorbidity of postural orthostatic tachycardia syndrome and chronic fatigue syndrome in an Australian cohort. *Journal of Internal Medicine* 275(4):409-417.

Royal College. 2004. *Evidence based guideline for the management of CFS/ME in children and young people.* http://www.rcpch.ac.uk/system/files/protected/page/RCPCH%20CFS. pdf (accessed January 12, 2015).

Social Security Ruling. 2014. Social Security Ruling, SSR 14-1p; Titles II and XVI: Evaluating claims involving chronic fatigue syndrome (CFS). *Federal Register* 79(64):18750-18754.

Tseng, C.-L., and B. H. Natelson. 2004. Few gender differences exist between women and men with chronic fatigue syndrome. *Journal of Clinical Psychology in Medical Settings* 11(1):55-62.

Twisk, F. N. 2014. The status of and future research into myalgic encephalomyelitis and chronic fatigue syndrome: The need of accurate diagnosis, objective assessment, and acknowledging biological and clinical subgroups. *Frontiers in Physiology* 5:109.

Vakil, N., S. V. van Zanten, P. Kahrilas, J. Dent, R. Jones, and Group Global Consensus. 2006. The Montreal definition and classification of gastroesophageal reflux disease: A global evidence-based consensus. *American Journal of Gastroenterology* 101(8):1900-1920; quiz 1943.

van der Meer, J. W., and A. R. Lloyd. 2012. A controversial consensus—comment on article by Broderick et al. *Journal of Internal Medicine* 271(1):29-31.

Watson, S., A. S. Ruskin, V. Simonis, L. Jason, M. Sunnquist, and J. Furst. 2014. Identifying defining aspects of chronic fatigue syndrome via unsupervised machine learning and feature selection. *International Journal of Machine Learning and Computing* 4(2):133-138.

Wojcik, W., D. Armstrong, and R. Kanaan. 2011. Chronic fatigue syndrome: Labels, meanings and consequences. *Journal of Psychosomatic Research* 70(6):500-504.

4

Review of the Evidence on Major ME/CFS Symptoms and Manifestations

This review of the evidence on major ME/CFS symptoms and manifestations begins with a discussion of the limitations of the research base in this area. The chapter then examines in turn the evidence on fatigue, post-exertional malaise (PEM), sleep-related symptoms, neurocognitive manifestations, and orthostatic intolerance and autonomic dysfunction in ME/CFS.

LIMITATIONS OF THE RESEARCH BASE

One of the most significant challenges to achieving a better understanding of ME/CFS results from the methodological limitations of the current research base. Issues related to external and internal validity and to reliability frequently have led to inconsistent results across studies, as well as other shortcomings. Despite these limitations, however, the committee was able to glean evidence of symptoms, signs, and objective measures for ME/CFS. The evidence with respect to major symptoms and manifestations is presented in this chapter, while that related to other symptoms and manifestations and to pediatric ME/CFS is reviewed in Chapters 5 and 6, respectively. This review of the evidence serves as the basis for the committee's proposed diagnostic criteria for ME/CFS, which are presented in Chapter 7.

External Validity

Studies on ME/CFS used different inclusion criteria and different sources of ME/CFS patients and control participants. The end result is heterogeneity in both patient and control cohorts, creating an unclear picture of the symptoms and signs of the disorder and its outcomes. Findings are based on samples with a large majority of middle-aged women (late 40s to early 50s) who are Caucasian and of higher educational status, perhaps limiting the generalizability of the studies. Very few studies focused on other population subsets, such as pediatric or geriatric patients, or included ethnic and racial minority patients. Some studies recruited patients from specialized ME/CFS treatment centers, while others used community-based samples. These different sampling methods may result in patient groups that differ in demographic characteristics and symptom type and severity. Furthermore, those most severely affected by ME/CFS may be bedridden or homebound and may not have been included in any of these studies (Wiborg et al., 2010). Thus, there are selection biases in the studies' sample composition.

Some limitations also stem from issues regarding the case definitions or diagnostic criteria used in the studies (see Chapter 3 for a review). Although a strong majority of studies used the Fukuda definition, a small number used various other definitions, thus complicating comparisons of the results. A major limitation of the Fukuda and other ME/CFS case definitions is their polythetic diagnostic criteria. Thus, two patients could have very little symptom overlap yet both be diagnosed with ME/CFS. Therefore, there is potential heterogeneity within and across patient samples in the literature that cannot be assessed because of the lack of reporting of symptom prevalence in most studies (Jason et al., 2012b). This problem is inherent in the study of any illness with polythetic diagnostic criteria. Finally, because most studies used the Fukuda definition to select cases, it is not possible to fully assess the evidence for the other diagnostic criteria for ME/CFS.

Internal Validity

In many cases, studies lacked properly matched controls to account for confounders. The majority of published studies compared a small number of ME/CFS patients with healthy controls. Control groups including people with other illnesses, sedentary individuals, or people who meet different case definitions of ME/CFS have not commonly been used. Because almost all controls were healthy and most were physically active, the findings from those studies do not shed light on which symptoms and signs distinguish ME/CFS from other disorders with some overlapping symptoms.

Some contradictory findings may also be due to the use of various scales, instruments, and measures for symptoms, some of which are imprecise, not comprehensive, or not validated. ME/CFS symptoms were derived mainly from patient self-reports, which raises questions about the internal validity of the study results. Moreover, relatively few studies were longitudinal, so little light has been shed on the natural history of ME/CFS (Jason et al., 2011b). There also were few studies of the early stages of the illness. This is understandable given that the diagnosis can be made only after 6 months of symptoms (see Chapter 3 and below), but nevertheless is a barrier to understanding the natural history of the illness.

Reliability

A lack of replication and validation in many studies limits the ability to assess the study findings critically. Few attempts have been made to follow up on or replicate intriguing findings in the literature to date.

FATIGUE AND ITS IMPACT ON FUNCTION

The dictionary definition of fatigue as a noun is "weariness from bodily or mental exertion." Fatigue is not typically considered a disease but is commonly used in medicine to represent a broad spectrum of tiredness, from the physical, cognitive, or emotional feeling at the end of a long day to the emotional or physical toll of acute, chronic, or terminal illness (Gambert, 2005).

Fatigue is one of the most common and nonspecific presenting complaints in primary care. Unfortunately, the word "fatigue" does not convey information about the cause, severity, or chronicity of fatigue or its impact on functionality. Although fatigue is a common experience, it has no unique physiological explanations or objective markers. A broad range of physical, medical, and mental health conditions and stressors may result in the complaint of fatigue (Matthews et al., 1991). Aging alone is associated with a gradual increase in fatigue and reduction in functional capacity for a variety of reasons (National Institute on Aging, 2007). Although overlap exists, fatigue usually can be distinguished from somnolence (also called drowsiness or sleepiness), which often is attributed to deprivation of sleep, primary sleep disorders, or sedating medications (Hossain et al., 2005). Thus, clinicians are challenged to integrate the subjective and objective evidence that can help identify the neurologic, malignant, infectious, inflammatory, cardiopulmonary, metabolic, endocrinologic, physical deconditioning, pharmacologic, or mental health factors that may underlie the presenting complaint of fatigue. (Note that a complete discussion of the differential diagnosis of fatigue is beyond the scope of this report.)

Description of Fatigue in ME/CFS

Patients with ME/CFS almost always suffer from fatigue, and the importance of the symptom is illustrated by its central role in most of the case criteria developed to date (see Chapter 3). Regardless of what criteria are used, however, ME/CFS patients often have a level of fatigue that is more profound, more devastating, and longer lasting than that observed in patients with other fatiguing disorders. In addition, fatigue in ME/CFS is not the result of ongoing exertion, not lifelong, and not particularly responsive to rest (Jason and Taylor, 2002). Patients describe their fatigue as "exhaustion, weakness, a lack of energy, feeling drained, an inability to stand for even a few minutes, an inability to walk even a few blocks without exhaustion, and an inability to sustain an activity for any significant length of time" (FDA, 2013, p. 7). Some of the more extreme examples include "too exhausted to change clothes more than every 7-10 days"; "exhaustion to the point that speaking is not possible"; and "exertion of daily toileting, particularly bowel movements, sends me back to bed struggling for breath and feeling like I just climbed a mountain." A few patients describe a "tired but wired" feeling (FDA, 2013, p. 14). Numerous efforts have been made to measure the nature and extent of fatigue in this population (Furst, 1999; Whitehead, 2009). Some patients improve, but most continue to experience some level of fatigue, physical and/or mental, ranging from mild to profound (Wilson et al., 1994).

Jason and colleagues (2009) found that those with ME/CFS frequently report the occurrence of several distinct fatigue states that may diverge from commonplace perceptions of fatigue among the general population. They examined dimensions of fatigue in ME/CFS using a unique 22-item ME/CFS Fatigue Types Questionnaire administered to 130 patients and 251 healthy controls. Factor analysis demonstrated a five-factor structure of fatigue for ME/CFS patients and a one-factor solution for controls. The five types of fatigue that differentiated ME/CFS patients from controls were post-exertional, wired, brain fog, energy, and flu-like fatigue (Jason et al., 2009, 2010a), clearly showing the complex nature of fatigue in ME/CFS. Earlier efforts to assess fatigue were made (Jason et al., 2011a), among others, by Chalder and colleagues (1993), who developed the Fatigue Scale; by Ray and colleagues (1992), who created the Profile of Fatigue-Related Symptoms; by Smets and colleagues (1995), who developed the Multidimensional Fatigue Inventory (MFI-20); and by Krupp and colleagues (1989), who developed the Fatigue Severity Scale.

Regarding the duration of fatigue, the Fukuda definition and the Canadian Consensus Criteria (CCC) require 6 months for a diagnosis of ME/CFS. This 6-month requirement is supported by Nisenbaum and colleagues (1998), who showed that unexplained fatigue lasting for more than 6 months was related to symptoms included in the ME/CFS case definitions and that most other causes of similar fatigue do not last beyond 6 months.

In their review of 39 measures of fatigue, Whitehead and colleagues (2009) found that although some measures were better than others, none were ideal. Most measures have insufficient sensitivity and specificity to encompass all of the various and important aspects of fatigue in ME/CFS (Jason et al., 2011a). In addition, health care providers should note that a single assessment of fatigue severity may not provide a full understanding of the patterns of fatigue presenting over 1 day in ME/CFS patients (Jason and Brown, 2013).

Impact of Fatigue on Function

Fatigue may be most relevant when assessed relative to its impact on function. However, disability caused by fatigue may not reflect the levels of fatigue a patient is experiencing. For instance, despite feeling extremely fatigued, a person may continue working to survive economically and stop only when functionally impaired (Jason and Brown, 2013). Appendix C provides additional examples and rates of functional impairment due to ME/CFS symptoms. In general, patients with ME/CFS experience a marked decrease in function across an array of domains, frequently attributed, at least in part, to their fatigue (Komaroff et al., 1996a).

Efforts have been made to assess the impact of the disease on patients' function, but most such efforts have been research based. One of the more commonly used tools in medical research as well as in ME/CFS studies is the Short Form 36-Item Questionnaire (SF-36) of the Medical Outcomes Study (MOS) (McHorney et al., 1993; Ware, 2002), a standardized and validated 36-item patient-report questionnaire with eight principal components or subscales used to determine the impact of illness on functionality. Early studies used this tool to distinguish ME/CFS from major depression, multiple sclerosis, acute infectious mononucleosis, hypertension, congestive heart failure, type II diabetes mellitus, acute myocardial infarction, unexplained chronic fatigue, and healthy controls (Buchwald et al., 1996; Komaroff et al., 1996a).

The VT (vitality) subscale of the MOS SF-36, for example, a questionnaire used to assess function, is thought to reflect both mental and physical function (McHorney et al., 1993) and includes the sum of four questions about having a lot of energy, being full of life/pep, feeling worn out, or feeling tired, with higher scores reflecting greater vitality (Ware, 2002). VT scores are consistently much lower in ME/CFS patients with and without comorbidities than in healthy controls and patients with other chronic illnesses, including fibromyalgia. Examples of mean VT scores on the MOS SF-36 from various published studies for the general population and those with ME/CFS and other chronic fatiguing illnesses are summarized in Table 4-1 to demonstrate the profoundly low scores for ME/CFS compared with the other conditions. Several of the studies in the table do not specify the scoring algorithm (raw versus normalized t score) for the MOS SF-36,

TABLE 4-1 Mean VT Score on the MOS SF-36 for ME/CFS Versus Other Fatigue Conditions

	HC	CHF NYHA III	HD	HepC	MD	SSc
Score	60-70	29	49	48	40	45
Reference	Buchwald et al., 1996; Komaroff et al., 1996a	Juenger et al., 2002	Merkus et al., 1997	Foster et al., 1998	Komaroff et al., 1996a	Harel et al., 2012

NOTES: CHF NYHA III = congestive heart failure New York Heart Association Class III; FM = fibromyalgia; HC = healthy control; HD = hemodialysis; HepC = chronic hepatitis C (without cirrhosis); MCS = multiple chemical sensitivity; MD = major depression; MSD 4+ = at least 4 musculoskeletal diseases; RA = rheumatoid arthritis; SSc = scleroderma/systemic sclerosis; VT = vitality subscale of the MOS SF-36.

so that bias may exist in comparing VT scores across the studies. However, this bias is unlikely to explain the clear differences seen between the ME/CFS and non-ME/CFS groups in Table 4-1.

While Jason and Brown (2013) demonstrated that the VT scores of ME/CFS patients ranged from 15 to 25 depending on subtyping strategies, other domains often are affected as well. Nacul and colleagues (2011a) found that scores on the role-physical (RP)[1] subscale of the SF-36 were even more affected than scores on the VT subscale (version 2) but that all domains were impaired, with mental health being the best preserved. Jason and colleagues (2011c) found that impairments in VT, social functioning, and RP had the greatest sensitivity and specificity in identifying patients who met the Fukuda definition of ME/CFS. In one early study, all eight subscores of the SF-36 were lower in ME/CFS patients than in the general population and other disease comparison controls, with the exception of the mental health and role-emotional subscales in the controls with major depression (Komaroff et al., 1996a).

It should be noted that, while widely used in research, the SF-36 may not be well suited to general clinical use because of user fees and the gen-

---

[1] The RP subscale combines the scores of four questions related to physical activity.

MSD 4+	RA	FM	ME/CFS	ME/CFS + FM	ME/CFS + MCS	ME/CFS + FM + MCS
48	43-52	39-40	15-25	20	15	11
Picavet and Hoeymans, 2004	Picavet and Hoeymans, 2004; Salaffi et al., 2009	Picavet and Hoeymans, 2004; Salaffi et al., 2009	Brown and Jason, 2007; Buchwald et al., 1996; Jason and Brown, 2013; Komaroff et al., 1996a	Brown and Jason, 2007	Brown and Jason, 2007	Brown and Jason, 2007

eral process of having to submit test results to the sponsor for scoring. The RAND-36 is an alternative version that is freely accessible, but it has a complex scoring algorithm (RAND, 1984).

Summary

Fatigue, chronic fatigue, and particularly the impact of fatigue on function should be assessed in making a diagnosis of ME/CFS. Health care providers may use a range of questions and instruments to evaluate fatigue and its impact on function in these patients (see Chapter 7, Table 7-1). However, ME/CFS should not be considered merely a point on the fatigue spectrum or as being simply about fatigue. Experienced clinicians and researchers, as well as patients and their supporters, have emphasized for years that this complex illness presentation entails much more than the chronic presence of fatigue. Other factors, such as orthostatic intolerance, widespread pain, unrefreshing sleep, cognitive dysfunction, and immune dysregulation, along with secondary anxiety and depression, contribute to the burden imposed by fatigue in this illness. The challenge in understanding this acquired chronic debility, unfortunately named "chronic fatigue syndrome" for more than two decades, will be to unravel those complexities.

Conclusion: There is sufficient evidence that fatigue in ME/CFS is profound, not the result of ongoing excessive exertion, and not substantially alleviated by rest. This fatigue results in a substantial reduction or impairment in the ability to engage in pre-illness levels of occupational, educational, social, or personal activities and persists for more than 6 months.

POST-EXERTIONAL MALAISE (PEM)

Description of PEM in ME/CFS

PEM is an exacerbation of some or all of an individual's ME/CFS symptoms that occurs after physical or cognitive exertion and leads to a reduction in functional ability (Carruthers et al., 2003). As described by patients and supported by research, PEM is more than fatigue following a stressor. Patients may describe it as a post-exertional "crash," "exhaustion," "flare-up," "collapse," "debility," or "setback."[2] PEM exacerbates a patient's baseline symptoms and, in addition to fatigue and functional impairment (Peterson et al., 1994), may result in flu-like symptoms (e.g., sore throat, tender lymph nodes, feverishness) (VanNess et al., 2010); pain (e.g., headaches, generalized muscle/joint aches) (Meeus et al., 2014; Van Oosterwijck et al., 2010); cognitive dysfunction (e.g., difficulty with comprehension, impaired short-term memory, prolonged processing time) (LaManca et al., 1998; Ocon et al., 2012; VanNess et al., 2010); nausea/gastrointestinal discomfort; weakness/instability; lightheadedness/vertigo; sensory changes (e.g., tingling skin, increased sensitivity to noise) (VanNess et al., 2010); depression/anxiety; sleep disturbances (e.g., trouble falling or staying asleep, hypersomnia, unrefreshing sleep) (Davenport et al., 2011a); and difficulty recovering capacity after physical exertion (Davenport et al., 2011a,b). In some cases, patients experience new symptoms as part of the PEM response. The following quote reflects the breadth and severity of symptoms associated with PEM in these patients:

> when I do any activity that goes beyond what I can do—I literally collapse—my body is in major pain, it hurts to lay in bed, it hurts to think, I can't hardly talk—I can't find the words, I feel my insides are at war. My autonomic system is so out of whack! I can't see farsighted and glasses won't help—only rest. My GI system is so messed up. Any food hurts it. I tried everything from elimination diets to all the GI meds. Nothing is working. My body jerks. The list goes on. There are days that I just want to cry because I can't take care of myself—I need help. But, I have no help

---

[2] Personal communication; public comments submitted to the IOM Committee on the Diagnostic Criteria for Myalgic Encephalomyelitis/Chronic Fatigue Syndrome for meeting 1, 2014.

because of the term CFS and not understanding PEM. I am sorry that I am not dying in the short-term, but I am living life waiting to die because no one takes this disease seriously.[3]

The types and thresholds of triggers of PEM, its onset, and its duration may vary among individuals and over the course of illness.

Triggers

PEM may occur after physical (Bazelmans et al., 2005; Davenport et al., 2011b; Nijs et al., 2010) or cognitive exertion (Arroll et al., 2014; Cockshell and Mathias, 2014; Smith et al., 1999). Patients also have described other potential triggers, such as emotional distress (Davenport et al., 2011a), physical trauma, decreased sleep quantity/quality, infection, and standing or sitting up for an extended period (FDA, 2013; Ocon et al., 2012). The type, severity, and duration of symptoms may be unexpected or seem out of proportion to the initiating trigger, which may be as mild as talking on the phone or being at the computer (Spotila, 2010). Patients report that PEM can be severe enough to render them bedridden (FDA, 2013).

Onset

Although PEM may begin immediately following a trigger, patients report that symptom exacerbation often may develop hours or days after the trigger has ceased or resolved.[4] Likewise, some studies have shown that PEM may occur quickly, within 30 minutes of exertion (Blackwood et al., 1998), while others have found that patients may experience a worsening of symptoms 1 to 7 days after exertion (Nijs et al., 2010; Sorensen et al., 2003; Van Oosterwijck et al., 2010; White et al., 2010; Yoshiuchi et al., 2007). The delayed onset and functional impairment associated with PEM also is supported by actigraphy data. ME/CFS participants enrolled in a walking program designed to increase their steps by about 30 percent daily were able to reach this goal initially, but after 4 to 10 days their steps decreased precipitously (Black and McCully, 2005).

Duration

PEM is unpredictable in duration, potentially lasting hours, days, weeks, and even months (FDA, 2013; Nijs et al., 2010). After maximal exercise

---

[3] Personal communication; public comments submitted to the IOM Committee on the Diagnostic Criteria for Myalgic Encephalomyelitis/Chronic Fatigue Syndrome for meeting 3, 2014.
[4] Ibid.

tests, ME/CFS patients experience greater fatigue compared with healthy controls (Bazelmans et al., 2005; LaManca et al., 1999b), and their fatigue and other symptoms last much longer relative to healthy active (Bazelmans et al., 2005) and sedentary controls (Davenport et al., 2011a,b; LaManca et al., 1999b; VanNess et al., 2010). In several studies, healthy controls declared themselves recovered within 24 to 48 hours after physical or cognitive exertion, whereas fewer than 31 percent of ME/CFS subjects had returned to their prestressor baseline state by this time, and as many as 60 percent were still experiencing multiple symptoms after 1 week (Cockshell and Mathias, 2014; Davenport et al., 2011b; VanNess et al., 2010).

Prevalence of PEM in ME/CFS Patients

The prevalence of PEM among ME/CFS patients as diagnosed by existing criteria varies from 69 to 100 percent (Chu et al., 2013; De Becker et al., 2001; Jason et al., 2011b; Kerr et al., 2010; Nacul et al., 2011b; Vermeulen and Scholte, 2003; Zhang et al., 2010). In a longitudinal study that followed a random, community-based sample for 10 years, 100 percent of participants fulfilling the Fukuda definition reported PEM as a symptom at some point during their illness (Jason et al., 2011b), even though the Fukuda definition does not require PEM for diagnosis. Prevalence estimates of PEM vary for two major reasons: (1) some studies use ME/CFS case definitions that require PEM, while others list it as an optional symptom; and (2) the way PEM is defined, operationalized, or queried for can affect how patients interpret the concept of PEM and whether they endorse it (Jason et al., 1999, 2004, 2014).

The prevalence of PEM in healthy control subjects is considerably lower than in ME/CFS patients, ranging from 4 to 8 percent (Hawk et al., 2006b; Jason et al., 2011b; Kerr et al., 2010; Komaroff et al., 1996b; Zhang et al., 2010). Jason and colleagues (2013b) found that a greater percentage of ME/CFS patients than healthy controls experienced PEM symptoms (see Figure 4-1). After moderate thresholds for frequency and severity were applied, the percentage of controls who endorsed PEM decreased further, from 7 to 19 percent to 2 to 7 percent.[5] Thus, applying increased severity or frequency thresholds for PEM may assist in identifying patients with ME/CFS (Hawk et al., 2006b).

A few studies that compared ME/CFS with other diseases found that, although PEM was experienced by 19 to 20 percent of subjects with major

---

[5] Jason and colleagues (2013b) compared 236 ME/CFS patients with 86 healthy controls who completed the DePaul Symptom Questionnaire, rating the frequency and severity of 54 symptoms. Patient data were obtained from the SolveCFS BioBank, which includes patients diagnosed by a licensed physician using either the Fukuda definition or the CCC.

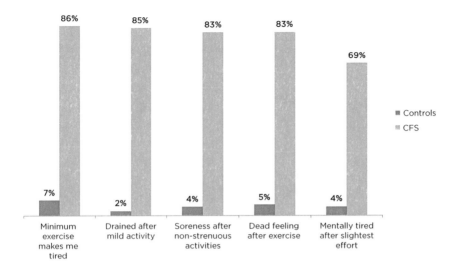

FIGURE 4-1 Percentage of ME/CFS patients and healthy controls reporting PEM symptoms of at least moderate severity that occurred at least half of the time during the past 6 months.
NOTE: All patients fulfilled the Fukuda definition for CFS.
SOURCE: Jason et al., 2013b.

depressive disorder (Hawk et al., 2006a; Komaroff et al., 1996b) and 52 percent of patients with multiple sclerosis (Komaroff et al., 1996b), it was still much more common in ME/CFS patients than in comparison groups. One study found that 64 percent of patients with major depressive disorder experienced PEM, but the authors did not describe how PEM was assessed (Zhang et al., 2010). As mentioned earlier, these prevalence estimates may vary depending on how PEM was defined and queried for, and thus they need to be interpreted with caution.

Assessment of PEM in ME/CFS

PEM can be assessed subjectively by clinical history. It also can be assessed by standardized symptom questionnaires specific to ME/CFS and by comparison of self-reported symptoms and objective measures (such as functional impairment) before and after exertion or other types of stressors. Instruments and tools for individually assessing various symptoms exacerbated by PEM triggers are discussed in other sections of this chapter. This section is focused on questionnaires and objective tests used to determine whether a patient experiences PEM. Self-report questionnaires currently are the more readily available way to assess whether a patient experiences PEM. Objective testing for PEM generally is costly and not easily accessible, and it may worsen the patient's condition (Diamond, 2007; Nijs et al., 2010).

Self-Report Measures of PEM

Standardized symptom questionnaires with self-report items used to assess PEM include the CFS Medical Questionnaire (Komaroff et al., 1996c), CFS Screening Questionnaire (Jason et al., 1997), Centers for Disease Control and Prevention (CDC) Symptom Inventory (SI) (CDC, 2005), ME/CFS Fatigue Types Questionnaire (MFTQ) (Jason et al., 2009), and DePaul Symptom Questionnaire (DePaul Research Team, 2010). These questionnaires, which include items designed to measure the presence, duration, frequency, or severity of PEM, were developed from patient input to query specifically about PEM, and some were tested for psychometric properties (Hawk et al., 2006b; Wagner et al., 2005). However, they have been used primarily for subject recruitment in research, for comparison of diagnoses in research protocols, or for epidemiological assessments.

Use of a standardized instrument is critical to measuring PEM accurately because slight differences in wording on various self-report items have been shown to change the prevalence of PEM in the same group of patients (Jason et al., in press); thus, how one asks about PEM can influence the responses. As indicated earlier in this chapter, individual experiences of PEM may vary widely in terms of triggers, onset, duration, severity, impairment, and symptoms that are exacerbated. For example, patients for whom normal daily activities, such as unloading the dishwasher, trigger PEM may not engage in exercise. Thus, an item that asks about fatigue after exercise will not capture these patients' experiences with PEM. Similarly, responses to this item will not indicate PEM in patients who experience symptom exacerbation after cognitive exertion (Jason et al., in press). Thus, development of a sufficiently inclusive but probing clinical instrument is essential.

Objective Measures of PEM

Emerging evidence for objective indicators that may help us understand the presentation of PEM in ME/CFS patients centers on the two commonly reported domains in the PEM complex: recovery after physical exertion and cognitive function. Objective assessment of cognitive function is discussed in the section on neurocognitive manifestations later in this chapter.

One common characteristic of PEM is delayed ability to return to prior levels of physical capacity after physical exertion. One way to have them demonstrate this delayed lack of recovery in patients with ME/CFS is to have them perform two cardiopulmonary exercise tests (CPETs) separated by 24 hours—the first to assess current level of function and elicit illness relapse (CPET 1) and the second to measure changes in exercise capacity due to the challenge (CPET 2) (Keller et al., 2014; Snell et al., 2013; Vermeulen et al., 2010). However, the committee emphasizes that the CPET is not required to diagnose patients with ME/CFS. Further, this test carries substantial risk for these patients as it may worsen their condition (Nijs et al., 2010; VanNess et al., 2010).

The CPET is used clinically to assess exercise capacity (maximal oxygen consumption or VO_2max) and predict outcomes in cardiac patients. VO_2max measured during repeated CPETs is both reliable (test-retest difference < 7 percent) (Katch et al., 1982; Taylor et al., 1955; Weltman et al., 1990) and reproducible (r > 0.95-0.99) (Balady et al., 2010; Bruce et al., 1973; Taylor et al., 1955). Several studies have found that, despite meeting objective indicators of maximal effort during both CPETs, ME/CFS patients have significantly lower results on CPET 2 than on CPET 1 on one or more of the following parameters: VO_2max (Keller et al., 2014; VanNess et al., 2007; Vermeulen et al., 2010), VO_2 at ventilatory threshold (Keller et al., 2014), and maximal workload or workload at ventilatory threshold (Keller et al., 2014; Snell et al., 2013). These findings support the 2-day CPET protocol as an objective indicator that physical exertion may decrease subsequent function in some ME/CFS patients.

By contrast, a single CPET may be insufficient to document the abnormal response of ME/CFS patients to exercise (Keller et al., 2014; Snell et al., 2013). Although some ME/CFS subjects show very low VO_2max results on a single CPET, others may show results similar to or only slightly lower than those of healthy sedentary controls (Cook et al., 2012; De Becker et al., 2000; Farquhar et al., 2002; Inbar et al., 2001; Sargent et al., 2002; VanNess et al., 2007). Thus, the functional capacity of a patient may be erroneously overestimated and decreased values attributed only to deconditioning. Repeating the CPET will guard against such misperceptions given that deconditioned but healthy persons are able to replicate their results, even if low, on the second CPET.

Evidence for PEM in ME/CFS

The committee conducted a targeted literature search to identify research comparing self-reported or objectively assessed PEM in ME/CFS subjects and in those without the illness. The methodology used is described in Chapter 1. The findings from the literature are described below, but there are several limitations to consider when interpreting the evidence base, as described at the beginning of this chapter.

Exacerbation of Fatigue Following Exertion

Many studies found that fatigue increased and was prolonged after a physical stressor to a greater extent in ME/CFS patients than in healthy or sedentary controls. Findings of increased fatigue were consistent across different types of physical stressors, including subsequent maximal exercise tests (Davenport et al., 2011a,b), single maximal exercise tests (Bazelmans et al., 2005; Kishi et al., 2013; LaManca et al., 1998, 1999b, 2001; Meyer et al., 2013; Togo et al., 2010; VanNess et al., 2010), and other physical stressors (Black et al., 2005; Gibson et al., 1993; Nijs et al., 2010). When studies differentiated between mental and physical fatigue, both were found to have worsened in ME/CFS patients (Light et al., 2009, 2012; White et al., 2010, 2012).

As noted earlier, cognitive exertion also may trigger increased mental and physical fatigue in ME/CFS patients (Arroll et al., 2014; Cockshell and Mathias, 2014). Mental fatigue tracks closely with physical fatigue (Light et al., 2009, 2012; Meyer et al., 2013; White et al., 2012). Subjected to a 3-hour standardized neuropsychological battery, healthy subjects experienced mental fatigue during and up to 3 hours after testing but recovered full mental energy, on average, by 7 hours posttest. In contrast, at 24 hours posttest, ME/CFS subjects continued to experience significant mental fatigue and did not return to their pretest mental energy levels for an average of 57 hours (Cockshell and Mathias, 2014).

Exacerbation of Cognitive Symptoms Following Exertion or Orthostatic Challenge

Although cognitive problems are common in ME/CFS patients, few studies have examined the effect of exertion on cognitive function. Some studies have demonstrated that a physical or orthostatic stressor may cause exacerbation of cognitive symptoms, including difficulty with concentration (Nijs et al., 2010); deficits in the speed of information processing (LaManca et al., 1998); and other self-reported cognitive problems (Meyer et al., 2013; VanNess et al., 2010). Studies also have shown decreased cognitive performance, such as on tests of focused and sustained attention, the Symbol Digit Modalities Test, the Stroop test, and the N-back task (Blackwood et al., 1998; LaManca et al., 2001; Ocon et al., 2012). Findings of other studies, however, suggest that cognitive problems do not worsen after physical exertion (Claypoole et al., 2001; Cook et al., 2005; Yoshiuchi et al., 2007).

Cognitive exertion also may trigger cognitive symptoms (Capuron et al., 2006; Ocon et al., 2012). For example, one study asked ME/CFS subjects and healthy controls to complete computerized tests of memory, attention, and psychomotor function and found that as the tests progressed, the performance of the ME/CFS subjects worsened significantly more than that of controls (Smith et al., 1999). On the other hand, the findings of some studies suggest that cognitive exertion alone may not necessarily trigger cognitive problems (LaManca et al., 1998; Marshall et al., 1997). These inconsistent results may be attributable to variations in subject selection, exercise testing procedures, and cognitive testing, which inhibit direct comparisons among studies.

Exacerbation of Pain Following Exertion

Many studies have demonstrated that pain is increased and prolonged after a physical stressor in ME/CFS subjects compared with healthy or sedentary controls. Similar to the evidence base for fatigue, reports of increased pain among ME/CFS subjects are consistent across maximal exercise tests (Davenport et al., 2011a,b; VanNess et al., 2010) and other physical stressors (Black et al., 2005; Nijs et al., 2010). In at least two studies, though, the increase in pain after exertion among ME/CFS subjects was not statistically significant compared with controls (Bazelmans et al., 2005; Kishi et al., 2013).

Effect of Exertion on Other Outcomes

In addition to the strong evidence demonstrating post-exertional effects on fatigue status, cognitive function, and pain, evidence is mounting for other symptoms and outcomes, albeit from a lesser number of studies to date. After an exercise stressor, ME/CFS patients compared with healthy controls demonstrated delayed recovery of muscle function and pH (Jones et al., 2010, 2012; Paul et al., 1999), increased depression or mood disturbances (Arroll et al., 2014; Meyer et al., 2013), inappropriate autonomic responses (Cordero et al., 1996; LaManca et al., 2001), and amplification of problems with sleep (Davenport et al., 2011a,b; Kishi et al., 2013; Togo et al., 2010). Further studies confirming the different expression of genes (Light et al., 2009, 2012; Meyer et al., 2013; White et al., 2012) and immune biomarkers (Maes et al., 2012; Nijs et al., 2010, 2014; Sorensen et al., 2003; White et al., 2010) in patients with ME/CFS in response to physical exertion may help us to better understanding the pathophysiology of PEM.

PEM as a Characteristic Symptom of ME/CFS

The existence of PEM can help physicians confirm a diagnosis of ME/CFS earlier rather than only after extensive exclusion of other conditions. Several studies have found that PEM best distinguishes ME/CFS from idiopathic chronic fatigue (Baraniuk et al., 2013; Jason et al., 2002a) and may help distinguish it from other fatiguing conditions with a lower frequency of PEM, such as multiple sclerosis and major depressive disorder (Hawk et al., 2006a; Komaroff et al., 1996b). Further, PEM may be an important prognostic indicator because its continued presence or increased duration predicts a poorer outcome for ME/CFS patients (Taylor et al., 2002).

Summary

PEM is a worsening of a patient's symptoms and function after exposure to physical or cognitive stressors that were normally tolerated before disease onset. Subjective reports of PEM and prolonged recovery are supported by objective evidence, including failure to normally reproduce exercise test results (2-day CPET) and impaired cognitive function. These objective indices track strongly with the presence, severity, and duration of PEM.

Patients' experience of PEM varies, and some patients may have adapted their lifestyle and activity level to avoid triggering symptoms. As a result, health care providers should ask a range of questions (see Chapter 7, Table 7-1) to determine whether PEM is present. Minimally, patients should be asked to describe baseline symptoms, the effects of physical or cognitive exertion, the time needed to recover to the pre-exertion state, and how they have limited their activities to avoid these effects. If the patient is unable to answer these questions clearly, health care providers may also ask the patient to track symptoms, activities, and rest in a diary—for example, in order to identify PEM patterns.

Conclusion: There is sufficient evidence that PEM is a primary feature that helps distinguish ME/CFS from other conditions.

SLEEP-RELATED SYMPTOMS

Description of Sleep-Related Symptoms in ME/CFS

Patients with ME/CFS frequently experience sleep-related problems such as insomnia, sleep disturbances, unrefreshing sleep, and nonrestorative sleep (FDA, 2013; Fossey et al., 2004). These symptoms are included in all existing ME/CFS case definitions and diagnostic criteria (see Chapter 3). Unrefreshing sleep, or feeling as tired upon waking as before going to bed, is among the most common symptoms reported by ME/CFS patients, and only a small percentage of patients diagnosed with ME/CFS fail to report some type of sleep dysfunction (Carruthers et al., 2003; IACFS/ME, 2014; Jason et al., 2013b). This section summarizes the evidence on sleep-related signs and symptoms in ME/CFS reviewed by the committee to determine whether such symptoms should be a component of its recommended diagnostic criteria for ME/CFS.

ME/CFS patients are more likely than healthy controls to experience sleep-related symptoms occurring at least half of the time and of at least moderate severity (see Figure 4-2) (Jason et al., 2013b). Although sleep-related symptoms also are reported by healthy persons and by chronically fatigued persons who do not fulfill ME/CFS criteria, a greater percentage of people fulfilling ME/CFS criteria report unrefreshing sleep, sleep disturbances, and difficulties falling asleep or waking up early in the morning (Komaroff et al., 1996a; Krupp et al., 1993; Nisenbaum et al., 2004) relative to these other groups.

Sleep-related complaints may change throughout the course of the illness. For example, one study found that in the first few months of the illness, ME/CFS patients complain of hypersomnia, but as the disease progresses, they have trouble staying asleep (Morriss et al., 1997). A cross-sectional study of randomly selected patients found that sleep-related symptoms may become less frequent over the course of the illness (Nisenbaum et al.,

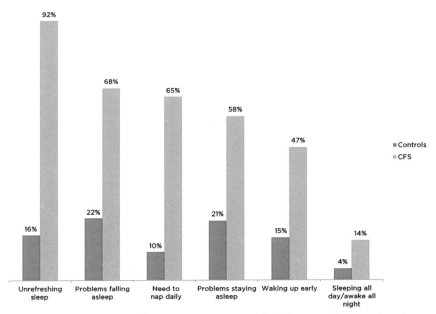

FIGURE 4-2 Percentage of ME/CFS patients and healthy controls reporting sleep-related symptoms of at least moderate severity that occurred at least half of the time during the past 6 months.
NOTE: All patients fulfilled the Fukuda definition for CFS.
SOURCE: Jason et al., 2013b.

2003); however, this may be due to behavioral adaptation or changes in sleep medication.

Sleep-related symptoms are listed differently in the various diagnostic criteria for ME/CFS (see Box 4-1), and there is conflicting evidence on whether ME/CFS patients fulfilling different diagnostic criteria experience sleep-related symptoms differently. Those fulfilling the CCC reported significantly worse (in terms of frequency and severity, $p < 0.05$) unrefreshing sleep (Jason et al., 2012a, 2013a) and more difficulty falling asleep (Jason et al., 2012a) relative to those fulfilling the Fukuda definition. Similarly, another

---

BOX 4-1
Sleep-Related Symptoms in Case Definitions and
Diagnostic Criteria for ME/CFS

1994 Fukuda Case Definition of CFS (Fukuda et al., 1994)

- Unrefreshing sleep is a minor criterion (not required).
- Sleep apnea and narcolepsy are exclusionary conditions (as they are conditions that explain chronic fatigue).

Canadian Consensus Criteria for ME/CFS (Carruthers et al., 2003, p. 16)

- Sleep dysfunction, including unrefreshing sleep or sleep quantity or rhythm disturbances such as reversed or chaotic diurnal sleep rhythms, is a required criterion for diagnosis. "Loss of the deeper phases of sleep is especially characteristic, with frequent awakenings, and loss of restorative feelings in the morning. Restless leg syndrome and periodic limb movement disorder often accompany sleep disturbance."
- "It is important to rule out treatable sleep disorders such as upper airway resistance syndrome, obstructive and central sleep apnea and restless leg syndrome."

2011 International Consensus Criteria for ME (Carruthers et al., 2011, p. 330)

- Sleep disturbance is a minor criterion (not required), which includes
  – disturbed sleep patterns, such as insomnia, prolonged sleep including naps, sleeping most of the day and being awake most of the night, frequent awakenings, awaking much earlier than before illness onset, and vivid dreams/nightmares; and
  – unrefreshing sleep, such as awakening feeling exhausted regardless of duration of sleep and daytime sleepiness.
- "Sleep disturbances are typically expressed by prolonged sleep, sometimes extreme, in the acute phase and often evolve into marked sleep reversal in the chronic stage."

study found that patients fulfilling the International Consensus Criteria for ME (ME-ICC) reported significantly worse symptom scores for unrefreshing sleep, need to nap during each day, difficulty falling asleep, and difficulty staying asleep relative to those fulfilling the Fukuda definition (Brown et al., 2013). In contrast to these results, however, are those from two other studies. One study found that more patients fulfilling the Fukuda definition reported greater difficulty staying asleep than those fulfilling the CCC (Jason et al., 2004), while a second study reported no significant differences in sleep-related symptom scores between patients fulfilling the Fukuda definition and those fulfilling the ME-ICC (Jason et al., 2014). Regardless, it is clear that all the major diagnostic criteria include sleep-related symptoms.

Chronic fatigue may be caused by sleep disorders; thus, most diagnostic criteria for ME/CFS require ruling out primary or treatable sleep disorders before a diagnosis of ME/CFS can be made (see Box 4-1). Sleep apnea— whether obstructive, central, or undefined—is an exclusionary condition in several criteria, but there is less consistency regarding whether other sleep disorders, such as narcolepsy or the spectrum of obstructive or central sleep disorders, truly exclude ME/CFS (Carruthers et al., 2003; Fukuda et al., 1994; Jason et al., 2010b; NICE, 2007). Some researchers have noted that the inclusion of unrefreshing or nonrestorative sleep as a case-defining symptom, combined with listing sleep disorders as exclusionary conditions, may confuse the diagnosis and management of ME/CFS (Mariman et al., 2012; Unger et al., 2004).

Assessment of Sleep-Related Symptoms in ME/CFS

Taking a careful history of sleep complaints can help a clinician identify whether objective testing of patients with such complaints is indicated. As noted above, sleep-related symptoms may change over time in ME/CFS patients, and it is possible for sleep disorders to develop over the course of the illness (Morriss et al., 1997; Nisenbaum et al., 2003; Reeves et al., 2006). Furthermore, it is plausible that the development of other symptoms, such as pain or headache, over time may cause or contribute to sleep disorders, or that the development of a primary sleep disorder leads to widespread pain. Also, many ME/CFS patients are prescribed medications that may improve or worsen sleep-related symptoms (Armitage, 1999; Foral et al., 2011; Kierlin and Littner, 2011; Trivedi et al., 1999).

Patients reporting symptoms of primary sleep disorders should be thoroughly evaluated to identify or rule out these conditions, as diagnosis and treatment of primary sleep disorders may be effective in reducing or relieving such symptoms (Qanneta, 2013; Reeves et al., 2006). Identifying insomnia in some patients may be useful therapeutically because techniques known to alleviate insomnia have been shown to be effective in fibromyalgia, a comorbid condition occurring in some ME/CFS patients (Edinger et al., 2005).

Several questionnaires exist with which to capture patient-reported sleep symptoms and assess the subjective quality of sleep or sleep-related symptoms, although readily accessible clinical tools are not easy to find. The DePaul Symptom Questionnaire includes several items that can be used to assess the frequency and severity of symptoms that indicate sleep dysfunction in ME/CFS patients (DePaul Research Team, 2010). The Sleep Assessment Questionnaire© also has been found to describe sleep abnormalities experienced by ME/CFS patients (Unger et al., 2004). And although not developed specifically for ME/CFS, the Pittsburgh Sleep Quality Index (PSQI) is a validated tool for assessing subjective sleep quality (Buysse et al., 1989).

It is important to consider frequency and severity thresholds when assessing subjective sleep complaints. In a study using the DePaul Symptom Questionnaire, for example, 65 percent of healthy controls reported unrefreshing sleep that occurred with mild severity at least a little of the time, yet only 16 percent of healthy controls reported unrefreshing sleep that occurred with moderate severity at least half of the time (Jason et al., 2013b). The percentages of ME/CFS patients reporting unrefreshing sleep at the same thresholds were 99 and 92 percent, respectively.

Complaints of sleepiness or fatigue so severe as to result in a substantial decrease in activity often lead to referral to a sleep laboratory for evaluation of underlying sleep pathology. Polysomnography (PSG), the continuous monitoring of variables that define sleep states and stages, is a type of sleep study used to diagnose sleep disorders such as sleep apnea and narcolepsy (Kasper et al., 2005; Kushida et al., 2005). Sleepiness usually is the driving symptom for referral for PSG, yet many ME/CFS patients do not undergo sleep studies because they report being fatigued rather than being sleepy (Spitzer and Broadman, 2010a). And although PSG can be useful for diagnosing primary sleep disorders that are often comorbid with ME/CFS, many ME/CFS patients have normal sleep studies despite complaining of nonrestorative sleep (Reeves et al., 2006).

Recently, new ways of assessing sleep quality have emerged and have been applied to assess these abnormalities in ME/CFS patients. The classic method for assessing sleep is to record the electroencephalogram (EEG) of a patient every 30 seconds to determine the stage of sleep (Kushida et al., 2005). In contrast, one new method uses the actual waveform of the EEG and determines power at different frequencies (Armitage et al., 2007; Duffy et al., 2011). Another new approach assesses transitions between sleep stages and determines the probability of occurrence of each transition (Kishi et al., 2008).

PSG requires spending the night in a sleep laboratory, which limits its use to those who are willing and able to travel to the laboratory for testing. PSG also may be less accessible in nonurban areas or too costly to include in a routine assessment (Oliveira et al., 2014; Rosen et al., 2012). However, home-based recording is a possibility. Moreover, the development of ambulatory monitoring methods, such as wrist actigraphy, may increase access to these diagnostic tests (Blackman et al., 2010; Corral-Peñafiel et al., 2013; Libman et al., 2009). However, this method has been normed only for healthy people (Marino et al., 2013), and its use in people with sleep problems still needs to be validated. And, of course, wrist actigraphy cannot be used to evaluate patients for conditions such as sleep apnea (Morgenthaler et al., 2007).

Evidence for Sleep-Related Symptoms in ME/CFS

The committee conducted a targeted literature search to identify research comparing self-reported or objectively assessed sleep-related symptoms and signs in ME/CFS subjects and in those without the illness. Details of the search methodology are described in Chapter 1. The findings from the literature are described below, but there are several limitations to consider when interpreting the evidence base, in addition to those discussed earlier.

In general, the design and implementation of these studies was highly heterogeneous. Most articles document case-control studies in which symptoms or signs were compared in groups of subjects with and without ME/CFS. Most studies used healthy controls as a comparison group, and several compared twin pairs in which one twin was diagnosed with ME/CFS and the other was healthy. Fewer studies used controls affected by other illnesses. The studies assessed varied outcomes of interest. Self-reported symptoms were assessed with many different questionnaires and scales. Several studies used PSG, but many used different testing protocols or diagnostic thresholds for sleep disorders.

As with other literature on ME/CFS, the use of different diagnostic criteria for patient selection limits comparisons across studies. In particular, because of the variations in diagnostic criteria for ME/CFS, some studies excluded patients with primary sleep disorders, while others included them. The following subsections describe in turn the evidence for primary sleep disorders in patients with ME/CFS and the evidence for sleep abnormalities in patients with ME/CFS that do not have primary sleep disorders. Note that for many studies, it was unclear whether ME/CFS patients with sleep disorders were included or excluded; these studies are not discussed below.

Sleep Disorders in ME/CFS Patients

Many of the sleep-related symptoms reported by ME/CFS patients—difficulty falling asleep, frequent or sustained awakenings, early-morning awakenings, and nonrestorative or unrefreshing sleep (persistent sleepiness despite sleep of adequate duration)—are types of insomnia (Kasper et al., 2005; Watson et al., 2003). Insomnia can have many causes, including other sleep disorders, such as sensory motor disorders (restless leg syndrome and periodic limb movement disorder), narcolepsy, and sleep disordered breathing (SDB). SDB constitutes a spectrum of breathing problems during sleep that range from subtle changes in the pattern of breathing to more severe snoring and obstructive sleep apnea. These disorders may result in multiple arousals during sleep, which can produce the daytime symptoms of sleepiness or fatigue (Cowan et al., 2014).

Primary sleep disorders are fairly common in ME/CFS patients, with prevalence ranging from 19 to 69 percent (Creti et al., 2010; Gotts et al., 2013; Le Bon et al., 2000; Reeves et al., 2006). Studies have found sleep apnea/hypopnea syndrome to be present in 13 to 65 percent of patients, followed by periodic limb movement disorder (4 to 25 percent), narcolepsy (5 to 7 percent), and restless leg syndrome (4 percent) (Creti et al., 2010; Gotts et al., 2013; Le Bon et al., 2000; Reeves et al., 2006). Effective treatments are available for many of these sleep disorders, but there is little evidence on the effectiveness of these interventions in reducing the sleep-related symptoms of ME/CFS aside from those caused by the sleep disorder. Continuous positive airway pressure (CPAP) is a common treatment for SDB, and while it has been shown to reduce fatigue and sleepiness in people with obstructive sleep apnea (Tomfohr et al., 2011), reports of its improving ME/CFS symptoms are limited (Qanneta, 2014). One study of CPAP treatment in ME/CFS patients with sleep apnea/hypopnea syndrome (SAHS), a condition within the spectrum of SDB, found no difference in sleep-related symptoms between patients who were and were not compliant with the CPAP treatment. Further, there were no significant differences in symptoms, quality of life, or activity levels between ME/CFS patients with and without SAHS (Libman et al., 2009).

One inference from these few studies is that sleep disorders can be considered an exclusionary diagnosis for ME/CFS only if treatment of the sleep disorder cures the ME/CFS symptoms. Some researchers have suggested that sleep disorders should be considered comorbid conditions rather than exclusionary criteria for a diagnosis of ME/CFS (Jackson and Bruck, 2012; Libman et al., 2009). Studies comparing clinical presentation in ME/CFS patients with and without sleep disorders have found no differences between the two groups (Le Bon et al., 2000; Libman et al., 2009), but greater functional impairment has been reported in ME/CFS patients with some sleep disorders (Morriss et al., 1993).

Studies that included ME/CFS patients with sleep disorders have found other objective abnormalities during sleep studies. One study found mean sleep latency to be greater in ME/CFS patients than in healthy controls (Bailes et al., 2006). Another found that ME/CFS patients spent less total time than controls in rapid eye movement (REM) sleep (Whelton et al., 1992). And in another study, ME/CFS patients compared with controls experienced significantly lower sleep efficiency—the ratio between sleep time and total recording time—and significantly more time awake after falling asleep (Morriss et al., 1993); these results have been replicated (Togo et al., 2008).

ME/CFS Patients Without Sleep Disorders

The studies described below excluded ME/CFS subjects that had previously been diagnosed with a sleep disorder. The authors of most of these studies explicitly describe their exclusion criteria, but studies also are included below if they selected participants that fulfilled the Fukuda definition for CFS, because sleep apnea and narcolepsy are exclusionary conditions. The selection criteria also may have differed in other ways (e.g., medication status), and the study designs (e.g., the type of control group) may have varied as well.

Subjective evidence Most of these studies found that ME/CFS patients without sleep disorders reported significantly more subjective sleep complaints than controls, but as described later, many failed to find major differences in objective measures of sleep (Majer et al., 2007; Reeves et al., 2006; Watson et al., 2004). More ME/CFS patients than controls reported unrefreshing sleep (Majer et al., 2007; Reeves et al., 2006) and problems sleeping (Majer et al., 2007). Self-reported sleep quality was significantly worse in ME/CFS patients than in healthy controls as measured by the PSQI (Le Bon et al., 2012; Neu et al., 2007, 2011; Rahman et al., 2011) and other questionnaires (Majer et al., 2007; Watson et al., 2004). PSQI sleep quality scores, however, were not associated with objective measures of sleep quality (Neu et al., 2007). ME/CFS patients also reported significantly more fatigue and sleepiness than healthy controls (Le Bon et al., 2012).

Objective evidence A number of studies have compared sleep parameters measured through PSG in ME/CFS patients and healthy controls; however, comparisons across studies are difficult to make because of the use of various case definitions and methods of measurement. One study examined pairs of twins in which one twin had ME/CFS and the other was healthy.

Compared with the healthy twins, the twins with ME/CFS reported more subjective complaints of insomnia, but objective measures of sleep were "remarkably similar" (Watson et al., 2003). Other studies generally have found only minor objective differences between ME/CFS patients and suitable comparison groups (Armitage et al., 2009; Majer et al., 2007; Neu et al., 2007; Reeves et al., 2006) or differences that were not statistically significant (Ball et al., 2004; Le Bon et al., 2007; Sharpley et al., 1997). These studies found that ME/CFS patients had decreased total sleep time, resulting in decreased sleep efficiency and less time spent in deep sleep, with some evidence for disturbed sleep in the form of more arousals and longer periods of being awake after sleep onset.

There is growing evidence that ME/CFS patients experience abnormal sleep continuation compared with healthy controls. In one study, ME/CFS patients had higher levels of microarousal, despite the study's exclusion of sleep disorders normally associated with microarousals (Neu et al., 2008). A study of sleep transitions also found that ME/CFS patients were more likely than normal controls to awaken during sleep, especially during the later hours of sleep (Kishi et al., 2008).

The use of stratification strategies may help. One study stratified on sleep latency and sleep time to propose different sleep phenotypes (Gotts et al., 2013). Another stratified patients according to whether they felt more or less sleepy the morning after versus the night before the sleep study (Togo et al., 2008). The patients who reported feeling less sleepy had normal PSG, while those who reported feeling more sleepy showed evidence of more disrupted sleep. Also, in a follow-up study conducted after subjects had performed a stress test, patients who reported being less sleepy after a night of sleep had normal PSG, while those who reported feeling more sleepy were the group with sleep disruption (Togo et al., 2010).

Multiple sleep latency tests (MSLTs) may be used to measure objective daytime sleepiness, which is characteristic of narcolepsy. Subjects are asked to nap, and the time it takes them to fall asleep—latency to nap—is measured several times during the day and averaged to determine a mean sleep latency for naps (Johns, 2000). A shortened latency to nap is indicative of increased sleepiness. One group of researchers found shortened latency to nap in ME/CFS patients compared with healthy controls (Neu et al., 2008; Watson et al., 2004), while others have failed to find significant differences (Majer et al., 2007; Reeves et al., 2006). The results of these studies suggest that narcolepsy is not a significant factor in ME/CFS. Supporting that conclusion is one study reporting an opposite result after a night of sleep deprivation. While one would expect this manipulation to result in short sleep latencies, the researchers found that one-third of the patients had difficulty falling asleep (Nakamura et al., 2010b). Such an outcome is consistent with the idea that the sleep disruption of some ME/CFS patients may reflect a problem with sleep initiation and maintenance. It is important to note that MSLT can be used reliably to diagnose narcolepsy only when patients are in a stable state off potentially sedating medications (Thorpy, 1992).

Subsets

To study more homogeneous groups of patients, some researchers have examined sleep characteristics in different subgroups of ME/CFS patients. As an example, ME/CFS patients who also had postural orthostatic tachycardia syndrome (POTS) were found to have reduced daytime hypersomnolence compared with those without POTS (Lewis et al., 2013).

Chronic pain is a common factor in sleep disorders resulting from a medical condition (Fishbain et al., 2010). A frequent cause of chronic widespread pain is fibromyalgia (FM)—a diagnosis that has substantial overlap with ME/CFS (Ciccone and Natelson, 2003). Several studies have compared evidence in ME/CFS patients with FM (CFS+FM) and those without FM (CFS only). In one study, FM was less frequent among ME/CFS patients with objective sleepiness as measured by short MSLT (< 10 minutes) (Le Bon et al., 2000). Some studies have found no differences in sleep parameters as measured through PSG between CFS+FM and CFS-only patients (Fischler et al., 1997; Spitzer and Broadman, 2010a,b).[6] A study examining sleep-stage dynamics found differences between CFS+FM and CFS-only groups in transition probabilities and rates among sleep stages (Kishi et al., 2011). In CFS-only patients, the probability of transition from REM sleep to awake was significantly greater than in healthy controls. CFS+FM patients experienced significantly greater probabilities and rates of transition from waking, REM sleep, and S1 to S2, as well as greater probabilities and rates of transition from slow wave sleep (SWS) to waking and S1. Thus, CFS-only patients differed from those with CFS+FM. Another study found evidence of increased IL-10, an anti-inflammatory cytokine that may contribute to disrupted sleep, during the sleep of CFS-only but not CFS+FM patients (Nakamura et al., 2010a); however, the magnitude of the difference was small. The role of cytokines in regulating sleep in ME/CFS remains a research question.

Summary

Standard sleep studies are not substantially abnormal in people with ME/CFS. Several studies have found differences in sleep architecture in subsets of people with ME/CFS and in people with ME/CFS compared with healthy controls (Whelton et al., 1992), yet the current evidence base is not

---

[6] Fischler and colleagues (1997) did not exclude sleep disorders.

strong enough to identify ME/CFS-specific sleep pathology. It is clear, however, that people with ME/CFS universally report experiencing unrefreshing sleep, and further research will be important to determine whether there is a specific sleep abnormality common to ME/CFS patients or a heterogeneity of abnormalities that may define subsets of ME/CFS patients.

In several case definitions and diagnostic criteria for ME/CFS, primary treatable sleep disorders such as sleep apnea and narcolepsy are listed as exclusionary criteria for an ME/CFS diagnosis. However, there is evidence to suggest that primary sleep disorders should be considered important comorbid conditions in the differential diagnosis and that sleep complaints are complex. Further, there is little evidence that treatment of primary sleep disorders improves ME/CFS symptoms rather than simply reduces symptoms of the comorbid disorder.

> **Conclusion:** *Despite the absence of an objective alteration in sleep architecture, the data are strong that the complaint of unrefreshing sleep is universal among patients with ME/CFS when questions about sleep specifically address this issue. While PSG is not required to diagnose ME/CFS, its use to screen for treatable sleep disorders when indicated is appropriate. Diagnosis of a primary sleep disorder does not rule out a diagnosis of ME/CFS.*

NEUROCOGNITIVE MANIFESTATIONS

Description of Neurocognitive Manifestations in ME/CFS

Impairments in cognitive functioning are one of the most frequently reported symptoms of ME/CFS. Patients describe these symptoms as debilitating and as affecting function as much as the physical symptoms that accompany this disease. During a survey of ME/CFS patients, descriptions of neurocognitive manifestations included, among others, "brain fog," "confusion," disorientation," "hard to concentrate, can't focus," "inability to process information," "inability to multitask," and "short-term memory loss" (FDA, 2013). The short-term memory problems of ME/CFS patients include difficulty remembering something they just read. Patients usually report slowed information processing and impaired psychomotor functioning in more general terms as overall mental fatigue or slowed thinking (Constant et al., 2011; Larun and Malterud, 2007). In more severe cases, patients have difficulty completing tasks that require sustained attention and report problems performing even relatively simple activities such as watching television (FDA, 2013). Studies of the exact nature of neurocognitive deficits reported by patients with ME/CFS have shown that some patients meeting various current criteria for ME/CFS have different or more severe impairments than others, but also that self-reported severity of impairments is not always associated with severity based on objective measures (Cockshell and Mathias, 2013).

Prevalence of Neurocognitive Manifestations in ME/CFS Patients

Estimates of the prevalence of neurocognitive manifestations in ME/CFS patients vary as a result of the different definitions used in research and the assessment of these manifestations using patient reports. The 2003 CCC, 2010 Revised CCC, and 2011 ME-ICC require the presence of neurological/cognitive manifestations for a diagnosis of ME/CFS, while the 1994 Fukuda definition and 2007 British National Institute for Health and Clinical Excellence (NICE) Clinical Guidelines do not. Moreover, these various case definitions and diagnostic criteria are inconsistent in the manifestations or symptoms listed for this category. For instance, the Fukuda definition includes only "impaired memory or concentration" as one optional criterion, while the CCC requires the presence of two or more difficulties from a more extensive list of cognitive (confusion, impairment of concentration and short-term memory consolidation, disorientation, difficulty with information processing) or neurologic (perceptual and sensory disturbances, ataxia, muscle weakness, and fasciculations) manifestations.

A study conducted in Belgium in a population of patients with chronic fatigue found a prevalence of 93 percent for attention deficit, 85.6 percent for memory disturbance, and 75.5 percent for difficulties with words for those fulfilling the Fukuda definition (De Becker et al., 2001). When applying frequency and severity scores of at least 2, Jason and colleagues (2013b) found that a greater percentage of ME/CFS patients than healthy controls reported neurocognitive symptoms of at least moderate severity that occurred at least half of the time (see Figure 4-3).

Assessment of Neurocognitive Manifestations in ME/CFS

Measurement of cognitive functioning is a challenge for researchers. While theoretical distinctions often are made among areas of cognition, such as memory, attention, and motor functioning, there presently are no "pure" measures that can directly test different areas of cognition individually rather than in the aggregate. Thus, while results of a specific neuropsychological test may be interpreted as evidence of a particular cognitive deficit, such as poor working memory, it is likely that any given test is actually measuring multiple aspects of cognitive function simultaneously.

Additionally, an important distinction must be made between objective measures of cognitive deficits, which measure participants' performance on cognitively demanding tasks, and subjective measures of cognitive func-

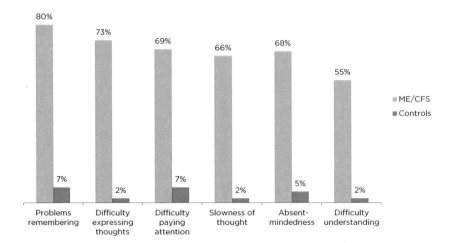

FIGURE 4-3 Percentage of ME/CFS patients and healthy controls reporting neuro-cognitive manifestations of at least moderate severity that occurred at least half of the time during the past 6 months.
NOTE: All patients fulfilled the Fukuda definition for CFS.
SOURCE: Jason et al., 2013b.

tioning that ask individuals to report cognitive difficulties they encounter in their daily lives. Both objective and subjective measures are important in understanding ME/CFS, but in the following discussion of evidence on the neurocognitive characteristics of ME/CFS, the committee has chosen to focus primarily on objective tests that may provide some indication of the cognitive processes and possible causal mechanisms involved in ME/CFS. It is worth noting, however, that from the clinical perspective, neuropsychological testing has shown significant overlap between ME/CFS and control populations, and that self-report of cognitive issues offers a more reliable means of discriminating between these two groups (Cockshell and Mathias, 2010).

Most studies focused on memory impairments test patients' working memory (the ability to retain and make use of information in the short term) as measured by a range of neuropsychological tests. Researchers also divide memory tasks into various categories based on whether a task requires immediate (also related to working memory), short-term, or long-term memory; remembering something that has already happened (retrospective memory); or remembering to do something in the future (prospective memory). Tasks are divided as well by the type of content that is recalled (verbal or visual memory) (Attree et al., 2014; DeLuca et al., 1995). Subjective measures used for memory testing include a range of different assessments, such as the Prospective and Retrospective Memory Questionnaire, the Cognitive Failures Questionnaire, or self-observation using a structured diary (Attree et al., 2014; Knoop et al., 2007). A meta-analysis of studies of cognitive functioning by Cockshell and Mathias (2010) found that the majority of objective tests used to assess memory function in ME/CFS asked participants to remember either verbal or written word lists, while some tested visual memory by having participants reproduce a complex figure from memory or remember visual patterns. Examples of verbal tests reported in the meta-analysis include the Selective Reminding Test, the Wechsler Memory Scale-Revised (WMS-R), and the California Verbal Learning Test. Tests of visual memory reviewed included, among others, the Rey Osterrieth Complex Figure and the Pattern Recognition Test. Some tests included both verbal and visual components and fell in both categories.

In addition, researchers use the n-back procedure to investigate the neurologic substrates of the working memory processes. The n-back task is a continuous performance measure whereby the subject is presented with stimulus sequences (i.e., visual, auditory, and olfactory) and is required to indicate when the current stimulus matches the one presented in "n" trials previously. This task requires the subject to maintain, update, and manipulate information and therefore is considered a demanding task. The n usually varies from 1 to 3. The responses of the n-back task can be correlated with neuroimaging reports of the activation of several brain regions (Owen et al., 2005).

In the neuropsychological literature, attempts are made to distinguish between information processing speed (as measured by reaction time) and motor speed (movement time or tests of fine motor speed [e.g., finger tapping test]). Recent studies assessing psychomotor functioning in ME/CFS have separated these components, but together these tests evaluate reaction time as part of the motor component (Schrijvers et al., 2009; Van Den Eede et al., 2011). The Paced Auditory Serial Addition Test (PASAT), the Attention Network Test (ANT), the Cambridge Neuropsychological Test Automated Battery (CANTAB), and similar measures or testing batteries are used to assess attention deficits and reaction times. Reaction times on these tests frequently are used to judge information processing speed independent of motor speed (Majer et al., 2008; Michiels and Cluydts, 2001). Impairment in psychomotor functioning is demonstrated by both increased simple reaction time, in which subjects respond to a verbal or visual stimulus, and choice reaction time, which measures length of time responding to a stimulus involving multiple potential options (Den Eede et al., 2011). The PASAT and ANT can additionally be used to assess slowed information processing (Davis and Claypoole, 1997; Togo et al., 2013).

Evidence for Neurocognitive Manifestations in ME/CFS

The committee conducted a targeted literature search to identify research papers comparing the presence of neurocognitive manifestations in ME/CFS cases versus controls. The researchers assessed presentation of neurocognitive impairments either by self-report questionnaires or by objective testing using neurocognitive test batteries. The committee's targeted search was limited to the past 10 years because of the large number of results but considered older research that was reviewed and cited in the introduction or discussion of more recent literature. The approach the committee used to review the literature is described in Chapter 1. The findings of the targeted literature review are presented below, with the caveats regarding the research base described at the beginning of this chapter.

The literature shows with some consistency that neurocognitive problems such as memory impairment, slowed information processing, attention deficits, and impaired psychomotor function are highly prevalent in ME/CFS patients, as discussed in this section. Slowed information processing is the neurocognitive symptom of ME/CFS most consistently reported in objective neuropsychological testing, with evidence from twin studies showing that individuals with ME/CFS tend to process information more slowly than healthy individuals with similar intellectual abilities (Claypoole et al., 2007; Mahurin et al., 2004; Togo et al., 2013). Numerous papers both support and refute the existence of memory impairment in individuals with ME/CFS. Studies that do report impairment show a wide range in the measured severity of memory problems, with small to moderate and significant deficits in memory having been found for a range of cognitive tests, but not all (Cockshell and Mathias, 2010; Constant et al., 2011; Dickson et al., 2009; Majer et al., 2008). A large number of studies also have found impaired attention (Capuron et al., 2006; Cockshell and Mathias, 2010; Constant et al., 2011; Dickson et al., 2009; Hou et al., 2008, 2014; Hutchinson and Badham, 2013) and slowed reaction and movement times in people with ME/CFS (Den Eede et al., 2011; Majer et al., 2008; Schrijvers et al., 2009). Comparisons with other illnesses, such as sleep apnea and depression, suggest that psychomotor impairment in ME/CFS may be less severe than in those other illnesses (Neu et al., 2011; Schrijvers et al., 2009).

Memory Impairment

In objective neuropsychological testing, individuals meeting criteria for ME/CFS have displayed deficits in working memory compared with healthy controls. These patients have been found to be impaired on tests that assess working memory over a sustained period of time (Cockshell and Mathias, 2010; DeLuca et al., 2004b). Attree and colleagues (2009) found that ME/CFS patients rated themselves as more forgetful than controls on both prospective and retrospective memory. However, objective memory impairment was limited to retrospective not prospective memory in these patients. Michiels and colleagues (1996) found that reduced verbal and visual memory was the most consistent finding in individuals with ME/CFS compared with normal controls.

With regard to verbal memory, moderate to large deficits were found on tests of list learning, including immediate recall, delayed recall, and recognition, while nonverbal memory for complex figures and spatial location was not impaired (Cockshell and Mathias, 2010). Numerous studies provide evidence that verbal memory impairment (often measured using the California Verbal Learning Test) likely is associated with ME/CFS (Cockshell and Mathias, 2010). However, because of the methodological weaknesses in much ME/CFS research, particularly the comparison of mean scores on neuropsychological tests rather than reporting of the number of impaired individuals, it is difficult to determine whether this impairment is characteristic of the illness or present only in a subset of patients (Vercoulen et al., 1998).

ME/CFS patients compared with controls perform significantly worse on free-recall retrospective memory. Research findings offer some support for the deficient acquisition hypothesis, which proposes that retrospective memory deficits in ME/CFS patients are attributable to difficulties with encoding information due to slower information processing (impaired delayed recall) (Attree et al., 2009). This interpretation appears to be supported by findings that the verbal memory problems of these patients stem from delayed acquisition of information rather than inaccuracy in recall (DeLuca et al., 2004a). Furthermore, in studies of working memory, researchers have found that difficulties emerge only when ME/CFS subjects are required to perform time-dependent tasks (DeLuca et al., 2004a; Togo et al., 2013), implying that ME/CFS patients' cognitive processes may be slower than but not otherwise different from those of healthy control patients.

Memory impairment does appear to distinguish ME/CFS from such psychiatric disorders as depression and anxiety. The majority of studies examining severity of cognitive impairment, including memory problems, failed to find a relationship between such impairment and depression, even though ME/CFS patients have high rates of depression (Busichio et al., 2004; DeLuca et al., 1995; Short et al., 2002). In studies that divided ME/CFS patients according to whether they had a comorbid psychiatric condition, those without such a comorbidity showed more severe memory impairment (DeLuca et al., 2004b; Tiersky et al., 2003).

It is less clear whether memory impairment may distinguish ME/CFS from other fatiguing illnesses. However, mental fatigue is an important correlate of working memory in ME/CFS patients, with a population-based sample of these patients showing a clear association between subjective complaints of mental fatigue and objective measurements of memory (Capuron et al., 2006). Patients with ME/CFS who specifically reported mental fatigue were found to show significant impairment of working memory in the task of sustained attention/vigilance (a spatial working memory task of the CANTAB), suggesting higher cognitive fatigability (Capuron et al., 2006). Cognitive impairment in ME/CFS patients with mental fatigue was not attributable to mood disorders or psychotropic medication (Capuron et al., 2006).

Slowed Information Processing

Slowed information processing appears to be one of the most easily distinguishable features of ME/CFS (Cockshell and Mathias, 2010, 2013; Michiels and Cluydts, 2001; Tiersky et al., 1997). Despite some contradictory evidence, a large number of papers have emerged supporting the idea that individuals with ME/CFS often display slowed information processing (Claypoole et al., 2007; DeLuca et al., 2004a; Togo et al., 2013).

Positive evidence is provided by twin-control studies in which individuals with ME/CFS were compared with their twins who did not have the illness. These studies frequently revealed similar premorbid intellectual functioning (Claypoole et al., 2007; Mahurin et al., 2004) and no differences in content-dependent untimed testing, but significant differences in time-dependent tasks (Mahurin et al., 2004). Multiple studies have found that individuals with ME/CFS perform poorly compared with controls only in time-dependent tasks, with ME/CFS subjects showing no impairment in accuracy of information processing when given as much time as necessary to complete a task (DeLuca et al., 2004a; Mahurin et al., 2004). Also, in a meta-analysis of research studies, measures of both simple (reaction time task) and complex (PASAT) information processing speed showed moderate to large significant impairments in persons with ME/CFS compared with healthy controls (Cockshell and Mathias, 2010).

As with memory impairment, ME/CFS patients without psychiatric comorbidity show greater delays in information processing. Moreover, some evidence suggests that slower information processing is not related to reduced effort, depression, anxiety, fatigue, or sleep problems, nor is it dependent on slowed motor functioning, psychological status, number or severity of ME/CFS symptoms, or overall functioning (Cockshell and Mathias, 2012, 2013). Researchers in the field consider this symptom to be a possible cause of other neurocognitive impairments, including difficulties with attention and memory (DeLuca et al., 2004a; Togo et al., 2013). For that reason, it may be useful to compare ME/CFS patients with this symptom with other control groups (e.g., besides those with depression), as slowed information processing speed has also been identified in other clinical groups, such as patients with multiple sclerosis and traumatic brain injury (DeLuca and Kalmar, 2008).

Attention Deficits

Considerable evidence shows that reduced attention is associated with ME/CFS (Cockshell and Mathias, 2010; Constant et al., 2011; Hou et al., 2014), although some research indicates that attentional deficits may be due to reduced information processing speed (Cockshell and Mathias, 2013). Cognition has been found to be weaker among patients with ME/CFS, who demonstrated an impaired ability to maintain attention and alertness (Constant et al., 2011). Several studies also have shown impairments in executive attention relative to healthy controls, with ME/CFS patients demonstrating greater difficulty concentrating on a particular element when confronted with potential distractions (Hou et al., 2014; Hutchinson and Badham, 2013). Some studies have confirmed the presence of objective impairments of attention in patients with ME/CFS compared with controls (Cockshell and Mathias, 2010; Hou et al., 2014). Differences have remained after patients showing low effort have been removed, suggesting that the differences cannot be explained by lack of effort (Constant et al., 2011).

Some studies have demonstrated that ME/CFS patients display greater attentional bias toward linguistic and pictorial health-related threat stimuli (i.e., any factor that represents a danger to one's health) (Hou et al., 2008, 2014). Other studies have failed to find attentional bias but have found greater mood volatility with rumination (Martin and Alexeeva, 2010), suggesting variability in the ability of ME/CFS patients to control and sustain attention.

It is unclear whether this symptom can be used to distinguish ME/CFS from other disorders. Doing so would be difficult given that depression and anxiety can cause similar problems with attention (Moffoot et al., 1994) and have high comorbidity with ME/CFS (Attree et al., 2014). However, executive attention may be an option for distinguishing among subsets of the ME/CFS population, given some evidence of variability of this symptom in people with the illness (Hou et al., 2014). Studies of executive attention in children have shown that changes in the surface area of the anterior cingulate cortex account for a significant proportion of the variance in functioning on a test of cognitive control, suggesting that structural differences in this region of the brain could be a biomarker of conditions such as ME/CFS (Fjell et al., 2012). Deficits in patients may lead to poor activation or reduced connectivity of the anterior cingulate cortex. Exploring this possibility could further the effort to identify biomarkers of the disorder. More research comparing attentional deficits in fatiguing disorders and psychiatric conditions is necessary for this question to be answered.

Impaired Psychomotor Function

The literature offers conflicting evidence for the presence of impaired psychomotor function in ME/CFS patients. Some studies have found no difference in motor coordination and motor speed between ME/CFS patients and controls (reaction time test) (Cockshell and Mathias, 2013). Moreover, a meta-analysis found that fine motor speed was not impaired in subjects with ME/CFS (Cockshell and Mathias, 2010). However, there are significant differences in the movement time of reaction time tests between people with ME/CFS and healthy controls (Cockshell and Mathias, 2010). These findings suggest that information processing deficits contributed to the noted deficits in the movement time of reaction time tasks, which reportedly are not pure measures of motor speed (Smith and Carew, 1987; Vercoulen et al., 1998). Moreover, because fine motor speed was not found to be impaired in persons with ME/CFS, motor functioning is unlikely to be the primary cause of slower reaction times. This conclusion is consistent with the findings of more recent studies previously mentioned (Schrijvers et al., 2009; Van Den Eede et al., 2011) that reaction time but not movement time was impaired in ME/CFS patients.

On the other hand, considerable evidence that this symptom is associated with ME/CFS has been published (Davey et al., 2001; Lawrie et al., 2000; Marshall et al., 1997; Michiels et al., 1996). Results from a population-based study confirm and quantify alterations in motor speed in ME/CFS patients that are independent of psychiatric disorders or medication usage (Majer et al., 2008). In this study, ME/CFS patients recruited from the general population presented motor slowing after the researchers controlled for level of depressive symptoms. ME/CFS subjects also exhibited decreased motor speed, demonstrated by slower response times on the movement component of simple and choice reaction time tasks, a finding suggesting that these are primary features of cognitive changes in ME/CFS patients. The consistency of these results may provide clues to the involvement of neural circuits (i.e., basal ganglia) in ME/CFS. Further evidence of slowed psychomotor functioning is provided by twin-control studies in which individuals with ME/CFS were compared with their twins who did not have the illness (Claypoole et al., 2007; Mahurin et al., 2004).

Brain Studies

Studies of the brain in relation to ME/CFS have been performed for two purposes: to document any possible objective finding in ME/CFS and to develop diagnostic criteria for the disease. While in general these studies have been small (most with fewer than 20 patients with ME/CFS, usually fulfilling the Fukuda definition), most have shown statistically significant differences between patients with the condition and controls using a wide range of technologies and in a variety of brain regions. One study found that ME/CFS patients had 8 percent less gray matter relative to healthy controls, and that this difference was correlated with lower levels of physical activity (De Lange et al., 2005). Puri and colleagues (2012) found similar losses of both white and gray matter in patients with ME/CFS. Another study found that cognitive-behavioral therapy for ME/CFS patients increased prefrontal cortical volume after 16 sessions, suggesting that changes in brain volume and structure associated with the illness may be reversible with treatment (De Lange et al., 2008). However, the authors do not indicate whether such changes cause or result from neurocognitive symptoms of ME/CFS.

Recently, Nakatomi and colleagues (2014) found evidence of neuroinflammation in a small group of ME/CFS patients. While this was a small study (patients = 9, healthy controls = 10), it showed a significant increase in activated microglia or astrocytes using positron emission tomography (PET) in patients compared with controls. This study also found a positive correlation between activated microglia or astrocytes in the amygdala, thalamus, and midbrain and the cognitive impairment score of these subjects. The involvement of microglia could point to connectivity issues similar to those proposed with respect to the role of the anterior cingulate in maintaining attention. Spin-echo magnetic resonance imaging (MRI) revealed midbrain white matter and gray matter volume changes in these patients at fatigue onset, which the authors found to be consistent with an insult to the midbrain affecting multiple feedback control loops (Barnden et al., 2011).

In other brain studies, Yamamoto and colleagues (2003) used PET scanning to show that serotonin transporters were significantly reduced in the rostral subdivision of the anterior cingulate in ME/CFS patients. Functional MRI (fMRI) has been used to show an association between the subjective feeling of mental fatigue and brain responses during fatiguing cognition (Cook et al., 2007); reduced basal ganglia activation (caudate and globus pallidus) also may contribute to fatigue (Unger et al., 2012). Murrough and colleagues (2010) found increased ventricular lactate in ME/CFS patients based on proton magnetic resonance spectroscopy (MRS) imaging. The same group later found further evidence that increased oxidative stress may play a role in ME/CFS pathophysiology (Shungu et al., 2012). In another study, ME/CFS patients who were not medicated were reliably differentiated from healthy controls and those with depression using EEG spectral coherence (Duffy et al., 2011).

Some studies have found reduced activity in ME/CFS patients in regions of the brain associated with working memory during completion of a working memory task (Caseras et al., 2006), while others have found that individuals with ME/CFS appear to use more of their brain during working memory tasks (Lange et al., 2005). In addition, increased activation has been seen by fMRI in ME/CFS patients in the occipito-parietal cortex, posterior cingulate gyrus, and parahippocampal gyrus, with decreased activation seen in the dorsolateral and dorsomedial prefrontal cortices (Caseras et al., 2008).

Findings suggest that ME/CFS patients require additional neural resources (more activation) to achieve the same level of behavioral performance as controls on the PASAT and other neuropsychological tests (Cook et al., 2007; Schmaling et al., 2003). During high-demand tasks, ME/CFS patients showed reduced activation in dorsolateral prefrontal and parietal cortices, showing differences only at the neurophysiological level. ME/CFS patients activated a large cluster in the right inferior/medial temporal cortex while undergoing 3-back condition testing—probably a compensatory strategy when working memory is dysfunctional or saturated as a result of ME/CFS (Caseras et al., 2006). Results are similar to those found in sleep-deprived healthy adults, so these findings could also be the consequence of sleep deprivation in ME/CFS patients (Caseras et al., 2006).

These objective findings based on multiple technologies support the concept that ME/CFS patients, at least those meeting Fukuda definition, have objective brain differences from healthy controls. However, the varying locations of these findings make insights into etiology and possible treatments less clear, and subsets of patients have not yet been defined.

Exacerbation of Cognitive Symptoms Following Exertion

Evidence on the effect of exertion on cognitive function was provided earlier in the section on PEM.

Summary

Collectively, the studies reviewed here support the notion that ME/CFS patients present with neurocognitive impairment. Slowed information processing, demonstrated by objective neuropsychological testing and potentially related to problems with white matter integrity, is one of the strongest neurocognitive indicators in support of a diagnosis of ME/CFS, particularly if there is evidence of normal functioning on untimed tests and impaired functioning on time-dependent tasks.

The greater severity of memory and other neurocognitive deficits in ME/CFS patients without psychiatric comorbidity suggests that these deficits may be a distinguishing feature of the disease, or at the very least a means of defining subgroups within the ME/CFS population. Confirming the presence of this symptom using objective neuropsychological testing would support diagnosis of ME/CFS and possibly support diagnosis of a specific subset of ME/CFS patients, but it is not necessary for the diagnosis.

The presence of attention deficits or impaired psychomotor function could support diagnosis of ME/CFS or potentially a subset of the ME/CFS population, but only in combination with other neurocognitive impairments.

> *Conclusion: There is sufficient evidence that slowed information processing is common in patients with ME/CFS, and a growing body of evidence shows that it may play a central role in overall neurocognitive impairment associated with the disease. Such a deficit may be responsible for the disability that results in loss of employment and loss of functional capacity in social environments.*

ORTHOSTATIC INTOLERANCE AND AUTONOMIC DYSFUNCTION

Description of Orthostatic Intolerance in ME/CFS

Orthostatic intolerance is defined as a clinical condition in which symptoms worsen upon assuming and maintaining upright posture and are ameliorated (although not necessarily abolished) by recumbency (Gerrity et al., 2002; Low et al., 2009). Symptoms in orthostatic intolerance syndromes are those caused primarily by (1) cerebral underperfusion (such as lightheadedness, near-syncope or syncope, impaired concentration, headaches, and dimming or blurring of vision), or (2) sympathetic nervous system activation (such as forceful beating of the heart, palpitations, tremulousness, and chest pain) (Low et al., 2009). Other common signs and symptoms of orthostatic intolerance are fatigue, a feeling of weakness, intolerance of low-impact exercise, nausea, abdominal pain, facial pallor, nervousness, and shortness of breath (Kanjwal et al., 2003; Legge et al., 2008; Raj, 2013).

Orthostatic intolerance can occur as an isolated syndrome or in association with a variety of other comorbid disorders, including ME/CFS (Benarroch, 2012). The most prevalent forms of orthostatic intolerance in the general population, as well as among those with ME/CFS, are POTS and neurally mediated hypotension (NMH), with delayed variants of orthostatic hypotension and orthostatic tachycardia also being seen. Some individuals simply have low tolerance for upright posture without evidence of these objective circulatory changes (Bush et al., 2000; Rowe and Calkins, 1998).

Symptoms that occur upon assuming or maintaining upright posture are among the most commonly reported clinical features of ME/CFS. In surveys of ME/CFS patients, along with dizziness, a drop in blood pressure, spatial disorientation, and fainting, many participants "reported an inability to stand for even a few minutes" (FDA, 2013, p. 7). Some individuals described to the committee having difficulty standing, eating, and showering.[7] Orthostatic symptoms also are a component of PEM: "[A crash is] not just the physical pain or it's not just the head pain, it's also more cognitive impairment, more orthostatic intolerance, more neurological issues . . . they're very interrelated" (FDA, 2013, p. 8) (see the earlier section on PEM for more detail).

The symptoms and triggers for orthostatic intolerance syndromes are similar regardless of the associated diagnoses, although severity typically is greater in those with ME/CFS and POTS than in those with POTS alone (Okamoto et al., 2012a; Stewart et al., 1999). Orthostatic intolerance can begin acutely following a viral illness (Freeman and Komaroff, 1997), other infections (Kanjwal et al., 2011), pregnancy, or trauma, or it can have an insidious onset (Raj, 2013). It is made worse by deconditioning (Parsaik et al., 2012). Symptoms of orthostatic intolerance often are exacerbated by prolonged periods of upright posture; low-impact exercise; exposure to warm environments; and, less commonly, meals. Circumstances in daily life that can act as triggers include standing in line, shopping, hot showers or baths, hot weather, overheated rooms, and even prolonged quiet sitting (Raj, 2013; Schondorf et al., 1999). Some patients with orthostatic intolerance feel somewhat better and more energized while exercising, but they often are much worse afterward, especially if they are standing in the "cool-down" period (Calkins et al., 1995). Women with orthostatic intolerance can have worse symptoms during their menstrual periods (Low et al., 2009).

Prevalence of Orthostatic Intolerance and Autonomic Dysfunction in ME/CFS Patients

The committee's literature review identified six research articles in which orthostatic and autonomic symptoms are reported. The prevalence of orthostatic symptoms in ME/CFS varies widely in these publications, but in all of them is higher in ME/CFS subjects than in controls (Bou-Holaigah et al., 1995; Miwa, 2014; Newton et al., 2007; Poole et al., 2000; Soetekouw et al., 1999; Timmers et al., 2002).

The study by Bou-Holaigah and colleagues (1995) included 23 U.S. adolescents and adults with ME/CFS, 96 percent of whom reported lightheadedness, 96 percent nausea, 83 percent diaphoresis, 78 percent abdominal discomfort, 78 percent blurred vision, and 43 percent prior syncope. Orthostatic stresses reported as exacerbating fatigue included a hot shower (78 percent), prolonged standing (78 percent), a warm environment (74 percent), and episodes of lightheadedness (43 percent). Autonomic symp-

---

[7] Personal communication; public comments submitted to the IOM Committee on the Diagnostic Criteria for Myalgic Encephalomyelitis/Chronic Fatigue Syndrome for meeting 3, 2014.

toms were assessed in 37 adult ME/CFS patients from the Netherlands compared with 38 controls of similar age and sex (Soetekouw et al., 1999). Those with ME/CFS had significantly higher rates of increased perspiration (57 percent versus 13 percent), decreased salivation (24 percent versus 3 percent), dysphagia (24 percent versus 0 percent), and constipation (22 percent versus 3 percent). Poole and colleagues (2000) evaluated 21 monozygotic twins discordant for CFS. Symptoms of orthostatic intolerance in the week before head-up tilt testing were graded on a 0 (none) to 5 (severe) scale. The CFS twins had significantly more severe dizziness (1.4 versus 0), lightheadedness (1.4 versus 0.3), nausea (0.6 versus 0), abdominal discomfort (0.7 versus 0.3), sweating (1.3 versus 0.4), chest pain (0.7 versus 0.3), and shortness of breath (0.8 versus 0.2). In a study of 36 Dutch adults with ME/CFS and 36 healthy controls, 28 percent of ME/CFS adults but no controls reported symptoms related to or avoidance of prolonged standing (Timmers et al., 2002). Newton and colleagues (2007) examined autonomic symptoms as measured by the detailed Composite Autonomic Symptom Score (COMPASS) questionnaire in 40 British adults with ME/CFS and 40 controls. The ME/CFS adults had significantly higher scores on domains assessing orthostatic tolerance, vasomotor, secretomotor, gastrointestinal, pupillomotor, and sleep problems, as well as higher total scores (mean [standard deviation] score 43.7 [16.6] versus 12.1 [10.2]; $p < 0.0001$). Finally, among 40 Japanese adults with ME/CFS, 28 (70 percent) reported symptoms of orthostatic intolerance, defined as the following symptoms while standing: disabling fatigue, dizziness, diminished concentration, tremulousness, sweating, lightheadedness, visual disturbances, palpitations, and nausea (Miwa, 2014).

The above variability in symptom reporting is related in part to the methods and comprehensiveness of the ascertainment for orthostatic intolerance, but also to temporal changes. While some older studies refer to autonomic and circulatory abnormalities in those with neuromyasthenia (MacLean et al., 1944), papers drawing attention to orthostatic intolerance in ME/CFS did not appear until 1995 (Bou-Holaigah et al., 1995; Rowe et al., 1995), the year after the Fukuda definition was published. As an example of the temporal changes in reporting, in a summary of clinical experience, Komaroff and Buchwald (1991) estimated that dizziness was present in 30-50 percent of patients. In a study published a decade later, Jason and colleagues (2002b) reported dizziness *after standing* in 47 percent of adults with ME/CFS, 21 percent of those with depression, and 9 percent of nonfatigued participants. And Nacul and colleagues (2011b) reported a prevalence of "intolerance to be on your feet" of 61 percent among 265 ME/CFS subjects in England.

A second source of variability in prevalence reports is the way in which orthostatic intolerance *symptoms* are classified. In the non-ME/CFS literature on orthostatic intolerance, symptoms of cerebral underperfusion (e.g., cognitive symptoms such as difficulty concentrating) were attributed to the circulatory dysfunction (Low et al., 2009). In the ME/CFS literature, those problems often are reported as independent symptoms. While orthostatic stress was reported to cause worse fatigue and cognitive function in those with ME/CFS as compared with those without ME/CFS (Stewart et al., 2012; Streeten and Anderson, 1992), it is impossible to determine which component of the overall ME/CFS symptom complex is due to the circulatory disorder or to some other aspect of ME/CFS physiology. Few studies specified the postures in which people reported triggering of their ME/CFS symptoms, and few distinguished orthostatic headaches or orthostatic cognitive difficulties from general causes of these symptoms. The dilemma is illustrated by the prevalence of symptoms documented by Nacul and colleagues (2011b): 61 percent of British adult ME/CFS patients reported intolerance of being on their feet, but 94 percent also reported memory or concentration problems, 82 percent difficulty thinking, 72 percent intolerance to exercise, 66 percent sweatiness/cold hands and feet, and 65 percent headaches. How many of these other symptoms were related to orthostatic stress is impossible to discern from the paper.

The Fukuda definition of CFS includes no mention of disorders in the regulation of heart rate and blood pressure in the differential diagnosis or management of ME/CFS symptoms (Fukuda et al., 1994). In the 2003 CCC, the diagnosis of ME/CFS can be made if—in addition to an illness of at least 6 months' duration characterized by fatigue, PEM, sleep dysfunction, pain, and neurologic or cognitive manifestations—the individual also has one symptom from two of three of the following categories: autonomic manifestations, neuroendocrine manifestations, and immune manifestations. These categories are not mutually exclusive, but autonomic manifestations include the following: orthostatic intolerance, NMH, POTS, delayed postural hypotension, lightheadedness, extreme pallor, nausea and irritable bowel syndrome, urinary frequency and bladder dysfunction, palpitations with or without cardiac arrhythmias, and exertional dyspnea (Carruthers et al., 2003). In contrast, the NICE guidelines devote very little attention to circulatory dysfunction either in the differential diagnosis of fatigue as a symptom of ME/CFS or as a comorbid condition. The NICE guidelines recommend against performing a tilt table test routinely to aid in making a diagnosis of ME/CFS, but they do not comment on the potential utility of head-up tilt or standing tests for diagnosing comorbid orthostatic intolerance (NICE, 2007). The 2011 ME-ICC criteria list orthostatic intolerance as one of several qualifying abnormalities under the rubric of energy production/transportation impairments (Carruthers et al., 2011).

Assessment of Orthostatic Intolerance and Autonomic Dysfunction in ME/CFS

Clinical History

When querying for orthostatic intolerance, clinicians should pose questions about the frequency and severity of lightheadedness, near-fainting (presyncope), syncope, sweating, palpitations, chest pain, orthostatic dyspnea, and related symptoms when individuals are sitting or standing for prolonged periods of time. Chronic fatigue, difficulty concentrating, exercise intolerance, nausea, and tremulousness are common across a variety of forms of orthostatic intolerance. Not all individuals report lightheadedness; some simply report feeling unwell when upright and they avoid these situations. Questions with a high yield include asking how individuals feel in the following circumstances: while waiting in line, at receptions, in choir, while shopping or at the mall, while sitting still for long periods, and when exposed to warm/stressful circumstances (e.g., summer weather; after hot showers, baths, and saunas; after episodes of fear, pain, or exposure to blood) (Grubb, 2005; Raj, 2013; Thieben et al., 2007).

Formal Questionnaires

Several questionnaires are validated for use in adults with autonomic dysfunction or orthostatic intolerance syndromes, but they have not been evaluated specifically among those with ME/CFS. They include the Orthostatic Grading Scale (OGS) (Schrezenmaier et al., 2005); the Orthostatic Hypotension Questionnaire (OHQ) (Kaufmann et al., 2012); and a series of questionnaires developed at the Mayo Clinic, beginning with the 169-item Autonomic Symptom Profile (ASP) (Suarez et al., 1999), followed by the 84-question COMPASS. The COMPASS has been further abbreviated to a 31-item questionnaire (COMPASS 31) (Sletten et al., 2012).

Objective Measures

Orthostatic vital signs—measured by taking heart rate and blood pressure in supine, sitting, and standing positions—often are measured within 2 minutes or less, and thus are insufficient to identify most forms of chronic orthostatic intolerance. Prolonged testing of at least 10 minutes usually is needed for a sufficient orthostatic challenge. Two forms of prolonged orthostatic testing (standing test and upright tilt test) are commonly employed (see Box 4-2). The recommended duration of upright posture for detecting POTS is 10 minutes (Raj, 2013). Although neurally mediated hypotension can occur within the first 10 minutes of upright posture, an orthostatic

---

BOX 4-2
Prolonged Orthostatic Testing

Standing Test (Rowe et al., 1999)

This test can be performed in any clinic. The individual lies supine for 5 minutes to yield a steady baseline, then stands quietly, leaning against a wall, for 10 minutes. The individual is instructed to avoid moving, shifting his or her weight, or engaging in leg and other muscle contraction maneuvers. Symptoms such as fatigue, lightheadedness, nausea, warmth, shortness of breath, headache, pain, and impaired concentration/mental fogginess are recorded on a 0-10 scale while the individual is supine and every 1-2 minutes while he/she is standing. Individuals also are encouraged to report changes in symptoms as they occur. Heart rate and blood pressure recordings are made every 1-2 minutes. The test must be observed because of the potential for syncope and injury. The standing test, while helpful in some cases, is not a substitute for prolonged head-up tilt testing, and has limited ability to identify those with neurally mediated hypotension, most of whom develop hypotension beyond the 10-minute duration of a typical standing test.

Upright Tilt Tests (Bou-Holaigah et al., 1995)

The head-up tilt table test requires specialized equipment. The individual lies supine on the tilt table for 5-15 minutes. The table is then brought upright, usually to 70 degrees, for 10 to 60 minutes (usually 45 minutes if the goal is to evaluate for neurally mediated hypotension). Patient movement is discouraged. Heart rate is monitored continuously, and blood pressure is measured either continuously, using beat-to-beat measurements, or every 1-2 minutes for the first 10 minutes upright and every 5 minutes thereafter. Symptom reports usually are elicited every 2 minutes for the first 10 minutes upright and every 5 minutes thereafter, and recorded whenever major changes are reported by the individual. Passive tilt testing provokes a larger heart rate change in those with postural orthostatic tachycardia syndrome (POTS) than does active standing beyond 5 minutes of upright posture (Plash et al., 2013). During prolonged head-up tilt, a variety of pharmacological agents, including isoproterenol and nitroglycerine, are employed to provoke syncope. However, these challenges can lead to abnormal tests in some healthy individuals, so they must be interpreted with caution, as is described elsewhere (Moya et al., 2009). Moreover, head-up tilt testing is no longer thought to be necessary to diagnose all forms of neurally mediated syncope (Moya et al., 2009).

---

stress of more than 10 minutes of upright posture more commonly is required (Benditt et al., 1991). The median time to develop hypotension among adults with ME/CFS is 30 minutes in some studies (Bou-Holaigah et al., 1995). Among those with ME/CFS, orthostatic symptoms during tilt testing emerge within minutes, long before hemodynamic changes are documented (Razumovsky et al., 2003).

Some investigators prefer to simulate orthostatic stress using lower-body negative pressure (LBNP), but these methods are used mainly in research settings (Wyller et al., 2008). Other methods used to capture physiological changes during upright tilt include transcranial Doppler ultrasound to measure cerebral blood flow velocity, capnography to measure expired CO_2, and near infrared spectroscopy to measure changes in cerebral tissue oxygenation (Naschitz et al., 2000; Ocon et al., 2012; Tanaka et al., 2002).

Clinicians who evaluate those with orthostatic intolerance recognize that individuals with ME/CFS can develop an exacerbation of their typical symptoms not just during the head-up tilt test but for several days afterward. The committee's literature search did not identify any publications describing this observation more formally, although administration of 1 liter of normal saline following the tilt test to reverse the post-tilt test exacerbation in symptoms is part of the tilt testing protocol in some centers (Rowe et al., 2001). Intravenous saline has been shown to improve orthostatic tolerance and to modify autonomic tone in those with neurally mediated syncope (Burklow et al., 1999) and after experimental prolonged bed rest (Takenaka et al., 2002).

Evidence for Orthostatic Intolerance and Autonomic Abnormalities in ME/CFS

This section examines the evidence for orthostatic intolerance and autonomic abnormalities in adults with ME/CFS. The methodology used for the committee's literature review is described in Chapter 1. A full search for all forms of autonomic dysfunction (e.g., bladder dysfunction, gastrointestinal motility disorders) was not conducted. Instead, the committee elected to focus on circulatory abnormalities, as these are the most frequently reported autonomic abnormalities in ME/CFS. The most common forms of orthostatic intolerance are described in Box 4-3. Several studies reviewed were conducted by the same group of investigators. When it was not possible to ascertain from the description of the study methods whether the data were for independent study populations or some of the same patients on more than one occasion, the committee chose to select the most representative (or largest) of the studies for each group.

The studies reviewed vary widely on several methodological variables, notably in the following categories:

- patient characteristics (age, duration of ME/CFS, severity of ME/CFS, the ME/CFS case definition used, whether subjects were selected based on autonomic symptoms, referral biases, whether the testing was performed on patients seeking clinical care or those participating in a research study);

- preparation for the test (medications allowed, prior sodium intake, duration of pretest fast);
- the type of orthostatic testing (active standing, standing while leaning against a wall, head-up tilt table) and, with tilt testing, the protocol used (e.g., angle of the tilt table, time of day for the study, ambient room temperature, degree of movement permitted);
- duration of the orthostatic stress; and
- criteria for abnormal response to orthostatic stress (earlier studies tended to report only rates of NMH, without reporting rates of

---

BOX 4-3
Common Orthostatic Intolerance Syndromes

Postural orthostatic tachycardia syndrome (POTS)

POTS is defined by a heart rate increase between the supine position and 10 minutes of standing of more than 30 beats per minute (bpm) for adults or 40 bpm for adolescents, or a heart rate that reaches 120 bpm or higher over the first 10 minutes of upright posture in the absence of orthostatic hypotension. A diagnosis of POTS requires that the change in heart rate also be accompanied by characteristic orthostatic symptoms that include lightheadedness, blurred vision, headaches, difficulty concentrating, diaphoresis, nausea, palpitations, chest pain, and shortness of breath (Freeman et al., 2011).

Neurally mediated hypotension (NMH)

NMH refers to a reflex drop in blood pressure that occurs during upright posture, and is defined as a drop in systolic blood pressure of 25 mm Hg (compared with supine blood pressure) during standing or upright tilt table testing. It usually is preceded by orthostatic symptoms of lightheadedness, nausea, pallor, and warmth and accompanied at the time of hypotension by a slowing of the heart rate (Bou-Holaigah et al., 1995). NMH sometimes is termed "neurocardiogenic syncope," "vasodepressor syncope," or "vaso-vagal syncope" (Bou-Holaigah et al., 1995).

Orthostatic hypotension (OH)

OH involves an immediate and sustained drop of at least 20 mm Hg in systolic or 10 mm Hg in diastolic blood pressure in the first 3 minutes of standing or upright tilt (Freeman et al., 2011). This is uncommon in ME/CFS, but a delayed form of OH has been recognized in ME/CFS patients, in which blood pressure changes occur after 3 minutes upright (Moya et al., 2009; Streeten and Anderson, 1992).

POTS, and studies employing less than 10 minutes of orthostatic stress reported rates of POTS, as these tests were not sufficiently prolonged to be able to exclude NMH).

These methodological factors contributed to the variability in rates of orthostatic intolerance reported in the various studies.

Orthostatic Testing

Prolonged orthostatic testing (> 10 minutes) The literature search identified 14 studies of prolonged orthostatic testing in which adults with ME/CFS were compared with healthy controls (Bou-Holaigah et al., 1995; De Lorenzo et al., 1997; Duprez et al., 1998; Hollingsworth et al., 2010; Jones et al., 2005; LaManca et al., 1999a; Naschitz et al., 2000, 2002; Poole et al., 2000; Razumovsky et al., 2003; Schondorf et al., 1999; Streeten et al., 2000; Timmers et al., 2002; Yataco et al., 1997), as well as three studies of subjects with ME/CFS without controls (Freeman and Komaroff, 1997; Reynolds et al., 2013; Rowe et al., 2001). None of the studies with controls and only one of the three studies without controls (Freeman and Komaroff, 1997) recruited participants based on the presence of autonomic symptoms.

Of the 14 studies with healthy controls in which orthostatic testing lasted longer than 10 minutes, only 2 did not report a higher prevalence of either POTS or NMH among those with ME/CFS compared with controls (Duprez et al., 1998; Jones et al., 2005). The rates of reported abnormalities ranged from 0 percent (Duprez et al., 1998) to 96 percent (Bou-Holaigah et al., 1995). The median proportion with hemodynamic abnormalities during the first 30-45 minutes upright in these studies was 37 percent in ME/CFS versus 7.5 percent in controls. In the three additional studies without controls, the reported rates of orthostatic intolerance ranged from 11 to 66 percent of adults with ME/CFS. This number needs to be interpreted with caution given the varying durations of orthostatic stress (ranging from 20 to 60 minutes) and other methodological differences in testing.

Brief orthostatic testing (< 10 minutes) The literature search identified seven studies with brief durations of orthostatic stress (2-10 minutes) (De Becker et al., 1998; Freeman and Komaroff, 1997; Hoad et al., 2008; Miwa, 2014; Natelson et al., 2007; Soetekouw et al., 1999; Winkler et al., 2004). The samples sizes ranged from 20 to 62 subjects with ME/CFS (median N = 37). Two studies used head-up tilt testing and five active standing as the orthostatic stressor. The prevalence of orthostatic intolerance was not documented in two studies in which the main focus was formal autonomic testing (De Becker et al., 1998; Soetekouw et al., 1999). In all of the remaining studies, the prevalence of POTS was numerically higher in adults with ME/CFS than in controls (Freeman and Komaroff, 1997; Hoad et al., 2008; Miwa, 2014; Natelson et al., 2007; Winkler et al., 2004). Combining the data from these studies, the overall prevalence of POTS was 27 percent in adults with ME/CFS and 4.2 percent in healthy controls. The range of *overall* orthostatic abnormalities (including POTS, hypotension, and hypocapnia) in these studies with brief orthostatic testing varied widely—from 14 to 67 percent—in individual studies, reflecting differences in study measures, subject selection, and duration of orthostatic stress.

Symptoms reported during orthostatic testing The literature review identified five studies reporting orthostatic or ME/CFS symptoms following standing or tilt table testing. Upright posture was associated with provocation of fatigue symptoms and higher rates of lightheadedness, nausea, and warmth in 55-100 percent of subjects with ME/CFS (Bou-Holaigah et al., 1995; Hollingsworth et al., 2010; Naschitz et al., 2000; Streeten et al., 2000). For example, during the first 45 minutes of head-up tilt, 100 percent of 23 ME/CFS participants reported worse fatigue, 91 percent lightheadedness, 91 percent increased warmth, 73 percent nausea, and 18 percent diaphoresis. Controls made no reports of similar symptoms (Bou-Holaigah et al., 1995). One small study found a normalization of heart rate and blood pressure changes and improvement in ME/CFS symptoms after the acute application of a 45-mm Hg external compression device while subjects continued to stand (Streeten et al., 2000). In a study of 64 British adults with ME/CFS, 6 participants were unable to tolerate head-up tilt because of weakness. Of the remaining 58 with ME/CFS, 32 (55 percent) were symptomatic during the test, compared with 17/64 (27 percent) healthy controls. The types of symptoms were not specified (Hollingsworth et al., 2010). Research also has shown that the severity of orthostatic symptoms may predict the functional status of those with ME/CFS (Costigan et al., 2010).

Treatment of orthostatic intolerance Open (nonblinded) treatment studies of ME/CFS subjects found improvement in function after increased sodium intake or pharmacological treatment of orthostatic intolerance (Bou-Holaigah et al., 1995; De Lorenzo et al., 1997; Kawamura et al., 2003; Naschitz et al., 2004). However, randomized trials of fludrocortisone failed to confirm the efficacy of this treatment in adults as monotherapy or combined with hydrocortisone (Blockmans et al., 2003; Peterson et al., 1998; Rowe et al., 2001).

Autonomic Testing

More formal autonomic testing—using such measures as the cold pressor test, heart rate responses to deep breathing, handgrip tests, the Valsalva maneuver, and quantitative sudomotor axon reflex tests—has not been conducted as extensively as have tests of the heart rate and blood pressure response to orthostatic stress. The majority of studies reporting the Valsalva ratio found no differences between ME/CFS and control groups (De Becker et al., 1998; Schondorf et al., 1999; Soetekouw et al., 1999; Winkler et al., 2004). Measures of heart rate variability have been used to examine the effects of autonomic tone on the heart noninvasively. ME/CFS is associated with enhanced sympathetic nervous system tone and reduced parasympathetic tone at baseline (Freeman and Komaroff, 1997; Frith et al., 2012; Sisto et al., 1995), in response to cognitive and orthostatic challenges (Beaumont et al., 2012; Yamamoto et al., 2003; Yataco et al., 1997), after walking (Cordero et al., 1996), and during sleep (Boneva et al., 2007; Rahman et al., 2011; Togo and Natelson, 2013; Yamaguti et al., 2013).

Ambulatory blood pressure measurements in subjects with ME/CFS have had conflicting results. One study found significantly lower systolic, diastolic, and mean arterial pressure in ME/CFS patients compared with controls, and a second found nighttime hypotension in ME/CFS patients (Newton et al., 2009; Van de Luit et al., 1998). Duprez and colleagues (1998), however, found no differences in daytime or nighttime blood pressure in ME/CFS patients. Of interest, although blood pressure did not differ in that study, there were significant differences in heart rate between ME/CFS cases and healthy controls throughout the 24-hour period.

Blood Volume and Cardiac Function Testing

Studies measuring blood volume have found lower values in ME/CFS subjects than in controls. Hurwitz and colleagues (2010) found a total blood volume deficit of 15.1 percent in ME/CFS patients compared with controls. Streeten and Bell (1998) identified low red blood cell mass in 16 of 19 patients with ME/CFS and an overall total lower blood volume in 63 percent of ME/CFS patients. Okamoto and colleagues (2012b) identified a 10.4 percent lower total blood volume in subjects with ME/CFS and POTS compared with controls studied at the same center.

Hurwitz and colleagues (2010) confirmed a lower cardiac index in ME/CFS patients (due to a 10.2 percent lower stroke index compared with sedentary and nonsedentary controls) and a cardiac contractility deficit of 25.1 percent. In a series of studies possibly involving some of the same patients, a high prevalence of orthostatic intolerance, associated with smaller heart on cardiothoracic ratios, was found in ME/CFS patients (Miwa, 2014; Miwa and Fujita, 2008, 2009, 2011). Hollingsworth and colleagues (2010) found a greater left ventricular work index with standing in ME/CFS patients compared with controls, suggesting that when the patients were standing, their hearts were working harder. These findings were associated with the presentation of symptoms with standing in 95 percent of ME/CFS patients.

Orthostatic Hypocapnia

Three studies examined orthostatic hypocapnia in subjects with CFS. Naschitz and colleagues (2000) found that end-tidal CO_2 was similar for ME/CFS patients and controls when supine, consistent with the absence of hyperventilation at baseline, but end-tidal CO_2 was lower for the ME/CFS subjects during upright tilt testing. These results were confirmed by Razumovsky and colleagues (2003) during prolonged head-up tilt testing and by Natelson and colleagues (2007) during 8 minutes of active standing.

Microcirculatory Flow

Three studies examined abnormalities in peripheral blood flow in ME/CFS patients using different physiologic or pharmacologic challenges. ME/CFS patients had abnormally prolonged vasodilation in response to transdermally applied acetylcholine (Khan et al., 2003), reduced oxygen delivery to muscles after exercise and after cuff ischemia (McCully and Natelson, 1999), and a strikingly increased venous contractile sensitivity to infused epinephrine (Streeten, 2001). These studies have yet to be replicated.

Overlap of ME/CFS with Other Conditions Associated with Orthostatic Intolerance

A small number of studies have examined the prevalence of ME/CFS symptoms in those diagnosed with POTS (Okamoto et al., 2012b) or vasovagal syncope (Kenny and Graham, 2001; Legge et al., 2008). Okamoto and colleagues (2012b) examined the prevalence of the ME/CFS symptoms of the Fukuda definition among those with POTS who did not satisfy the criteria for ME/CFS, comparing this group with those who had POTS together with ME/CFS. Those with POTS alone often reported an elevated prevalence of severe fatigue, unrefreshing sleep, impaired memory or concentration, muscle pain, and post-exertional fatigue, although they did not have a sufficient number of symptoms to satisfy the Fukuda definition. By definition, the prevalence of Fukuda symptoms was higher in ME/CFS subjects who also had POTS than in those with POTS alone, but the pattern of symptoms was similar between the two groups (Okamoto et al., 2012b).

A high prevalence of hypotension and tachycardia is seen in FM, which, as noted earlier, is a clinical condition often comorbid with ME/CFS. Sympathetic predominance of heart rate variability also is seen in FM studies (Martinez-Lavin, 2007; Martinez-Martinez et al., 2014).

The prevalence of Ehlers-Danlos syndrome and joint hypermobility is higher in ME/CFS patients than in healthy controls (Barron et al., 2002; Rowe et al., 1999). Studies also confirm high rates of fatigue as well as orthostatic and autonomic symptoms in those with hypermobility (Gazit et al., 2003) and the hypermobile form of Ehlers-Danlos syndrome (De Wandele et al., 2014a,b).

Summary

There is consistent evidence that upright posture is associated with a worsening of ME/CFS symptoms, as well as the onset of other symptoms such as lightheadedness, nausea, and palpitations. While there is variability in the reported prevalence of orthostatic intolerance in ME/CFS, heart rate and blood pressure abnormalities during standing or head-up tilt testing are more common in those with ME/CFS than in those without ME/CFS. Heart rate variability analyses demonstrate a sympathetic predominance of autonomic tone in those with ME/CFS, including during sleep.

Conclusion: Sufficient evidence indicates a high prevalence of orthostatic intolerance in ME/CFS, as measured by objective heart rate and blood pressure abnormalities during standing or head-up tilt testing or by patient-reported exacerbation of orthostatic symptoms with standing in day-to-day life. These findings indicate that orthostatic intolerance is a common and clinically important finding in ME/CFS.

REFERENCES

Armitage, R. 1999. The effects of nefazodone on sleep in depressed patients and healthy controls. *International Journal of Psychiatry in Clinical Practice* 3(2):73-79.

Armitage, R., C. Landis, R. Hoffmann, M. Lentz, N. F. Watson, J. Goldberg, and D. Buchwald. 2007. The impact of a 4-hour sleep delay on slow wave activity in twins discordant for chronic fatigue syndrome. *Sleep* 30(5):657-662.

Armitage, R., C. Landis, R. Hoffmann, M. Lentz, N. Watson, J. Goldberg, and D. Buchwald. 2009. Power spectral analysis of sleep EEG in twins discordant for chronic fatigue syndrome. *Journal of Psychosomatic Research* 66(1):51-57.

Arroll, M. A., E. A. Attree, J. M. O'Leary, and C. P. Dancey. 2014. The delayed fatigue effect in myalgic encephalomyelitis/chronic fatigue syndrome (ME/CFS). *Fatigue: Biomedicine, Health & Behavior* 2(2):57-63.

Attree, E. A., C. P. Dancey, and A. L. Pope. 2009. An assessment of prospective memory retrieval in women with chronic fatigue syndrome using a virtual-reality environment: An initial study. *Cyberpsychology and Behavior* 12(4):379-385.

Attree, E. A., M. A. Arroll, C. P. Dancey, C. Griffith, and A. S. Bansal. 2014. Psychosocial factors involved in memory and cognitive failures in people with myalgic encephalomyelitis/chronic fatigue syndrome. *Psychology Research and Behavior Management* 7:67-76.

Bailes, S., E. Libman, M. Baltzan, R. Amsel, R. Schondorf, and C. S. Fichten. 2006. Brief and distinct empirical sleepiness and fatigue scales. *Journal of Psychosomatic Research* 60(6):605-613.

Balady, G. J., R. Arena, K. Sietsema, J. Myers, L. Coke, G. F. Fletcher, D. Forman, B. Franklin, M. Guazzi, M. Gulati, S. J. Keteyian, C. J. Lavie, R. Macko, D. Mancini, and R. V. Milani. 2010. Clinician's guide to cardiopulmonary exercise testing in adults: A scientific statement from the American Heart Association. *Circulation* 122(2):191-225.

Ball, N., D. S. Buchwald, D. Schmidt, J. Goldberg, S. Ashton, and R. Armitage. 2004. Monozygotic twins discordant for chronic fatigue syndrome: Objective measures of sleep. *Journal of Psychosomatic Research* 56(2):207-212.

Baraniuk, J. N., O. Adewuyi, S. J. Merck, M. Ali, M. K. Ravindran, C. R. Timbol, R. Ray-Han, Y. Zheng, U. Le, R. Esteitie, and K. N. Petrie. 2013. A chronic fatigue syndrome (CFS) severity score based on case designation criteria. *American Journal of Translational Research* 5(1):53-68.

Barnden, L. R., B. Crouch, R. Kwiatek, R. Burnet, A. Mernone, S. Chryssidis, G. Scroop, and P. del Fante. 2011. A brain MRI study of chronic fatigue syndrome: Evidence of brainstem dysfunction and altered homeostasis. *NMR in Biomedicine* 24(10):1302-1312.

Barron, D. F., B. A. Cohen, M. T. Geraghty, R. Violand, and P. C. Rowe. 2002. Joint hypermobility is more common in children with chronic fatigue syndrome than in healthy controls. *Journal of Pediatrics* 141(3):421-425.

Bazelmans, E., G. Bleijenberg, M. J. M. Voeten, J. W. M. van der Meer, and H. Folgering. 2005. Impact of a maximal exercise test on symptoms and activity in chronic fatigue syndrome. *Journal of Psychosomatic Research* 59(4):201-208.

Beaumont, A., A. R. Burton, J. Lemon, B. K. Bennett, A. Lloyd, and U. Vollmer-Conna. 2012. Reduced cardiac vagal modulation impacts on cognitive performance in chronic fatigue syndrome. *PLoS ONE* 7(11):e49518.

Benarroch, E. E. 2012. Postural tachycardia syndrome: A heterogeneous and multifactorial disorder. *Mayo Clinic Proceedings* 87(12):1214-1225.

Benditt, D. G., S. Remole, S. Bailin, A. N. N. Dunnigan, A. Asso, and S. Milstein. 1991. Tilt table testing for evaluation of neurally-mediated (cardioneurogenic) syncope: Rationale and proposed protocols. *PACE Pacing and Clinical Electrophysiology* 14(10):1528-1537.

Black, C. D., and K. K. McCully. 2005. Time course of exercise induced alterations in daily activity in chronic fatigue syndrome. *Dynamic Medicine* 4(10).

Black, C. D., P. J. O'Connor, and K. K. McCully. 2005. Increased daily physical activity and fatigue symptoms in chronic fatigue syndrome. *Dynamic Medicine* 4(3).

Blackman, A., C. McGregor, R. Dales, H. S. Driver, I. Dumov, J. Fleming, K. Fraser, C. George, A. Khullar, J. Mink, M. Moffat, G. E. Sullivan, J. A. Fleetham, N. Ayas, T. D. Bradley, M. Fitzpatrick, J. Kimoff, D. Morrison, F. Ryan, R. Skomro, F. Series, and W. Tsai. 2010. Canadian Sleep Society/Canadian Thoracic Society position paper on the use of portable monitoring for the diagnosis of obstructive sleep apnea/hypopnea in adults. *Canadian Respiratory Journal* 17(5):229-232.

Blackwood, S. K., S. M. MacHale, M. J. Power, G. M. Goodwin, and S. M. Lawrie. 1998. Effects of exercise on cognitive and motor function in chronic fatigue syndrome and depression. *Journal of Neurology Neurosurgery and Psychiatry* 65(4):541-546.

Blockmans, D., P. Persoons, B. Van Houdenhove, M. Lejeune, and H. Bobbaers. 2003. Combination therapy with hydrocortisone and fludrocortisone does not improve symptoms in chronic fatigue syndrome: A randomized, placebo-controlled, double-blind, crossover study. *American Journal of Medicine* 114(9):736-741.

Boneva, R. S., M. J. Decker, E. M. Maloney, J. M. Lin, J. F. Jones, H. G. Helgason, C. M. Heim, D. B. Rye, and W. C. Reeves. 2007. Higher heart rate and reduced heart rate variability persist during sleep in chronic fatigue syndrome: A population-based study. *Autonomic Neuroscience: Basic and Clinical* 137(1-2):94-101.

Bou-Holaigah, I., P. C. Rowe, J. Kan, and H. Calkins. 1995. The relationship between neurally mediated hypotension and the chronic fatigue syndrome. *Journal of the American Medical Association* 274(12):961-967.

Brown, A. A., L. A. Jason, M. A. Evans, and S. Flores. 2013. Contrasting case definitions: The ME international consensus criteria vs. the Fukuda et al. CFS criteria. *North American Journal of Psychology* 15(1):103-120.

Brown, M. M., and L. A. Jason. 2007. Functioning in individuals with chronic fatigue syndrome: Increased impairment with co-occurring multiple chemical sensitivity and fibromyalgia. *Dynamic Medicine* 6(6).

Bruce, R. A., F. Kusumi, and D. Hosmer. 1973. Maximal oxygen intake and nomographic assessment of functional aerobic impairment in cardiovascular disease. *American Heart Journal* 85(4):546-562.

Buchwald, D., T. Pearlman, J. Umali, K. Schmaling, and W. Katon. 1996. Functional status in patients with chronic fatigue syndrome, other fatiguing illnesses, and healthy individuals. *American Journal of Medicine* 101(4):364-370.

Burklow, T. R., J. P. Moak, J. J. Bailey, and F. T. Makhlouf. 1999. Neurally mediated cardiac syncope: Autonomic modulation after normal saline infusion. *Journal of the American College of Cardiology* 33(7):2059-2066.

Bush, V. E., V. L. Wight, C. M. Brown, and R. Hainsworth. 2000. Vascular responses to orthostatic stress in patients with Postural Orthostatic Tachycardia Syndrome (POTS), in patients with low orthostatic tolerance, and in asymptomatic controls. *Clinical Autonomic Research* 10(5):279-284.

Busichio, K., L. A. Tiersky, J. DeLuca, and B. H. Natelson. 2004. Neuropsychological deficits in patients with chronic fatigue syndrome. *Journal of the International Neuropsychological Society* 10(2):278-285.

Buysse, D. J., C. F. Reynolds III, T. H. Monk, S. R. Berman, and D. J. Kupfer. 1989. The Pittsburgh Sleep Quality Index: A new instrument for psychiatric practice and research. *Psychiatry Research* 28(2):193-213.

Calkins, H., M. Seifert, and F. Morady. 1995. Clinical presentation and long-term follow-up of athletes with exercise-induced vasodepressor syncope. *American Heart Journal* 129(6):1159-1164.

Capuron, L., L. Welberg, C. Heim, D. Wagner, L. Solomon, D. A. Papanicolaou, R. C. Craddock, A. H. Miller, and W. C. Reeves. 2006. Cognitive dysfunction relates to subjective report of mental fatigue in patients with chronic fatigue syndrome. *Neuropsychopharmacology* 31(8):1777-1784.

Carruthers, B. M., A. K. Jain, K. L. De Meirleir, D. L. Peterson, N. G. Klimas, A. M. Lemer, A. C. Bested, P. Flor-Henry, P. Joshi, A. C. P. Powles, J. A. Sherkey, and M. I. van de Sande. 2003. Myalgic encephalomyelitis/chronic fatigue syndrome: Clinical working case definition, diagnostic and treatment protocols (Canadian case definition). *Journal of Chronic Fatigue Syndrome* 11(1):7-115.

Carruthers, B. M., M. I. van de Sande, K. L. De Meirleir, N. G. Klimas, G. Broderick, T. Mitchell, D. Staines, A. C. P. Powles, N. Speight, R. Vallings, L. Bateman, B. Baumgarten-Austrheim, D. S. Bell, N. Carlo-Stella, J. Chia, A. Darragh, D. Jo, D. Lewis, A. R. Light, S. Marshall-Gradisbik, I. Mena, J. A. Mikovits, K. Miwa, M. Murovska, M. L. Pall, and S. Stevens. 2011. Myalgic encephalomyelitis: International consensus criteria. *Journal of Internal Medicine* 270(4):327-338.

Caseras, X., D. Mataix-Cols, V. Giampietro, K. A. Rimes, M. Brammer, F. Zelaya, T. Chalder, and E. L. Godfrey. 2006. Probing the working memory system in chronic fatigue syndrome: A functional magnetic resonance imaging study using the n-back task. *Psychosomatic Medicine* 68(6):947-955.

Caseras, X., D. Mataix-Cols, K. A. Rimes, V. Giampietro, M. Brammer, F. Zelaya, T. Chalder, and E. Godfrey. 2008. The neural correlates of fatigue: An exploratory imaginal fatigue provocation study in chronic fatigue syndrome. *Psychological Medicine* 38(7):941-951.

CDC (Centers for Disease Control and Prevention). 2005. *CDC symptom inventory.* http://www.institutferran.org/documentos/cdc_full_symptom_inventory.pdf (accessed January 12, 2015).

Chalder, T., G. Berelowitz, T. Pawlikowska, L. Watts, S. Wessely, D. Wright, and E. P. Wallace. 1993. Development of a fatigue scale. *Journal of Psychosomatic Research* 37(2):147-153.

Chu, L., M. Sunnquist, S. So, and L. A. Jason. 2013. *Patient survey results for FDA drug development meeting for ME and CFS,* April 25-26. http://www.iacfsme.org/LinkClick.aspx?fileticket=E8i8MVWh%2bX0%3d&tabid=119 (accessed August 19, 2014).

Ciccone, D. S., and B. H. Natelson. 2003. Comorbid illness in women with chronic fatigue syndrome: A test of the single syndrome hypothesis. *Psychosomatic Medicine* 65(2):268-275.

Claypoole, K., R. Mahurin, M. E. Fischer, J. Goldberg, K. B. Schmaling, R. B. Schoene, S. Ashton, and D. Buchwald. 2001. Cognitive compromise following exercise in monozygotic twins discordant for chronic fatigue syndrome: Fact or artifact? *Applied Neuropsychology* 8(1):31-40.

Claypoole, K. H., C. Noonan, R. K. Mahurin, J. Goldberg, T. Erickson, and D. Buchwald. 2007. A twin study of cognitive function in chronic fatigue syndrome: The effects of sudden illness onset. *Neuropsychology* 21(4):507-513.

Cockshell, S. J., and J. L. Mathias. 2010. Cognitive functioning in chronic fatigue syndrome: A meta-analysis. *Psychological Medicine* 40(8):1253-1267.

Cockshell, S. J., and J. L. Mathias. 2012. Test effort in persons with chronic fatigue syndrome when assessed using the validity indicator profile. *Journal of Clinical and Experimental Neuropsychology* 34(7):679-687.

Cockshell, S. J., and J. L. Mathias. 2013. Cognitive deficits in chronic fatigue syndrome and their relationship to psychological status, symptomatology, and everyday functioning. *Neuropsychology* 27(2):230-242.

Cockshell, S. J., and J. L. Mathias. 2014. Cognitive functioning in people with chronic fatigue syndrome: A comparison between subjective and objective measures. *Neuropsychology* 28(3):394-405.

Constant, E. L., S. Adam, B. Gillain, M. Lambert, E. Masquelier, and X. Seron. 2011. Cognitive deficits in patients with chronic fatigue syndrome compared to those with major depressive disorder and healthy controls. *Clinical Neurology & Neurosurgery* 113(4):295-302.

Cook, D. B., P. R. Nagelkirk, A. Peckerman, A. Poluri, J. Mores, and B. H. Natelson. 2005. Exercise and cognitive performance in chronic fatigue syndrome. *Medicine & Science in Sports & Exercise* 37(9):1460-1467.

Cook, D. B., P. J. O'Connor, G. Lange, and J. Steffener. 2007. Functional neuroimaging correlates of mental fatigue induced by cognition among chronic fatigue syndrome patients and controls. *Neuroimage* 36(1):108-122.

Cook, D. B., A. J. Stegner, P. R. Nagelkirk, J. D. Meyer, F. Togo, and B. H. Natelson. 2012. Responses to exercise differ for chronic fatigue syndrome patients with fibromyalgia. *Medicine and Science in Sports and Exercise* 44(6):1186-1193.

Cordero, D. L., S. A. Sisto, W. N. Tapp, J. J. LaManca, J. G. Pareja, and B. H. Natelson. 1996. Decreased vagal power during treadmill walking in patients with chronic fatigue syndrome. *Clinical Autonomic Research* 6(6):329-333.

Corral-Penafiel, J., J. L. Pepin, and F. Barbe. 2013. Ambulatory monitoring in the diagnosis and management of obstructive sleep apnoea syndrome. *European Respiratory Review* 22(129):312-324.

Costigan, A., C. Elliott, C. McDonald, and J. L. Newton. 2010. Orthostatic symptoms predict functional capacity in chronic fatigue syndrome: Implications for management. *QJM: Monthly Journal of the Association of Physicians* 103(8):589-595.

Cowan, D. C., G. Allardice, D. Macfarlane, D. Ramsay, H. Ambler, S. Banham, E. Livingston, and C. Carlin. 2014. Predicting sleep disordered breathing in outpatients with suspected OSA. *BMJ Open* 4(4):e004519.

Creti, L., E. Libman, M. Baltzan, D. Rizzo, S. Bailes, and C. S. Fichten. 2010. Impaired sleep in chronic fatigue syndrome: How is it best measured? *Journal of Health Psychology* 15(4):596-607.

Davenport, T. E., S. R. Stevens, K. Baroni, J. M. Van Ness, and C. R. Snell. 2011a. Reliability and validity of Short Form 36 version 2 to measure health perceptions in a sub-group of individuals with fatigue. *Disability & Rehabilitation* 33(25-26):2596-2604.

Davenport, T. E., S. R. Stevens, K. Baroni, M. Van Ness, and C. R. Snell. 2011b. Diagnostic accuracy of symptoms characterising chronic fatigue syndrome. *Disability & Rehabilitation* 33(19-20):1768-1775.

Davey, N. J., B. K. Puri, A. V. Nowicky, J. Main, and R. Zaman. 2001. Voluntary motor function in patients with chronic fatigue syndrome. *Journal of Psychosomatic Research* 50(1):17-20.

Davis, J. M., and K. H. Claypoole. 1997. Neuropsychological functioning in a pre-screened sample of chronic fatigue syndrome patients. *Archives of Clinical Neuropsychology* 12(4):306.

De Becker, P., P. Dendale, K. De Meirleir, I. Campine, K. Vandenborne, and Y. Hagers. 1998. Autonomic testing in patients with chronic fatigue syndrome. *American Journal of Medicine* 105(3A):22S-26S.

De Becker, P., J. Roeykens, M. Reynders, N. McGregor, and K. De Meirleir. 2000. Exercise capacity in chronic fatigue syndrome. *Archives of Internal Medicine* 160(21):3270-3277.

De Becker, P., N. McGregor, and K. De Meirleir. 2001. A definition-based analysis of symptoms in a large cohort of patients with chronic fatigue syndrome. *Journal of Internal Medicine* 250(3):234-240.

De Lange, F. P., J. S. Kalkman, G. Bleijenberg, P. Hagoort, J. W. M. van der Meer, and I. Toni. 2005. Gray matter volume reduction in the chronic fatigue syndrome. *Neuroimage* 26(3):777-781.

De Lange, F. P., A. Koers, J. S. Kalkman, G. Bleijenberg, P. Hagoort, J. W. M. van der Meer, and I. Toni. 2008. Increase in prefrontal cortical volume following cognitive behavioural therapy in patients with chronic fatigue syndrome. *Brain* 131(8):2172-2180.

De Lorenzo, F., J. Hargreaves, and V. V. Kakkar. 1997. Pathogenesis and management of delayed orthostatic hypotension in patients with chronic fatigue syndrome. *Clinical Autonomic Research* 7(4):185-190.

De Wandele, I., P. Calders, W. Peersman, S. Rimbaut, T. De Backer, F. Malfait, A. De Paepe, and L. Rombaut. 2014a. Autonomic symptom burden in the hypermobility type of Ehlers-Danlos syndrome: A comparative study with two other EDS types, fibromyalgia, and healthy controls. *Seminars in Arthritis and Rheumatism* 44(3):353-361.

De Wandele, I., L. Rombaut, L. Leybaert, P. Van de Borne, T. De Backer, F. Malfait, A. De Paepe, and P. Calders. 2014b. Dysautonomia and its underlying mechanisms in the hypermobility type of Ehlers-Danlos syndrome. *Seminars in Arthritis and Rheumatism* 44(1):93-100.

DeLuca, J., and J. H. Kalmar. 2008. *Information processing speed in clinical populations.* New York: Taylor & Francis.

DeLuca, J., S. K. Johnson, D. Beldowicz, and B. H. Natelson. 1995. Neuropsychological impairments in chronic fatigue syndrome, multiple sclerosis, and depression. *Journal of Neurology, Neurosurgery & Psychiatry* 58(1):38-43.

DeLuca, J., C. Christodoulou, B. J. Diamond, E. D. Rosenstein, N. Kramer, and B. H. Natelson. 2004a. Working memory deficits in chronic fatigue syndrome: Differentiating between speed and accuracy of information processing. *Journal of the International Neuropsychological Society* 10(1):101-109.

DeLuca, J., C. Christodoulou, B. J. Diamond, E. D. Rosenstein, N. Kramer, J. H. Ricker, and B. H. Natelson. 2004b. The nature of memory impairment in chronic fatigue syndrome. *Rehabilitation Psychology* 49(1):62-70.

Den Eede, F. V., G. Moorkens, W. Hulstijn, Y. Maas, D. Schrijvers, S. R. Stevens, P. Cosyns, S. J. Claes, and B. G. C. Sabbe. 2011. Psychomotor function and response inhibition in chronic fatigue syndrome. *Psychiatry Research* 186(2-3):367-372.

DePaul Research Team. 2010. *Depaul symptom questionnaire.* http://condor.depaul.edu/ljason/cfs/measures.html (accessed August 20, 2014).

Diamond, E. 2007. Developing a cardiopulmonary exercise testing laboratory. *Chest* 132(6): 2000-2007.

Dickson, A., A. Toft, and R. E. O'Carroll. 2009. Neuropsychological functioning, illness perception, mood and quality of life in chronic fatigue syndrome, autoimmune thyroid disease and healthy participants. *Psychological Medicine* 39(9):1567-1576.

Duffy, F. H., G. B. McAnulty, M. C. McCreary, G. J. Cuchural, and A. L. Komaroff. 2011. EEG spectral coherence data distinguish chronic fatigue syndrome patients from healthy controls and depressed patients: A case control study. *BMC Neurology* 11.

Duprez, D. A., M. L. De Buyzere, B. Drieghe, F. Vanhaverbeke, Y. Taes, W. Michielsen, and D. L. Clement. 1998. Long- and short-term blood pressure and RR-interval variability and psychosomatic distress in chronic fatigue syndrome. *Clinical Science* 94(1):57-63.

Edinger, J. D., W. K. Wohlgemuth, A. D. Krystal, and J. R. Rice. 2005. Behavioral insomnia therapy for fibromyalgia patients: A randomized clinical trial. *Archives of Internal Medicine* 165(21):2527-2535.

Farquhar, W. B., B. E. Hunt, J. A. Taylor, S. E. Darling, and R. Freeman. 2002. Blood volume and its relation to peak O(2) consumption and physical activity in patients with chronic fatigue. *American Journal of Physiology. Heart and Circulatory Physiology* 282(1):H66-H71.

FDA (Food and Drug Administration). 2013. *The voice of the patient: Chronic fatigue syndrome and myalgic encephalomyelitis.* Bethesda, MD: Center for Drug Evaluation and Research (CDER), FDA.

Fischler, B., O. LeBon, G. Hoffmann, R. Cluydts, L. Kaufman, and K. DeMeirleir. 1997. Sleep anomalies in the chronic fatigue syndrome: A comorbidity study. *Neuropsychobiology* 35(3):115-122.

Fishbain, D. A., B. Cole, J. E. Lewis, and J. Gao. 2010. What is the evidence for chronic pain being etiologically associated with the DSM-IV category of sleep disorder due to a general medical condition? A structured evidence-based review. *Pain Medicine* 11:158-179.

Fjell, A. M., K. B. Walhovd, T. T. Brown, J. M. Kuperman, Y. Chung, D. J. Hagler, Jr., V. Venkatraman, J. C. Roddey, M. Erhart, C. McCabe, N. Akshoomoff, D. G. Amaral, C. S. Bloss, O. Libiger, B. F. Darst, N. J. Schork, B. J. Casey, L. Chang, T. M. Ernst, J. R. Gruen, W. E. Kaufmann, T. Kenet, J. Frazier, S. S. Murray, E. R. Sowell, P. van Zijl, S. Mostofsky, T. L. Jernigan, and A. M. Dale. 2012. Multimodal imaging of the self-regulating developing brain. *Proceedings of the National Academy of Sciences of the United States of America* 109(48):19620-19625.

Foral, P., J. Knezevich, N. Dewan, and M. Malesker. 2011. Medication-induced sleep disturbances. *The Consultant Pharmacist* 26(6):414-425.

Fossey, M., E. Libman, S. Bailes, M. Baltzan, R. Schondorf, R. Amsel, and C. S. Fichten. 2004. Sleep quality and psychological adjustment in chronic fatigue syndrome. *Journal of Behavioral Medicine* 27(6):581-605.

Foster, G. R., R. D. Goldin, and H. C. Thomas. 1998. Chronic hepatitis C virus infection causes a significant reduction in quality of life in the absence of cirrhosis. *Hepatology* 27(1):209-212.

Freeman, R., and A. L. Komaroff. 1997. Does the chronic fatigue syndrome involve the autonomic nervous system? *American Journal of Medicine* 102(4):357-364.

Freeman, R., W. Wieling, F. B. Axelrod, D. G. Benditt, E. Benarroch, I. Biaggioni, W. P. Cheshire, T. Chelimsky, P. Cortelli, C. H. Gibbons, D. S. Goldstein, R. Hainsworth, M. J. Hilz, G. Jacob, H. Kaufmann, J. Jordan, L. A. Lipsitz, B. D. Levine, P. A. Low, C. Mathias, S. R. Raj, D. Robertson, P. Sandroni, I. J. Schatz, R. Schondorf, J. M. Stewart, and J. G. van Dijk. 2011. Consensus statement on the definition of orthostatic hypotension, neurally mediated syncope and the postural tachycardia syndrome. *Autonomic Neuroscience* 161(1-2):46-48.

Frith, J., P. Zalewski, J. J. Klawe, J. Pairman, A. Bitner, M. Tafil-Klawe, and J. L. Newton. 2012. Impaired blood pressure variability in chronic fatigue syndrome: A potential biomarker. *QJM: Monthly Journal of the Association of Physicians* 105(9):831-838.

Fukuda, K., S. E. Straus, I. Hickie, M. C. Sharpe, J. G. Dobbins, A. Komaroff, A. Schluederberg, J. F. Jones, A. R. Lloyd, S. Wessely, N. M. Gantz, G. P. Holmes, D. Buchwald, S. Abbey, J. Rest, J. A. Levy, H. Jolson, D. L. Peterson, J. Vercoulen, U. Tirelli, B. Evengård, B. H. Natelson, L. Steele, M. Reyes, and W. C. Reeves. 1994. The chronic fatigue syndrome: A comprehensive approach to its definition and study. *Annals of Internal Medicine* 121(12):953-959.

Furst, G. 1999. Measuring fatigue in chronic fatigue syndrome why and how. *Journal of Chronic Fatigue Syndrome* 5(3-4):55-59.

Gambert, S. R. 2005. Fatigue: Finding the cause of a common complaint. *Clinical Geriatrics* 13(10):6-8.

Gazit, Y., A. M. Nahir, R. Grahame, and G. Jacob. 2003. Dysautonomia in the joint hypermobility syndrome. *American Journal of Medicine* 115(1):33-40.

Gerrity, T. R., J. Bates, D. S. Bell, G. Chrousos, G. Furst, T. Hedrick, B. Hurwitz, R. W. Kula, S. M. Levine, R. C. Moore, and R. Schondorf. 2002. Chronic fatigue syndrome: What role does the autonomic nervous system play in the pathophysiology of this complex illness? *Neuroimmunomodulation* 10(3):134-141.

Gibson, H., N. Carroll, J. E. Clague, and R. H. Edwards. 1993. Exercise performance and fatiguability in patients with chronic fatigue syndrome. *Journal of Neurology, Neurosurgery & Psychiatry* 56(9):993-998.

Gotts, Z. M., V. Deary, J. Newton, D. Van der Dussen, P. De Roy, and J. G. Ellis. 2013. Are there sleep-specific phenotypes in patients with chronic fatigue syndrome? A cross-sectional polysomnography analysis. *BMJ Open* 3(6):e002999.

Grubb, B. P. 2005. Clinical practice. Neurocardiogenic syncope. *New England Journal of Medicine* 352(10):1004-1010.

Harel, D., B. D. Thombs, M. Hudson, M. Baron, and R. Steele. 2012. Measuring fatigue in SSC: A comparison of the Short Form-36 Vitality Subscale and Functional Assessment of Chronic Illness Therapy-Fatigue Scale. *Rheumatology (Oxford)* 51(12):2177-2185.

Hawk, C., L. A. Jason, and S. Torres-Harding. 2006a. Differential diagnosis of chronic fatigue syndrome and major depressive disorder. *International Journal of Behavioral Medicine* 13(3):244-251.

Hawk, C., L. A. Jason, and S. Torres-Harding. 2006b. Reliability of a chronic fatigue syndrome questionnaire. *Journal of Chronic Fatigue Syndrome* 13(4):41-66.

Hoad, A., G. Spickett, J. Elliott, and J. Newton. 2008. Postural orthostatic tachycardia syndrome is an under-recognized condition in chronic fatigue syndrome. *QJM: Monthly Journal of the Association of Physicians* 101(12):961-965.

Hollingsworth, K. G., D. E. Jones, R. Taylor, A. M. Blamire, and J. L. Newton. 2010. Impaired cardiovascular response to standing in chronic fatigue syndrome. *European Journal of Clinical Investigation* 40(7):608-615.

Hossain, J. L., P. Ahmad, L. W. Reinish, L. Kayumov, N. K. Hossain, and C. M. Shapiro. 2005. Subjective fatigue and subjective sleepiness: Two independent consequences of sleep disorders? *Journal of Sleep Research* 14(3):245-253.

Hou, R., R. Moss-Morris, B. Bradley, R. Peveler, and K. Mogg. 2008. Attentional bias towards health-threat information in chronic fatigue syndrome. *European Neuropsychopharmacology* 18(Suppl. 4):S278.

Hou, R., R. Moss-Morris, A. Risdale, J. Lynch, P. Jeevaratnam, B. P. Bradley, and K. Mogg. 2014. Attention processes in chronic fatigue syndrome: Attentional bias for health-related threat and the role of attentional control. *Behaviour Research and Therapy* 52:9-16.

Hurwitz, B. E., V. T. Coryell, M. Parker, P. Martin, A. Laperriere, N. G. Klimas, G. N. Sfakianakis, and M. S. Bilsker. 2010. Chronic fatigue syndrome: Illness severity, sedentary lifestyle, blood volume and evidence of diminished cardiac function. *Clinical Science* 118(2):125-135.

Hutchinson, C. V., and S. P. Badham. 2013. Patterns of abnormal visual attention in myalgic encephalomyelitis. *Optometry and Vision Science* 90(6):607-614.

IACFS/ME (International Association for Chronic Fatigue Syndrome/Myalgic Encephalomyelitis). 2014. *ME/CFS: Primer for clinical practitioners.* Chicago, IL: IACFS/ME.

Inbar, O., R. Dlin, A. Rotstein, and B. J. Whipp. 2001. Physiological responses to incremental exercise in patients with chronic fatigue syndrome. *Medicine & Science in Sports & Exercise* 33(9):1463-1470.

Jackson, M. L., and D. Bruck. 2012. Sleep abnormalities in chronic fatigue syndrome/myalgic encephalomyelitis: A review. *Journal of Clinical Sleep Medicine* 8(6):719-728.

Jason, L. A., and M. M. Brown. 2013. Sub-typing daily fatigue progression in chronic fatigue syndrome. *Journal of Mental Health* 22(1):4-11.

Jason, L. A., and R. R. Taylor. 2002. Applying cluster analysis to define a typology of chronic fatigue syndrome in a medically-evaluated, random community sample. *Psychology and Health* 17(3):323-337.

Jason, L. A., M. T. Ropacki, N. B. Santoro, J. A. Richman, W. Heatherly, R. Taylor, J. R. Ferrari, T. M. Haney-Davis, A. Rademaker, J. Dupuis, J. Golding, A. V. Plioplys, and S. Plioplys. 1997. A screening instrument for chronic fatigue syndrome: Reliability and validity. *Journal of Chronic Fatigue Syndrome* 3(1):39-59.

Jason, L. A., C. P. King, E. L. Frankenberry, K. M. Jordan, W. W. Tryon, F. Rademaker, and C. F. Huang. 1999. Chronic fatigue syndrome: Assessing symptoms and activity level. *Journal of Clinical Psychology* 55(4):411-424.

Jason, L. A., R. R. Taylor, C. L. Kennedy, K. Jordan, C. F. Huang, S. Torres-Harding, S. Song, and D. Johnson. 2002a. A factor analysis of chronic fatigue symptoms in a community-based sample. *Social Psychiatry & Psychiatric Epidemiology* 37(4):183-189.

Jason, L. A., S. R. Torres-Harding, A. W. Carrico, and R. R. Taylor. 2002b. Symptom occurrence in persons with chronic fatigue syndrome. *Biological Psychology* 59(1):15-27.

Jason, L. A., S. R. Torres-Harding, A. Jurgens, and J. Helgerson. 2004. Comparing the Fukuda et al. criteria and the Canadian case definition for chronic fatigue syndrome. *Journal of Chronic Fatigue Syndrome* 12(1):37-52.

Jason, L. A., T. Jessen, N. Porter, A. Boulton, M. G. Njoku, and G. Friedberg. 2009. Examining types of fatigue among individuals with ME/CFS. *Disability Studies Quaterly* 29(3).

Jason, L. A., A. Boulton, N. S. Porter, T. Jessen, M. G. Njoku, and F. Friedberg. 2010a. Classification of myalgic encephalomyelitis/chronic fatigue syndrome by types of fatigue. *Behavioral Medicine* 36(1):24-31.

Jason, L. A., M. Evans, N. Porter, M. Brown, A. Brown, J. Hunnell, V. Anderson, A. Lerch, K. De Meirleir, and F. Friedberg. 2010b. The development of a revised Canadian myalgic encephalomyelitis chronic fatigue syndrome case definition. *American Journal of Biochemistry and Biotechnology* 6(2):120-135.

Jason, L. A., M. Evans, M. Brown, N. Porter, A. Brown, J. Hunnell, V. Anderson, and A. Lerch. 2011a. Fatigue scales and chronic fatigue syndrome: Issues of sensitivity and specificity. *Disability Studies Quarterly: DSQ* 31(1).

Jason, L. A., N. Porter, J. Hunnell, A. Brown, A. Rademaker, and J. A. Richman. 2011b. A natural history study of chronic fatigue syndrome. *Rehabilitation Psychology* 56(1):32-42.

Jason, L. A., M. Brown, M. Evans, V. Anderson, A. Lerch, A. Brown, J. Hunnell, and N. Porter. 2011c. Measuring substantial reductions in functioning in patients with chronic fatigue syndrome. *Disability and Rehabilitation* 33(7):589-598.

Jason, L. A., A. Brown, E. Clyne, L. Bartgis, M. Evans, and M. Brown. 2012a. Contrasting case definitions for chronic fatigue syndrome, myalgic encephalomyelitis/chronic fatigue syndrome and myalgic encephalomyelitis. *Evaluation and the Health Professions* 35(3):280-304.

Jason, L. A., E. R. Unger, J. D. Dimitrakoff, A. P. Fagin, M. Houghton, D. B. Cook, G. D. Marshall, N. Klimas, and C. Snell. 2012b. Minimum data elements for research reports on CFS. *Brain, Behavior, and Immunity* 26(3):401-406.

Jason, L. A., A. Brown, M. Evans, M. Sunnquist, and J. L. Newton. 2013a. Contrasting chronic fatigue syndrome versus myalgic encephalomyelitis/chronic fatigue syndrome. *Fatigue* 1(3):168-183.

Jason, L. A., M. Sunnquist, A. Brown, M. Evans, S. Vernon, J. Furst, and V. Simonis. 2013b. Examining case definition criteria for chronic fatigue syndrome and myalgic encephalomyelitis. *Fatigue: Biomedicine, Health & Behavior* 2(1).

Jason, L. A., M. Sunnquist, A. Brown, M. Evans, and J. L. Newton. 2014. Are myalgic encephalomyelitis and chronic fatigue syndrome different illnesses? A preliminary analysis. *Journal of Health Psychology* [Epub ahead of print].

Jason, L., M. Evans, S. So, J. Scott, and A. Brown. In press. Problems in defining postexertional malaise. *Journal of Prevention and Intervention in the Community*.

Johns, M. W. 2000. Sensitivity and specificity of the multiple sleep latency test (MSLT), the maintenance of wakefulness test and the epworth sleepiness scale: Failure of the MSLT as a gold standard. *Journal of Sleep Research* 9(1):5-11.

Jones, D. E., K. G. Hollingsworth, R. Taylor, A. M. Blamire, and J. L. Newton. 2010. Abnormalities in ph handling by peripheral muscle and potential regulation by the autonomic nervous system in chronic fatigue syndrome. *Journal of Internal Medicine* 267(4):394-401.

Jones, D. E., K. G. Hollingsworth, D. G. Jakovljevic, G. Fattakhova, J. Pairman, A. M. Blamire, M. I. Trenell, and J. L. Newton. 2012. Loss of capacity to recover from acidosis on repeat exercise in chronic fatigue syndrome: A case-control study. *European Journal of Clinical Investigation* 42(2):186-194.

Jones, J. F., A. Nicholson, R. Nisenbaum, D. A. Papanicolaou, L. Solomon, R. Boneva, C. Heim, and W. C. Reeves. 2005. Orthostatic instability in a population-based study of chronic fatigue syndrome. *American Journal of Medicine* 118(12):1415.

Juenger, J., D. Schellberg, S. Kraemer, A. Haunstetter, C. Zugck, W. Herzog, and M. Haass. 2002. Health related quality of life in patients with congestive heart failure: Comparison with other chronic diseases and relation to functional variables. *Heart* 87(3):235-241.

Kanjwal, K., B. Karabin, Y. Kanjwal, and B. P. Grubb. 2011. Postural orthostatic tachycardia syndrome following Lyme disease. *Cardiology Journal* 18(1):63-66.

Kanjwal, Y., D. A. N. Kosinski, and B. P. Grubb. 2003. The postural orthostatic tachycardia syndrome. *Pacing and Clinical Electrophysiology* 26(8):1747-1757.

Kasper, D. L., E. Braunwalkd, A. S. Fauci, S. L. Hauser, D. L. Longo, and J. L. Jameson, eds. 2005. *Harrison's principles of internal medicine*, 16th ed., Vol. 2. New York: McGraw-Hill.

Katch, V. L., S. S. Sady, and P. Freedson. 1982. Biological variability in maximum aerobic power. *Medicine & Science in Sports & Exercise* 14(1):21-25.

Kaufmann, H., R. Malamut, L. Norcliffe-Kaufmann, K. Rosa, and R. Freeman. 2012. The Orthostatic Hypotension Questionnaire (OHQ): Validation of a novel symptom assessment scale. *Clinical Autonomic Research* 22(2):79-90.

Kawamura, Y., M. Kihara, K. Nishimoto, and M. Taki. 2003. Efficacy of a half dose of oral pyridostigmine in the treatment of chronic fatigue syndrome: Three case reports. *Pathophysiology* 9(3):189-194.

Keller, B. A., J. L. Pryor, and L. Giloteaux. 2014. Inability of myalgic encephalomyelitis/chronic fatigue syndrome patients to reproduce VO_2 peak indicates functional impairment. *Journal of Translational Medicine* 12(1):104.

Kenny, R. A., and L. A. Graham. 2001. Chronic fatigue syndrome symptoms common in patients with vasovagal syncope. *American Journal of Medicine* 110(3):242-243.

Kerr, J. R., J. Gough, S. C. Richards, J. Main, D. Enlander, M. McCreary, A. L. Komaroff, and J. K. Chia. 2010. Antibody to parvovirus B19 nonstructural protein is associated with chronic arthralgia in patients with chronic fatigue syndrome/myalgic encephalomyelitis. *Journal of General Virology* 91(Pt. 4):893-897.

Khan, F., V. Spence, G. Kennedy, and J. J. Belch. 2003. Prolonged acetylcholine-induced vasodilatation in the peripheral microcirculation of patients with chronic fatigue syndrome. *Clinical Physiology & Functional Imaging* 23(5):282-285.

Kierlin, L., and M. R. Littner. 2011. Parasomnias and antidepressant therapy: A review of the literature. *Front Psychiatry* 2:71.

Kishi, A., Z. R. Struzik, B. H. Natelson, F. Togo, and Y. Yamamoto. 2008. Dynamics of sleep stage transitions in healthy humans and patients with chronic fatigue syndrome. *American Journal of Physiology—Regulatory Integrative & Comparative Physiology* 294(6):R1980-R1987.

Kishi, A., B. H. Natelson, F. Togo, Z. R. Struzik, D. M. Rapoport, and Y. Yamamoto. 2011. Sleep-stage dynamics in patients with chronic fatigue syndrome with or without fibromyalgia. *Sleep* 34(11):1551-1560.

Kishi, A., F. Togo, D. B. Cook, M. Klapholz, Y. Yamamoto, D. M. Rapoport, and B. H. Natelson. 2013. The effects of exercise on dynamic sleep morphology in healthy controls and patients with chronic fatigue syndrome. *Physiological Reports* 1(6):e00152.

Knoop, H., J. B. Prins, M. Stulemeijer, J. W. M. van der Meer, and G. Bleijenberg. 2007. The effect of cognitive behaviour therapy for chronic fatigue syndrome on self-reported cognitive impairments and neuropsychological test performance. *Journal of Neurology, Neurosurgery & Psychiatry* 78(4):434-436.

Komaroff, A. L., and D. Buchwald. 1991. Symptoms and signs of chronic fatigue syndrome. *Reviews of Infectious Diseases* 13(Suppl. 1):S8-S11.

Komaroff, A. L., L. R. Fagioli, T. H. Doolittle, B. Gandek, M. A. Gleit, R. T. Guerriero, I. R. J. Kornish, N. C. Ware, J. E. Ware, Jr., and D. W. Bates. 1996a. Health status in patients with chronic fatigue syndrome and in general population and disease comparison groups. *American Journal of Medicine* 101(3):281-290.

Komaroff, A. L., L. R. Fagioli, A. M. Geiger, T. H. Doolittle, J. Lee, J. Kornish, M. A. Gleit, and R. T. Guerriero. 1996b. An examination of the working case definition of chronic fatigue syndrome. *American Journal of Medicine* 100(1):56-64.

Komaroff, A. L., L. R. Fagioli, T. H. Doolittle, B. Gandek, M. A. Gleit, R. T. Guerriero, R. J. Kornish II, N. C. Ware, J. E. Ware, Jr., and D. W. Bates. 1996c. Chronic fatigue syndrome questionnaire. In Health status in patients with chronic fatigue syndrome and in general population and disease comparison groups. *American Journal of Medicine* 101(3):281-290.

Krupp, L. B., N. G. LaRocca, J. Muir-Nash, and A. D. Steinberg. 1989. The fatigue severity scale. Application to patients with multiple sclerosis and systemic lupus erythematosus. *Archives of Neurology* 46(10):1121-1123.

Krupp, L. B., L. Jandorf, P. K. Coyle, and W. B. Mendelson. 1993. Sleep disturbance in chronic fatigue syndrome. *Journal of Psychosomatic Research* 37(4):325-331.

Kushida, C. A., M. R. Littner, T. Morgenthaler, C. A. Alessi, D. Bailey, J. Coleman, Jr., L. Friedman, M. Hirshkowitz, S. Kapen, M. Kramer, T. Lee-Chiong, D. L. Loube, J. Owens, J. P. Pancer, and M. Wise. 2005. Practice parameters for the indications for polysomnography and related procedures: An update for 2005. *Sleep* 28(4):499-521.

LaManca, J. J., S. A. Sisto, J. DeLuca, S. K. Johnson, G. Lange, J. Pareja, S. Cook, and B. H. Natelson. 1998. Influence of exhaustive treadmill exercise on cognitive functioning in chronic fatigue syndrome. *American Journal of Medicine* 105(3A):59S-65S.

LaManca, J. J., A. Peckerman, J. Walker, W. Kesil, S. Cook, A. Taylor, and B. H. Natelson. 1999a. Cardiovascular response during head-up tilt in chronic fatigue syndrome. *Clinical Physiology* 19(2):111-120.

LaManca, J. J., S. A. Sisto, X. Zhou, J. E. Ottenweller, S. Cook, A. Peckerman, Q. W. Zhang, T. N. Denny, W. C. Gause, and B. H. Natelson. 1999b. Immunological response in chronic fatigue syndrome following a graded exercise test to exhaustion. *Journal of Clinical Immunology* 19(2):135-142.

LaManca, J. J., A. Peckerman, S. A. Sisto, J. DeLuca, S. Cook, and B. H. Natelson. 2001. Cardiovascular responses of women with chronic fatigue syndrome to stressful cognitive testing before and after strenuous exercise. *Psychosomatic Medicine* 63(5):756-764.

Lange, G., J. Steffener, D. B. Cook, B. M. Bly, C. Christodoulou, W. C. Liu, J. DeLuca, and B. H. Natelson. 2005. Objective evidence of cognitive complaints in chronic fatigue syndrome: A BOLD fMRI study of verbal working memory. *Neuroimage* 26(2):513-524.

Larun, L., and K. Malterud. 2007. Identity and coping experiences in chronic fatigue syndrome: A synthesis of qualitative studies. *Patient Education and Counseling* 69(1-3):20-28.

Lawrie, S. M., S. M. MacHale, J. T. O. Cavanagh, R. E. O'Carroll, and G. M. Goodwin. 2000. The difference in patterns of motor and cognitive function in chronic fatigue syndrome and severe depressive illness. *Psychological Medicine* 30(2):433-442.

Le Bon, O., B. Fischler, G. Hoffmann, J. R. Murphy, K. De Meirleir, R. Cluydts, and I. Pelc. 2000. How significant are primary sleep disorders and sleepiness in the chronic fatigue syndrome? *Sleep Research Online* 3(2):43-48.

Le Bon, O., D. Neu, F. Valente, and P. Linkowski. 2007. Paradoxical nrems distribution in "pure" chronic fatigue patients a comparison with sleep apnea-hypopnea patients and healthy control subjects. *Journal of Chronic Fatigue Syndrome* 14(2):45-59.

Le Bon, O., D. Neu, Y. Berquin, J.-P. Lanquart, R. Hoffmann, O. Mairesse, and R. Armitage. 2012. Ultra-slow delta power in chronic fatigue syndrome. *Psychiatry Research* 200(2-3):742-747.

Legge, H., M. Norton, and J. Newton. 2008. Fatigue is significant in vasovagal syncope and is associated with autonomic symptoms. *Europace* 10(9):1095-1101.

Lewis, I., J. Pairman, G. Spickett, and J. L. Newton. 2013. Clinical characteristics of a novel subgroup of chronic fatigue syndrome patients with postural orthostatic tachycardia syndrome. *Journal of Internal Medicine* 273(5):501-510.

Libman, E., L. Creti, M. Baltzan, D. Rizzo, C. S. Fichten, and S. Bailes. 2009. Sleep apnea and psychological functioning in chronic fatigue syndrome. *Journal of Health Psychology* 14(8):1251-1267.

Light, A. R., A. T. White, R. W. Hughen, and K. C. Light. 2009. Moderate exercise increases expression for sensory, adrenergic, and immune genes in chronic fatigue syndrome patients but not in normal subjects. *The Journal of Pain* 10(10):1099-1112.

Light, A. R., L. Bateman, D. Jo, R. W. Hughen, T. A. Vanhaitsma, A. T. White, and K. C. Light. 2012. Gene expression alterations at baseline and following moderate exercise in patients with chronic fatigue syndrome and fibromyalgia syndrome. *Journal of Internal Medicine* 271(1):64-81.

Low, P. A., P. Sandroni, M. Joyner, and W. Shen. 2009. Postural tachycardia syndrome. *Journal of Cardiovascular Electrophysiology* 20(3):352-358.

MacLean, A., E. Allen, and T. Magath. 1944. Orthostatic tachycardia and orthostatic hypotension: Defects in the return of venous blood to the heart. *American Heart Journal* 27(2):145-163.

Maes, M., F. N. M. Twisk, and C. Johnson. 2012. Myalgic encephalomyelitis (ME), chronic fatigue syndrome (CFS), and chronic fatigue (CF) are distinguished accurately: Results of supervised learning techniques applied on clinical and inflammatory data. *Psychiatry Research* 200(2-3):754-760.

Mahurin, R. K., J. H. Goldberg, K. H. Claypoole, L. Arguelles, S. Ashton, and D. Buchwald. 2004. Cognitive processing in monozygotic twins discordant for chronic fatigue syndrome. *Neuropsychology* 18(2):232-239.

Majer, M., J. F. Jones, E. R. Unger, L. S. Youngblood, M. J. Decker, B. Gurbaxani, C. Heim, and W. C. Reeves. 2007. Perception versus polysomnographic assessment of sleep in CFS and non-fatigued control subjects: Results from a population-based study. *BMC Neurology* 7.

Majer, M., L. A. M. Welberg, L. Capuron, A. H. Miller, G. Pagnoni, and W. C. Reeves. 2008. Neuropsychological performance in persons with chronic fatigue syndrome: Results from a population-based study. *Psychosomatic Medicine* 70(7):829-836.

Mariman, A., D. Vogelaers, I. Hanoulle, L. Delesie, and D. Pevernagie. 2012. Subjective sleep quality and daytime sleepiness in a large sample of patients with chronic fatigue syndrome (CFS). *Acta Clinica Belgica* 67(1):19-24.

Marino, M., Y. Li, M. N. Rueschman, J. W. Winkelman, J. M. Ellenbogen, J. M. Solet, H. Dulin, L. F. Berkman, and O. M. Buxton. 2013. Measuring sleep: Accuracy, sensitivity, and specificity of wrist actigraphy compared to polysomnography. *Sleep* 36(11):1747-1755.

Marshall, P. S., M. Forstot, A. Callies, P. K. Peterson, and C. H. Schenck. 1997. Cognitive slowing and working memory difficulties in chronic fatigue syndrome. *Psychosomatic Medicine* 59(1):58-66.

Martin, M., and I. Alexeeva. 2010. Mood volatility with rumination but neither attentional nor interpretation biases in chronic fatigue syndrome. *British Journal of Health Psychology* 15(4):779-796.

Martinez-Lavin, M. 2007. Biology and therapy of fibromyalgia. Stress, the stress response system, and fibromyalgia. *Arthritis Research & Therapy* 9(4):216.

Martinez-Martinez, L. A., T. Mora, A. Vargas, M. Fuentes-Iniestra, and M. Martinez-Lavin. 2014. Sympathetic nervous system dysfunction in fibromyalgia, chronic fatigue syndrome, irritable bowel syndrome, and interstitial cystitis: A review of case-control studies. *Journal of Clinical Rheumatology* 20(3):146-150.

Matthews, D. A., P. Manu, and T. J. Lane. 1991. Evaluation and management of patients with chronic fatigue. *American Journal of the Medical Sciences* 302(5):269-277.

McCully, K. K., and B. H. Natelson. 1999. Impaired oxygen delivery to muscle in chronic fatigue syndrome. *Clinical Science* 97(5):603-608; discussion 611-613.

McHorney, C. A., J. E. Ware, Jr., and A. E. Raczek. 1993. The MOS 36-item Short-Form Health Survey (SF-36): II. Psychometric and clinical tests of validity in measuring physical and mental health constructs. *Medical Care* 31(3):247-263.

Meeus, M., L. Hermans, K. Ickmans, F. Struyf, D. Van Cauwenbergh, L. Bronckaerts, L. S. De Clerck, G. Moorken, G. Hans, S. Grosemans, and J. Nijs. 2014. Endogenous pain modulation in response to exercise in patients with rheumatoid arthritis, patients with chronic fatigue syndrome and comorbid fibromyalgia, and healthy controls: A double-blind randomized controlled trial. *Pain Practice.* http://onlinelibrary.wiley.com/doi/10.1111/papr.12181/pdf (accessed January 14, 2015).

Merkus, M. P., K. J. Jager, F. W. Dekker, E. W. Boeschoten, P. Stevens, and R. T. Krediet. 1997. Quality of life in patients on chronic dialysis: Self-assessment 3 months after the start of treatment. The Necosad Study Group. *American Journal of Kidney Diseases* 29(4):584-592.

Meyer, J. D., A. R. Light, S. K. Shukla, D. Clevidence, S. Yale, A. J. Stegner, and D. B. Cook. 2013. Post-exertion malaise in chronic fatigue syndrome: Symptoms and gene expression. *Fatigue: Biomedicine, Health & Behavior* 1(4):190-209.

Michiels, V., and R. Cluydts. 2001. Neuropsychological functioning in chronic fatigue syndrome: A review. *Acta Psychiatrica Scandinavica* 103(2):84-93.

Michiels, V., R. Cluydts, B. Fischler, G. Hoffmann, O. Le Bon, and K. De Meirleir. 1996. Cognitive functioning in patients with chronic fatigue syndrome. *Journal of Clinical & Experimental Neuropsychology: Official Journal of the International Neuropsychological Society* 18(5):666-677.

Miwa, K. 2014. Cardiac dysfunction and orthostatic intolerance in patients with myalgic encephalomyelitis and a small left ventricle. *Heart Vessels* 1-6.

Miwa, K., and M. Fujita. 2008. Small heart syndrome in patients with chronic fatigue syndrome. *Clinical Cardiology* 31(7):328-333.

Miwa, K., and M. Fujita. 2009. Cardiovascular dysfunction with low cardiac output due to a small heart in patients with chronic fatigue syndrome. *Internal Medicine* 48(21):1849-1854.

Miwa, K., and M. Fujita. 2011. Small heart with low cardiac output for orthostatic intolerance in patients with chronic fatigue syndrome. *Clinical Cardiology* 34(12):782-786.

Moffoot, A. P., R. E. O'Carroll, J. Bennie, S. Carroll, H. Dick, K. P. Ebmeier, and G. M. Goodwin. 1994. Diurnal variation of mood and neuropsychological function in major depression with melancholia. *Journal of Affective Disorders* 32(4):257-269.

Morgenthaler, T., C. Alessi, L. Friedman, J. Owens, V. Kapur, B. Boehlecke, T. Brown, A. Chesson, Jr., J. Coleman, T. Lee-Chiong, J. Pancer, and T. J. Swick. 2007. Practice parameters for the use of actigraphy in the assessment of sleep and sleep disorders: An update for 2007. *Sleep* 30(4):519-529.

Morriss, R., M. Sharpe, A. L. Sharpley, P. J. Cown, K. Hawton, and J. Morris. 1993. Abnormalities of sleep in patients with the chronic fatigue syndrome. *British Medical Journal* 306(6886):1161-1164.

Morriss, R. K., A. J. Wearden, and L. Battersby. 1997. The relation of sleep difficulties to fatigue, mood and disability in chronic fatigue syndrome. *Journal of Psychosomatic Research* 42(6):597-605.

Moya, A., R. Sutton, F. Ammirati, J. J. Blanc, M. Brignole, J. B. Dahm, J. C. Deharo, J. Gajek, K. Gjesdal, A. Krahn, M. Massin, M. Pepi, T. Pezawas, R. Ruiz Granell, F. Sarasin, A. Ungar, J. G. van Dijk, E. P. Walma, and W. Wieling. 2009. Guidelines for the diagnosis and management of syncope (version 2009). *European Heart Journal* 30(21):2631-2671.

Murrough, J. W., X. Mao, K. A. Collins, C. Kelly, G. Andrade, P. Nestadt, S. M. Levine, S. J. Mathew, and D. C. Shungu. 2010. Increased ventricular lactate in chronic fatigue syndrome measured by 1H MRS imaging at 3.0 T. II: Comparison with major depressive disorder. *NMR in Biomedicine* 23(6):643-650.

Nacul, L. C., E. M. Lacerda, P. Campion, D. Pheby, M. D. Drachler, J. C. Leite, F. Poland, A. Howe, S. Fayyaz, and M. Molokhia. 2011a. The functional status and well being of people with myalgic encephalomyelitis/chronic fatigue syndrome and their carers. *BMC Public Health* 11.

Nacul, L. C., E. M. Lacerda, D. Pheby, P. Campion, M. Molokhia, S. Fayyaz, J. C. Leite, F. Poland, A. Howe, and M. L. Drachler. 2011b. Prevalence of myalgic encephalomyelitis/chronic fatigue syndrome (ME/CFS) in three regions of England: A repeated cross-sectional study in primary care. *BMC Medicine* 9:91.

Nakamura, T., S. K. Schwander, R. Donnelly, F. Ortega, F. Togo, G. Broderick, Y. Yamamoto, N. S. Cherniack, D. Rapoport, and B. H. Natelson. 2010a. Cytokines across the night in chronic fatigue syndrome with and without fibromyalgia. *Clinical and Vaccine Immunology* 17(4):582-587.

Nakamura, T., F. Togo, N. S. Cherniack, D. Rapoport, and B. H. Natelson. 2010b. A subgroup of patients with chronic fatigue syndrome may have a disorder of arousal. *The Open Sleep Journal* 3:6-11.

Nakatomi, Y., K. Mizuno, A. Ishii, Y. Wada, M. Tanaka, S. Tazawa, K. Onoe, S. Fukuda, J. Kawabe, K. Takahashi, Y. Kataoka, S. Shiomi, K. Yamaguti, M. Inaba, H. Kuratsune, and Y. Watanabe. 2014. Neuroinflammation in patients with chronic fatigue syndrome/myalgic encephalomyelitis: An 11C-(R)-PK11195 PET study. *Journal of Nuclear Medicine* 55(6):945-950.

Naschitz, J. E., I. Rosner, M. Rozenbaum, L. Gaitini, I. Bistritzki, E. Zuckerman, E. Sabo, and D. Yeshurun. 2000. The capnography head-up tilt test for evaluation of chronic fatigue syndrome. *Seminars in Arthritis & Rheumatism* 30(2):79-86.

Naschitz, J. E., E. Sabo, S. Naschitz, I. Rosner, M. Rozenbaum, M. Fields, H. Isseroff, R. M. Priselac, L. Gaitini, S. Eldar, E. Zukerman, and D. Yeshurun. 2002. Hemodynamics instability score in chronic fatigue syndrome and in non-chronic fatigue syndrome. *Seminars in Arthritis & Rheumatism* 32(3):141-148.

Naschitz, J., D. Dreyfuss, D. Yeshurun, and I. Rosner. 2004. Midodrine treatment for chronic fatigue syndrome. *Postgraduate Medical Journal* 80(942):230-232.

Natelson, B. H., R. Intriligator, N. S. Cherniack, H. K. Chandler, and J. M. Stewart. 2007. Hypocapnia is a biological marker for orthostatic intolerance in some patients with chronic fatigue syndrome. *Dynamic Medicine* 6.

National Institute on Aging. 2007. *Unexplained fatigue in the elderly—workshop summary.* http://www.nia.nih.gov/print/about/events/2011/unexplained-fatigue-elderly (accessed January 12, 2015).

Neu, D., O. Mairesse, G. Hoffmann, A. Dris, L. J. Lambrecht, P. Linkowski, P. Verbanck, and L. B. Olivier. 2007. Sleep quality perception in the chronic fatigue syndrome: Correlations with sleep efficiency, affective symptoms and intensity of fatigue. *Neuropsychobiology* 56(1):40-46.

Neu, D., G. Hoffmann, R. Moutrier, P. Verbanck, P. Linkowski, and O. Le Bon. 2008. Are patients with chronic fatigue syndrome just "tired" or also "sleepy"? *Journal of Sleep Research* 17(4):427-431.

Neu, D., H. Kajosch, P. Peigneux, P. Verbanck, P. Linkowski, and O. Le Bon. 2011. Cognitive impairment in fatigue and sleepiness associated conditions. *Psychiatry Research* 189(1):128-134.

Newton, J. L., O. Okonkwo, K. Sutcliffe, A. Seth, J. Shin, and D. E. J. Jones. 2007. Symptoms of autonomic dysfunction in chronic fatigue syndrome. *QJM: Monthly Journal of the Association of Physicians* 100(8):519-526.

Newton, J. L., A. Sheth, J. Shin, J. Pairman, K. Wilton, J. A. Burt, and D. E. Jones. 2009. Lower ambulatory blood pressure in chronic fatigue syndrome. *Psychosomatic Medicine* 71(3):361-365.

NICE (National Institute for Health and Clinical Excellence). 2007. *Chronic fatigue syndrome/ myalgic encephalomyelitis (or encephalopathy): Diagnosis and management of CFS/ME in adults and children.* London, UK: NICE.

Nijs, J., J. Van Oosterwijck, M. Meeus, L. Lambrecht, K. Metzger, M. Fremont, and L. Paul. 2010. Unravelling the nature of postexertional malaise in myalgic encephalomyelitis/ chronic fatigue syndrome: The role of elastase, complement C4a and interleukin-1beta. *Journal of Internal Medicine* 267(4):418-435.

Nijs, J., A. Nees, L. Paul, M. De Kooning, K. Ickmans, M. Meeus, and J. Van Oosterwijck. 2014. Altered immune response to exercise in patients with chronic fatigue syndrome/ myalgic encephalomyelitis: A systematic literature review. *Exercise Immunology Review* 20:94-116.

Nisenbaum, R., M. Reyes, A. C. Mawle, and W. C. Reeves. 1998. Factor analysis of unexplained severe fatigue and interrelated symptoms: Overlap with criteria for chronic fatigue syndrome. *American Journal of Epidemiology* 148(1):72-77.

Nisenbaum, R., J. F. Jones, E. R. Unger, M. Reyes, and W. C. Reeves. 2003. A population-based study of the clinical course of chronic fatigue syndrome. *Health & Quality of Life Outcomes* 1:49.

Nisenbaum, R., M. Reyes, E. R. Unger, and W. C. Reeves. 2004. Factor analysis of symptoms among subjects with unexplained chronic fatigue: What can we learn about chronic fatigue syndrome? *Journal of Psychosomatic Research* 56(2):171-178.

Ocon, A. J., Z. R. Messer, M. S. Medow, and J. M. Stewart. 2012. Increasing orthostatic stress impairs neurocognitive functioning in chronic fatigue syndrome with postural tachycardia syndrome. *Clinical Science* 122(5):227-238.

Okamoto, L. E., S. R. Raj, and I. Biaggioni. 2012a. Chronic fatigue syndrome and the autonomic nervous system. In *Primer on the Autonomic Nervous System*, 3rd ed., edited by D. Robertson, I. Biaggioni, G. Burnstock, P. A. Low, and J. F. R. Paton. Oxford: Academic Press. Pp. 531-534.

Okamoto, L. E., S. R. Raj, A. Peltier, A. Gamboa, C. Shibao, A. Diedrich, B. K. Black, D. Robertson, and I. Biaggioni. 2012b. Neurohumoral and haemodynamic profile in postural tachycardia and chronic fatigue syndromes. *Clinical Science* 122(4):183-192.

Oliveira, M. G., S. Garbuio, E. C. Treptow, J. F. Polese, S. Tufik, L. E. Nery, and L. Bittencourt. 2014. The use of portable monitoring for sleep apnea diagnosis in adults. *Expert Review of Respiratory Medicine* 8(1):123-132.

Owen, A. M., K. M. McMillan, A. R. Laird, and E. Bullmore. 2005. N-back working memory paradigm: A meta-analysis of normative functional neuroimaging studies. *Human Brain Mapping* 25(1):46-59.

Parsaik, A., T. G. Allison, W. Singer, D. M. Sletten, M. J. Joyner, E. E. Benarroch, P. A. Low, and P. Sandroni. 2012. Deconditioning in patients with orthostatic intolerance. *Neurology* 79(14):1435-1439.

Paul, L., L. Wood, W. M. H. Behan, and W. M. Maclaren. 1999. Demonstration of delayed recovery from fatiguing exercise in chronic fatigue syndrome. *European Journal of Neurology* 6(1):63-69.

Peterson, P. K., S. A. Sirr, F. C. Grammith, C. H. Schenck, A. M. Pheley, S. Hu, and C. C. Chao. 1994. Effects of mild exercise on cytokines and cerebral blood flow in chronic fatigue syndrome patients. *Clinical and Diagnostic Laboratory Immunology* 1(2):222-226.

Peterson, P. K., A. Pheley, J. Schroeppel, C. Schenck, P. Marshall, A. Kind, J. M. Haugland, L. J. Lambrecht, S. Swan, and S. Goldsmith. 1998. A preliminary placebo-controlled crossover trial of fludrocortisone for chronic fatigue syndrome. *Archives of Internal Medicine* 158(8):908-914.

Picavet, H. S., and N. Hoeymans. 2004. Health related quality of life in multiple musculoskeletal diseases: SF-36 and EQ-5d in the DMC_3 study. *Annals of the Rheumatic Diseases* 63(6):723-729.

Plash, W. B., A. Diedrich, I. Biaggioni, E. M. Garland, S. Y. Paranjape, B. K. Black, W. D. Dupont, and S. R. Raj. 2013. Diagnosing postural tachycardia syndrome: Comparison of tilt testing compared with standing haemodynamics. *Clinical Science (London)* 124(2):109-114.

Poole, J., R. Herrell, S. Ashton, J. Goldberg, and D. Buchwald. 2000. Results of isoproterenol tilt table testing in monozygotic twins discordant for chronic fatigue syndrome. *Archives of Internal Medicine* 160(22):3461-3468.

Puri, B. K., P. M. Jakeman, M. Agour, K. D. Gunatilake, K. A. Fernando, A. I. Gurusinghe, I. H. Treasaden, A. D. Waldman, and P. Gishen. 2012. Regional grey and white matter volumetric changes in myalgic encephalomyelitis (chronic fatigue syndrome): A voxel-based morphometry 3 T MRI study. *British Journal of Radiology* 85(1015):e270-e273.

Qanneta, R. 2013. Obstructive sleep apnea syndrome manifested as a subset of chronic fatigue syndrome: A comorbidity or an exclusion criterion? *Rheumatology International* 1-2.

Qanneta, R. 2014. Obstructive sleep apnea syndrome manifested as a subset of chronic fatigue syndrome: A comorbidity or an exclusion criterion? *Rheumatology International* 34(3):441-442.

Rahman, K., A. Burton, S. Galbraith, A. Lloyd, and U. Vollmer-Conna. 2011. Sleep-wake behavior in chronic fatigue syndrome. *Sleep: Journal of Sleep and Sleep Disorders Research* 34(5):671-678.

Raj, S. R. 2013. Postural Orthostatic Tachycardia Syndrome (POTS). *Circulation* 127(23): 2336-2342.

RAND. 1984. *RAND 36-Item Health Survey.* http://www.rand.org/health/surveys_tools/mos/mos_core_36item_survey.html (accessed January 14, 2015).

Ray, C., W. R. C. Weir, S. Phillips, and S. Cullen. 1992. Development of a measure of symptoms in chronic fatigue syndrome: The Profile of Fatigue-Related Symptoms (PFRS). *Psychology & Health* 7(1):27-43.

Razumovsky, A. Y., K. DeBusk, H. Calkins, S. Snader, K. E. Lucas, P. Vyas, D. F. Hanley, and P. C. Rowe. 2003. Cerebral and systemic hemodynamics changes during upright tilt in chronic fatigue syndrome. *Journal of Neuroimaging* 13(1):57-67.

Reeves, W. C., C. Heim, E. M. Maloney, L. S. Youngblood, E. R. Unger, M. J. Decker, J. F. Jones, and D. B. Rye. 2006. Sleep characteristics of persons with chronic fatigue syndrome and non-fatigued controls: Results from a population-based study. *BMC Neurology* 6.

Reynolds, G. K., D. P. Lewis, A. M. Richardson, and B. A. Lidbury. 2013. Comorbidity of postural orthostatic tachycardia syndrome and chronic fatigue syndrome in an Australian cohort. *Journal of Internal Medicine* 275(4):409-417.

Rosen, C. L., D. Auckley, R. Benca, N. Foldvary-Schaefer, C. Iber, V. Kapur, M. Rueschman, P. Zee, and S. Redline. 2012. A multisite randomized trial of portable sleep studies and positive airway pressure autotitration versus laboratory-based polysomnography for the diagnosis and treatment of obstructive sleep apnea: The homepap study. *Sleep* 35(6):757-767.

Rowe, P. C., and H. Calkins. 1998. Neurally mediated hypotension and chronic fatigue syndrome. *American Journal of Medicine* 105(3A):15S-21S.

Rowe, P. C., I. Bou-Holaigah, J. S. Kan, and H. Calkins. 1995. Is neurally mediated hypotension an unrecognised cause of chronic fatigue? *Lancet* 345(8950):623-624.

Rowe, P. C., D. F. Barron, H. Calkins, I. H. Maumenee, P. Y. Tong, and M. T. Geraghty. 1999. Orthostatic intolerance and chronic fatigue syndrome associated with Ehlers-Danlos syndrome. *Journal of Pediatrics* 135(4):494-499.

Rowe, P. C., H. Calkins, K. DeBusk, R. McKenzie, R. Anand, G. Sharma, B. A. Cuccherini, N. Soto, P. Hohman, S. Snader, K. E. Lucas, M. Wolff, and S. E. Straus. 2001. Fludrocortisone acetate to treat neurally mediated hypotension in chronic fatigue syndrome: A randomized controlled trial. *Journal of the American Medical Association* 285(1):52-59.

Salaffi, F., P. Sarzi-Puttini, R. Girolimetti, F. Atzeni, S. Gasparini, and W. Grassi. 2009. Health-related quality of life in fibromyalgia patients: A comparison with rheumatoid arthritis patients and the general population using the SF-36 Health Survey. *Clinical and Experimental Rheumatology* 27(5, Suppl. 56):S67-S74.

Sargent, C., G. C. Scroop, P. M. Nemeth, R. B. Burnet, and J. D. Buckley. 2002. Maximal oxygen uptake and lactate metabolism are normal in chronic fatigue syndrome. *Medicine & Science in Sports & Exercise* 34(1):51-56.

Schmaling, K. B., D. H. Lewis, J. I. Fiedelak, R. Mahurin, and D. S. Buchwald. 2003. Single-photon emission computerized tomography and neurocognitive function in patients with chronic fatigue syndrome. *Psychosomatic Medicine* 65(1):129-136.

Schondorf, R., J. Benoit, T. Wein, and D. Phaneuf. 1999. Orthostatic intolerance in the chronic fatigue syndrome. *Journal of the Autonomic Nervous System* 75(2-3):192-201.

Schrezenmaier, C., J. A. Gehrking, S. M. Hines, P. A. Low, L. M. Benrud-Larson, and P. Sandroni. 2005. Evaluation of orthostatic hypotension: Relationship of a new self-report instrument to laboratory-based measures. *Mayo Clinic Proceedings* 80(3):330-334.

Schrijvers, D., F. Van Den Eede, Y. Maas, P. Cosyns, W. Hulstijn, and B. G. C. Sabbe. 2009. Psychomotor functioning in chronic fatigue syndrome and major depressive disorder: A comparative study. *Journal of Affective Disorders* 115(1-2):46-53.

Sharpley, A., A. Clements, K. Hawton, and M. Sharpe. 1997. Do patients with "pure" chronic fatigue syndrome (neurasthenia) have abnormal sleep? *Psychosomatic Medicine* 59(6):592-596.

Short, K., M. McCabe, and G. Tooley. 2002. Cognitive functioning in chronic fatigue syndrome and the role of depression, anxiety, and fatigue. *Journal of Psychosomatic Research* 52(6):475-483.

Shungu, D. C., N. Weiduschat, J. W. Murrough, X. Mao, S. Pillemer, J. P. Dyke, M. S. Medow, B. H. Natelson, J. M. Stewart, and S. J. Mathew. 2012. Increased ventricular lactate in chronic fatigue syndrome. III. Relationships to cortical glutathione and clinical symptoms implicate oxidative stress in disorder pathophysiology. *NMR in Biomedicine* 25(9):1073-1087.

Sisto, S. A., W. Tapp, S. Drastal, M. Bergen, I. DeMasi, D. Cordero, and B. Natelson. 1995. Vagal tone is reduced during paced breathing in patients with the chronic fatigue syndrome. *Clinical Autonomic Research* 5(3):139-143.

Sletten, D. M., G. A. Suarez, P. A. Low, J. Mandrekar, and W. Singer. 2012. COMPASS 31: A refined and abbreviated Composite Autonomic Symptom Score. *Mayo Clinic Proceedings* 87(12):1196-1201.

Smets, E. M., B. Garssen, B. Bonke, and J. C. De Haes. 1995. The Multidimensional Fatigue Inventory (MFI) psychometric qualities of an instrument to assess fatigue. *Journal of Psychosomatic Research* 39(3):315-325.

Smith, A. P., L. Borysiewicz, J. Pollock, M. Thomas, K. Perry, and M. Llewelyn. 1999. Acute fatigue in chronic fatigue syndrome patients. *Psychological Medicine* 29(2):283-290.

Smith, G. A., and M. Carew. 1987. Decision time unmasked: Individuals adopt different strategies. *Australian Journal of Psychology* 39(3):339-351.

Snell, C. R., S. R. Stevens, T. E. Davenport, and J. M. Van Ness. 2013. Discriminative validity of metabolic and workload measurements for identifying people with chronic fatigue syndrome. *Physical Therapy* 93(11):1484-1492.

Soetekouw, P., J. W. M. Lenders, G. Bleijenberg, T. Thien, and J. W. M. van der Meer. 1999. Autonomic function in patients with chronic fatigue syndrome. *Clinical Autonomic Research* 9(6):334-340.

Sorensen, B., J. E. Streib, M. Strand, B. Make, P. C. Giclas, M. Fleshner, and J. F. Jones. 2003. Complement activation in a model of chronic fatigue syndrome. *Journal of Allergy & Clinical Immunology* 112(2):397-403.

Spitzer, A. R., and M. Broadman. 2010a. A retrospective review of the sleep characteristics in patients with chronic fatigue syndrome and fibromyalgia. *Pain Practice* 10(4):294-300.

Spitzer, A. R., and M. Broadman. 2010b. Treatment of the narcoleptiform sleep disorder in chronic fatigue syndrome and fibromyalgia with sodium oxybate. *Pain Practice* 10(1): 54-59.

Spotila, J. 2010. *Post-exertional malaise in chronic fatigue syndrome.* Charlotte, NC: CFIDS Association of America.

Stewart, J. M., M. H. Gewitz, A. Weldon, and J. Munoz. 1999. Patterns of orthostatic intolerance: The orthostatic tachycardia syndrome and adolescent chronic fatigue. *Journal of Pediatrics* 135(2, Pt. 1):218-225.

Stewart, J. M., M. S. Medow, Z. R. Messer, I. L. Baugham, C. Terilli, and A. J. Ocon. 2012. Postural neurocognitive and neuronal activated cerebral blood flow deficits in young chronic fatigue syndrome patients with postural tachycardia syndrome. *American Journal of Physiology—Heart & Circulatory Physiology* 302(5):H1185-H1194.

Streeten, D. H. P. 2001. Role of impaired lower-limb venous innervation in the pathogenesis of the chronic fatigue syndrome. *American Journal of the Medical Sciences* 321(3):163-167.

Streeten, D. H., and G. H. Anderson, Jr. 1992. Delayed orthostatic intolerance. *Archives of Internal Medicine* 152(5):1066-1072.

Streeten, D. H. P., and D. S. Bell. 1998. Circulating blood volume in chronic fatigue syndrome. *Journal of Chronic Fatigue Syndrome* 4(1):3-11.

Streeten, D. H. P., D. Thomas, and D. S. Bell. 2000. The roles of orthostatic hypotension, orthostatic tachycardia, and subnormal erythrocyte volume in the pathogenesis of the chronic fatigue syndrome. *American Journal of the Medical Sciences* 320(1):1-8.

Suarez, G. A., T. L. Opfer-Gehrking, K. P. Offord, E. J. Atkinson, P. C. O'Brien, and P. A. Low. 1999. The autonomic symptom profile: A new instrument to assess autonomic symptoms. *Neurology* 52(3):523-528.

Takenaka, K., Y. Suzuki, K. Uno, M. Sato, T. Komuro, Y. Haruna, H. Kobayashi, K. Kawakubo, M. Sonoda, M. Asakawa, K. Nakahara, and A. Gunji. 2002. Effects of rapid saline infusion on orthostatic intolerance and autonomic tone after 20 days bed rest. *American Journal of Cardiology* 89(5):557-561.

Tanaka, H., R. Matsushima, H. Tamai, and Y. Kajimoto. 2002. Impaired postural cerebral hemodynamics in young patients with chronic fatigue with and without orthostatic intolerance. *Journal of Pediatrics* 140(4):412-417.

Taylor, H. L., E. Buskirk, and A. Henschel. 1955. Maximal oxygen intake as an objective measure of cardio-respiratory performance. *Journal of Applied Physiology* 8(1):73-80.

Taylor, R. R., L. A. Jason, and C. J. Curie. 2002. Prognosis of chronic fatigue in a community-based sample. *Psychosomatic Medicine* 64(2):319-327.

Thieben, M. J., P. Sandroni, D. M. Sletten, L. M. Benrud-Larson, R. D. Fealey, S. Vernino, V. A. Lennon, W. K. Shen, and P. A. Low. 2007. Postural orthostatic tachycardia syndrome: The Mayo Clinic experience. *Mayo Clinic Proceedings* 82(3):308-313.

Thorpy, M. J. 1992. The clinical use of the multiple sleep latency test. The standards of practice committee of the American sleep disorders association. *Sleep* 15(3):268-276.

Tiersky, L. A., S. K. Johnson, G. Lange, B. H. Natelson, and J. DeLuca. 1997. Neuropsychology of chronic fatigue syndrome: A critical review. *Journal of Clinical and Experimental Neuropsychology* 19(4):560-586.

Tiersky, L. A., R. J. Matheis, J. DeLuca, G. Lange, and B. H. Natelson. 2003. Functional status, neuropsychological functioning, and mood in chronic fatigue syndrome (CFS): Relationship to psychiatric disorder. *Journal of Nervous and Mental Disease* 191(5):324-331.

Timmers, H. J., W. Wieling, P. M. Soetekouw, G. Bleijenberg, J. W. van der Meer, and J. W. Lenders. 2002. Hemodynamic and neurohumoral responses to head-up tilt in patients with chronic fatigue syndrome. *Clinical Autonomic Research* 12(4):273-280.

Togo, F., and B. H. Natelson. 2013. Heart rate variability during sleep and subsequent sleepiness in patients with chronic fatigue syndrome. *Autonomic Neuroscience: Basic and Clinical* 176(1-2):85-90.

Togo, F., B. H. Natelson, N. S. Cherniack, J. FitzGibbons, C. Garcon, and D. M. Rapoport. 2008. Sleep structure and sleepiness in chronic fatigue syndrome with or without coexisting fibromyalgia. *Arthritis Research & Therapy* 10(3):R56.

Togo, F., B. H. Natelson, N. S. Cherniack, M. Klapholz, D. M. Rapoport, and D. B. Cook. 2010. Sleep is not disrupted by exercise in patients with chronic fatigue syndromes. *Medicine & Science in Sports & Exercise* 42(1):16-22.

Togo, F., G. Lange, B. H. Natelson, and K. S. Quigley. 2013. Attention network test: Assessment of cognitive function in chronic fatigue syndrome. *Journal of Neuropsychology.* http://onlinelibrary.wiley.com/doi/10.1111/jnp.12030/pdf (accessed January 14, 2015).

Tomfohr, L. M., S. Ancoli-Israel, J. S. Loredo, and J. E. Dimsdale. 2011. Effects of continuous positive airway pressure on fatigue and sleepiness in patients with obstructive sleep apnea: Data from a randomized controlled trial. *Sleep* 34(1):121-126.

Trivedi, M. H., A. J. Rush, R. Armitage, C. M. Gullion, B. D. Grannemann, P. J. Orsulak, and H. P. Roffwarg. 1999. Effects of fluoxetine on the polysomnogram in outpatients with major depression. *Neuropsychopharmacology* 20(5):447-459.

Unger, E. R., R. Nisenbaum, H. Moldofsky, A. Cesta, C. Sammut, M. Reyes, and W. C. Reeves. 2004. Sleep assessment in a population-based study of chronic fatigue syndrome. *BMC Neurology* 4.

Unger, E. R., A. H. Miller, J. F. Jones, D. F. Drake, H. Tian, and G. Pagnoni. 2012. Decreased basal ganglia activation in chronic fatigue syndrome subjects is associated with increased fatigue. *The FASEB Journal* 26.

Van de Luit, L., J. Van der Meulen, T. J. M. Cleophas, and A. H. Zwinderman. 1998. Amplified amplitudes of circadian rhythms and night time hypotension in patients with chronic fatigue syndrome; improvement by inopamil but not by melatonin. *European Journal of Internal Medicine* 9(2):99-103.

Van Den Eede, F., G. Moorkens, W. Hulstijn, Y. Maas, D. Schrijvers, S. R. Stevens, P. Cosyns, S. J. Claes, and B. G. C. Sabbe. 2011. Psychomotor function and response inhibition in chronic fatigue syndrome. *Psychiatry Research* 186(2-3):367-372.

Van Oosterwijck, J., J. Nijs, M. Meeus, I. Lefever, L. Huybrechts, L. Lambrecht, and L. Paul. 2010. Pain inhibition and postexertional malaise in myalgic encephalomyelitis/chronic fatigue syndrome: An experimental study. *Journal of Internal Medicine* 268(3):265-278.

VanNess, J. M., C. R. Snell, and S. R. Stevens. 2007. Diminished cardiopulmonary capacity during post-exertional malaise. *Journal of Chronic Fatigue Syndrome* 14:77-85.

VanNess, J. M., S. R. Stevens, L. Bateman, T. L. Stiles, and C. R. Snell. 2010. Postexertional malaise in women with chronic fatigue syndrome. *Journal of Women's Health* 19(2):239-244.

Vercoulen, J. H. M. M., E. Bazelmans, C. M. A. Swanink, J. M. D. Galama, J. F. M. Fennis, J. W. M. van der Meer, and G. Bleijenberg. 1998. Evaluating neuropsychological impairment in chronic fatigue syndrome. *Journal of Clinical and Experimental Neuropsychology* 20(2):144-156.

Vermeulen, R. C., and H. R. Scholte. 2003. Rupture of silicone gel breast implants and symptoms of pain and fatigue. *Journal of Rheumatology* 30(10):2263-2267.

Vermeulen, R. C. W., R. M. Kurk, F. C. Visser, W. Sluiter, and H. R. Scholte. 2010. Patients with chronic fatigue syndrome performed worse than controls in a controlled repeated exercise study despite a normal oxidative phosphorylation capacity. *Journal of Translational Medicine* 8(93).

Wagner, D., R. Nisenbaum, C. Heim, J. F. Jones, E. R. Unger, and W. C. Reeves. 2005. Psychometric properties of the CDC symptom inventory for assessment of chronic fatigue syndrome. *Population Health Metrics* 3:8.

Ware, J. E. 2002. SF-36 Health Survey. In Chronic fatigue and chronic fatigue syndrome: A co-twin control study of functional status. *Quality of Life Research* 11:463-471.

Watson, N. F., V. Kapur, L. M. Arguelles, J. Goldberg, D. F. Schmidt, R. Armitage, and D. Buchwald. 2003. Comparison of subjective and objective measures of insomnia in monozygotic twins discordant for chronic fatigue syndrome. *Sleep* 26(3):324-328.

Watson, N. F., C. Jacobsen, J. Goldberg, V. Kapur, and D. Buchwald. 2004. Subjective and objective sleepiness in monozygotic twins discordant for chronic fatigue syndrome. *Sleep* 27(5):973-977.

Weltman, A., D. Snead, P. Stein, R. Seip, R. Schurrer, R. Rutt, and J. Weltman. 1990. Reliability and validity of a continuous incremental treadmill protocol for the determination of lactate threshold, fixed blood lactate concentrations, and VO_2max. *International Journal of Sports Medicine* 11(1):26-32.

Whelton, C. L., I. Salit, and H. Moldofsky. 1992. Sleep, Epstein-Barr virus infection, musculoskeletal pain, and depressive symptoms in chronic fatigue syndrome. *Journal of Rheumatology* 19(6):939-943.

White, A. T., A. R. Light, R. W. Hughen, L. Bateman, T. B. Martins, H. R. Hill, and K. C. Light. 2010. Severity of symptom flare after moderate exercise is linked to cytokine activity in chronic fatigue syndrome. *Psychophysiology* 47(4):615-624.

White, A. T., A. R. Light, R. W. Hughen, T. A. VanHaitsma, and K. C. Light. 2012. Differences in metabolite-detecting, adrenergic, and immune gene expression after moderate exercise in patients with chronic fatigue syndrome, patients with multiple sclerosis, and healthy controls. *Psychosomatic Medicine* 74(1):46-54.

Whitehead, L. 2009. The measurement of fatigue in chronic illness: A systematic review of unidimensional and multidimensional fatigue measures. *Journal of Pain and Symptom Management* 37(1):107-128.

Wiborg, J. F., S. van der Werf, J. B. Prins, and G. Bleijenberg. 2010. Being homebound with chronic fatigue syndrome: A multidimensional comparison with outpatients. *Psychiatry Research* 177(1-2):246-249.

Wilson, A., I. Hickie, A. Lloyd, D. Hadzi-Pavlovic, C. Boughton, J. Dwyer, and D. Wakefield. 1994. Longitudinal study of outcome of chronic fatigue syndrome. *British Medical Journal* 308(6931):756-759.

Winkler, A. S., D. Blair, J. T. Marsden, T. J. Peters, S. Wessely, and A. J. Cleare. 2004. Autonomic function and serum erythropoietin levels in chronic fatigue syndrome. *Journal of Psychosomatic Research* 56(2):179-183.

Wyller, V. B., R. Barbieri, E. Thaulow, and J. P. Saul. 2008. Enhanced vagal withdrawal during mild orthostatic stress in adolescents with chronic fatigue. *Annals of Noninvasive Electrocardiology* 13(1):67-73.

Yamaguti, K., S. Tajima, and H. Kuratsune. 2013. Autonomic dysfunction in chronic fatigue syndrome. *Advances in Neuroimmune Biology* 4(4):281-289.

Yamamoto, Y., J. J. LaManca, and B. H. Natelson. 2003. A measure of heart rate variability is sensitive to orthostatic challenge in women with chronic fatigue syndrome. *Experimental Biology & Medicine* 228(2):167-174.

Yataco, A., H. Talo, P. Rowe, D. A. Kass, R. D. Berger, and H. Calkin. 1997. Comparison of heart rate variability in patients with chronic fatigue syndrome and controls. *Clinical Autonomic Research* 7(6):293-297.

Yoshiuchi, K., D. B. Cook, K. Ohashi, H. Kumano, T. Kuboki, Y. Yamamoto, and B. H. Natelson. 2007. A real-time assessment of the effect of exercise in chronic fatigue syndrome. *Physiology & Behavior* 92(5):963-968.

Zhang, L., J. Gough, D. Christmas, D. L. Mattey, S. C. Richards, J. Main, D. Enlander, D. Honeybourne, J. G. Ayres, D. J. Nutt, and J. R. Kerr. 2010. Microbial infections in eight genomic subtypes of chronic fatigue syndrome/myalgic encephalomyelitis. *Journal of Clinical Pathology* 63(2):156-164.

5

Review of the Evidence on Other ME/CFS Symptoms and Manifestations

This chapter reviews the evidence on symptoms and manifestations of ME/CFS other than the major ones addressed in Chapter 4. Discussed in turn are pain, immune impairment, neuroendocrine manifestations, and infection.

PAIN

Description of Pain in ME/CFS

Pain is a defining characteristic of ME/CFS and is listed as either a required or additional symptom in all case definitions and diagnostic criteria evaluated in this report. The existing ME/CFS case definitions include muscle pain, joint pain, headaches, tender lymph nodes, and sore throat as pain symptoms (Carruthers et al., 2003, 2011; Fukuda et al., 1994; Jason et al., 2010; NICE, 2007). The Canadian Consensus Criteria (CCC), the Revised CCC, and the 2011 International Consensus Criteria for ME (ME-ICC) mention additional symptoms—including abdominal pain, chest pain, hyperalgesia, and stiffness—and such descriptors as myofascial, radiating, and migratory pain. Patients also described chronic pain behind the eyes, neck pain, neuropathic or nerve pain, "full-body ice-cream-headache-like pains," and feeling like "my brain was going to explode" (FDA, 2013, p. 14).

The majority of ME/CFS patients experience some type of pain, although individual experiences with pain vary widely (FDA, 2013; Meeus et al., 2007; Unger, 2013). In one community-based study, 94 percent of respondents fulfilling the Fukuda definition reported muscle aches and pain,

141

and 84 percent reported joint pain (Jason et al., 1999). Recent preliminary data from the Centers for Disease Control and Prevention's (CDC's) Multi-Site Clinical Study of CFS indicate that 80 percent of patients enrolled had experienced pain in the past week (Unger, 2013). Muscle aches and pains were the most common pain complaint (reported by 72 to 79 percent of patients), followed by joint pain (reported by 58 to 60 percent of patients) and headaches (reported by 48 to 56 percent of patients). Less common pain complaints included tender lymph nodes (37 to 39 percent), abdominal pain (32 percent), sore throat (25 to 28 percent), eye pain (23 percent), and chest pain (15 percent).[1,2]

Pain interferes similarly in the life of someone with ME/CFS and someone with spinal cord injury, muscular dystrophy, or multiple sclerosis[3] (Unger, 2013). More severely disabled ME/CFS patients may experience more pain (Marshall et al., 2010). Regardless of the definitions used, the presence of chronic regional and widespread pain in individuals with ME/CFS is associated with poor general health, physical functioning, and sleep quality independently of ME/CFS (Aaron et al., 2002). In a systematic review of chronic musculoskeletal pain in ME/CFS (which included studies using various ME/CFS diagnostic criteria), Meeus and colleagues (2007) concluded that there is no consensus on the definition of chronic widespread pain in ME/CFS, and while there is no strong proof of its exact cause or prevalence, this pain is strongly disabling and not necessarily related to depression.

Patients diagnosed with ME/CFS experience more pain than the general population (Ickmans et al., 2013; Jason et al., 2013b). Employing moderate thresholds for frequency and severity, Jason and colleagues (2013b) found that a greater percentage of ME/CFS patients experienced pain symptoms relative to healthy controls (see Figure 5-1).[4]

Pain in ME/CFS often is a component of post-exertional malaise (PEM), a symptom constellation triggered or worsened by physical and/or mental activity (see the discussion of PEM in Chapter 4). Exercise has

---

[1] Personal communication from Elizabeth Unger, 2014. Preliminary analysis of CDC Multi-Site Clinical Study.

[2] The percentages in the preceding two sentences reflect patients reporting that each symptom occurred with moderate severity at least half of the time.

[3] The mean Patient-Reported Outcomes Measurement Information System (PROMIS) t scores for pain interference in the CDC Multi-Site Clinical Study were similar to or slightly higher than the scores published for spinal cord injury, muscular dystrophy, and multiple sclerosis (Unger, 2013).

[4] Jason and colleagues (2013b) compared 236 ME/CFS patients with 86 healthy controls who completed the DePaul Symptom Questionnaire, rating the frequency and severity of 54 symptoms. Patient data were obtained from the SolveCFS BioBank, which includes patients diagnosed by a licensed physician using either the Fukuda definition or CCC.

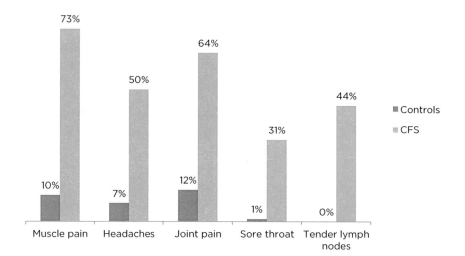

FIGURE 5-1 Percentage of ME/CFS patients and healthy controls reporting pain symptoms of at least moderate severity that occurred at least half of the time for the past 6 months.
NOTE: All patients fulfilled the Fukuda definition for CFS.
SOURCE: Jason et al., 2013b.

been shown to decrease pain threshold, increase pain severity, and worsen global symptoms in patients with ME/CFS compared with healthy controls (Van Oosterwijck et al., 2010; Whiteside et al., 2004) and in patients with both ME/CFS and fibromyalgia compared with patients with rheumatoid arthritis and healthy controls (Meeus et al., 2014).

Assessment of Pain in ME/CFS

Tools useful for evaluating pain clinically in ME/CFS include the 1990 and 2010 American College of Rheumatology (ACR) fibromyalgia criteria, numeric or visual analog scales (VASs), the Fibromyalgia Impact Questionnaire (FIQ), the Revised Fibromyalgia Impact Questionnaire (FIQR), and the Brief Pain Inventory (BPI) (Bennett et al., 2009; Boomershine, 2012). The VAS and the BPI are highly validated across many pain conditions, and the FIQ and FIQR are highly validated for fibromyalgia (Bennett et al., 2009; Herr and Garand, 2001; McCormack et al., 1988). Other tools used to assess pain include the Short Form 36-Item Questionnaire (SF-36) of the Medical Outcomes Study (MOS) and Patient-Reported Outcomes Measurement Information System (PROMIS) instruments for pain interference and pain behavior (Boomershine, 2012; Komaroff et al., 1996).[5] Preliminary data from the CDC Multi-Site Clinical Study of CFS were used to compare pain interference scores as measured by PROMIS and the BPI, revealing a 0.75 correlation. PROMIS instruments are used primarily for research, while the BPI is an assessment tool more readily accessible to clinicians (Unger, 2013). Several instruments that were validated for diagnosing ME/CFS—the DePaul Symptom Questionnaire, CDC Symptom Inventory (SI), and CFS Questionnaire—include measures of pain (Jason et al., 2012).

Evidence for Pain in ME/CFS

The literature does not provide evidence on the cause, nature, and relevance of pain in ME/CFS as compared with normal controls, other subjectively defined conditions such as fibromyalgia, or other chronic pain conditions. Although some studies have investigated pain in ME/CFS and fibromyalgia, the ability to make comparisons across studies is limited by the use of varying case definitions. It is also challenging to elicit the characteristics and severity of pain attributable solely to ME/CFS in patients with comorbid fibromyalgia and ME/CFS. Nonetheless, the severity and frequency of pain have been studied in ME/CFS patients.

Pain Symptoms in Different Diagnostic Categories

Although pain symptoms are listed in all recent diagnostic criteria for ME/CFS, some of the diagnostic criteria identify patients with more frequent and more debilitating pain symptoms. In various studies, persons fulfilling the CCC,[6] a revised definition of ME,[7] and ME-ICC were found to have significantly greater disability due to bodily pain (as measured by the bodily pain subscale of the SF-36) than those fulfilling the Fukuda definition (Brown et al., 2013; Jason et al., 2012, 2013a, 2014b). People fulfilling the CCC and revised definition of ME also reported significantly worse (in terms of frequency and severity) headaches, chest pain, abdomen pain, eye

---

[5] PROMIS "is a system of highly reliable, precise measures of patient-reported health status for physical, mental, and social well-being. PROMIS tools measure what patients are able to do and how they feel by asking questions. PROMIS'[s] measures can be used as primary or secondary endpoints in clinical studies of the effectiveness of treatment" (http://www.nihpromis.org/about/abouthome [accessed January 14, 2015]).

[6] In one study, frequency and severity were specified according to the Revised CCC (Jason et al., 2013a). In another, for key symptoms, individuals had to have a frequency score of 2 or higher and symptoms had to be moderate or severe (rated at 50 or higher) as reported on the CFS Questionnaire (Jason et al., 2012).

[7] Jason and colleagues (2012) created a revised case definition based on past case definitions, requiring PEM, neurological manifestation, and autonomic dysfunction.

pain, and tender/sore lymph nodes than those fulfilling the Fukuda defini-tion (Jason et al., 2012). Those fulfilling the ME-ICC reported significantly worse headaches, chest pain, eye pain, muscle pain, pain in multiple joints, and tender/sore lymph nodes than those fulfilling the Fukuda definition (Brown et al., 2013; Jason et al., 2014b). In one study, those fulfilling the ME-ICC also experienced significantly worse abdomen/stomach pain and bloating than those fulfilling the Fukuda definition (Jason et al., 2014b).

Pain Symptoms in Other Fatigue Conditions

Chest pain and lymph node pain are more frequent in persons fulfill-ing the CCC than in those with chronic fatigue explained by psychiatric illness. Persons fulfilling the Fukuda definition experience more abdominal pain than those with chronic fatigue explained by psychiatric illness (Jason et al., 2004).

Pain Symptoms in Other Chronic Pain Conditions

Some evidence indicates that pain experienced by those with ME/CFS is different from chronic pain experienced in other conditions. For example, severity of pain has been associated with impaired cognitive performance in other chronic pain conditions such as fibromyalgia, chronic whiplash-associated disorders, and chronic low back pain (Antepohl et al., 2003; Park et al., 2001; Weiner et al., 2006). Pain levels in ME/CFS are similar to pain levels in other chronic pain conditions, however, pain severity is not correlated with cognitive impairment in ME/CFS, a finding suggesting that the pain in ME/CFS may be unique (Ickmans et al., 2013).

ME/CFS and Fibromyalgia

Population-based studies predict the prevalence of fibromyalgia to be 3-5 percent and the prevalence of ME/CFS to be 0.5-1 percent. The overlap of fibromyalgia and ME/CFS ranges from 20 to 70 percent across a number of studies using the 1990 ACR fibromyalgia criteria (Meeus et al., 2007). The revised 2010 ACR fibromyalgia criteria—which exclude the tender point exam; score pain distribution numerically; and include severity scores for fatigue, brain fog, unrefreshing sleep, and multisystem complaints—may greatly increase the overlap between ME/CFS and fibromyalgia (Wolfe et al., 2010).

The reason for this overlap of ME/CFS with the ACR fibromyalgia criteria has not been rigorously discussed. Some researchers suggested that the reason for the overlap has to do with both syndromes being a mani-festation of somatic amplification (Clauw, 2014). There is a comparatively large evidence base supporting fibromyalgia as a process involving heightened central sensitivity, hyperalgesia, and sensory amplification, causing widespread pain and contributing to other associated symptoms such as fatigue, brain fog, and unrefreshing sleep (Clauw, 2014). Other researchers used the existence of separate case definitions to ask the empirical question of whether the two syndromes are the same or different. Unfortunately, most studies on the pathophysiology of ME/CFS do not evaluate ME/CFS subjects with fibromyalgia separately from those unaffected by fibromyalgia, nor do they compare them with patients with fibromyalgia who do not meet ME/CFS criteria (Abbi and Natelson, 2013). This is primarily because ME/CFS studies do not assess the bodily distribution of pain and presence of hyperalgesia as defined by the tender point exam, and fibromyalgia studies do not use published case definitions to identify those fibromyalgia patients with comorbid ME/CFS (Reeves et al., 2007; Reyes et al., 2003; White et al., 1999; Wolfe et al., 1995).

Studies that do examine the differences between ME/CFS + fibromyalgia and ME/CFS alone suggest that the addition of widespread pain with tenderness to the usual diagnostic symptoms of ME/CFS leads to qualitative differences between the two groups. The first of these differences relates to spinal fluid Substance P, which has been shown to be elevated in fibromyalgia but not in ME/CFS (Evengård et al., 1998; Russell et al., 1994). While these studies were done on separate groups of ME/CFS or fibromyalgia patients, more recent studies carefully identified patients with ME/CFS alone, fibromyalgia alone, or ME/CFS with coexisting fibromyalgia. The results of these studies suggest that the pathophysiology of each group may present differently. Naschitz and colleagues (2008) used tilt table testing to develop a "hemodynamic instability score" based on blood pressure and heart rate changes, which enabled them to differentiate patients with ME/CFS alone from those with fibromyalgia alone. Natelson and colleagues conducted a number of studies comparing patients with ME/CFS alone and those with ME/CFS and fibromyalgia (Ciccone and Natelson, 2003; Cook et al., 2005, 2006; Natelson, 2010). Except for deficits in cognitive function, which were more prominent in the ME/CFS-only group (Cook et al., 2005), having comorbid fibromyalgia was an illness multiplier for patients with ME/CFS: self-ratings of severity of muscle and joint pain were higher and physical function on the SF-36 lower in the ME/CFS + fibromyalgia group; in addition, the rate of lifetime major depressive disorder was 52 percent in the ME/CFS + fibromyalgia group, approximately twice that seen in the ME/CFS-only group (Ciccone and Natelson, 2003). While no differences between ME/CFS patients and controls were found in any cardiopulmonary variable studied during a maximal stress test, patients with ME/CFS + fibromyalgia, but not those with ME/CFS only, perceived the exercise to be both more painful and more effortful compared with controls (Cook et al., 2006).

Summary

Sufficient evidence shows that pain is common in ME/CFS, and its presentation supports the diagnosis. However, while pain worsens ME/CFS when present, there is no conclusive evidence that the pain experienced by ME/CFS patients can be distinguished from that experienced by healthy people or those with other illnesses. Further, pain may be experienced in many areas, and while comprehensively assessing a patient's pain symptoms is a challenging task, it is not specific to ME/CFS.

Conclusion: *The committee elected not to include pain as a required element of its recommended diagnostic criteria for ME/CFS.*

IMMUNE IMPAIRMENT

Description of Immune Impairment in ME/CFS

Symptoms related to inflammation are reported frequently by ME/CFS patients. When attempting to convey their illness experience to healthy persons, many patients describe it as similar to a perpetual flu-like state (Maupin, 2014). Patients also report persistent or recurrent sore throats, tender/swollen cervical and/or axillary lymph nodes, muscle pain, achy joints without swelling or redness, headaches, chills, "feverishness" (but not necessarily meeting objective criteria for fever), and new or worsened sensitivities to certain substances (e.g., foods, odors, medications) (FDA, 2013). Interestingly, "susceptibility to infections" was among the most common written-in symptoms submitted to the Food and Drug Administration during its April 2013 Drug Development Workshop for ME/CFS (FDA, 2013). These symptoms can fluctuate and may be unmasked or exacerbated with physical or cognitive activity as part of the constellation of symptoms associated with the individual patient's PEM (see the section on PEM in Chapter 4).

All of the case definitions evaluated in this report include some inflammatory symptoms and/or signs; however, whether such symptoms or signs are mandatory and which are included varies among the definitions. The clinical case definition most commonly used in the United States, the Fukuda definition of 1994, includes five symptoms that are sometimes associated with systemic inflammation (tender cervical/axillary lymph nodes, joint pain, muscle pain, headache, and sore throat), but no specific symptom or group of symptoms is required (Fukuda et al., 1994). It is not clear, moreover, whether these symptoms have an infectious or inflammatory etiology in ME/CFS.

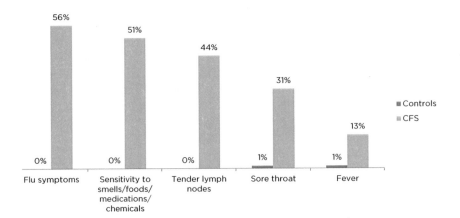

FIGURE 5-2 Percentage of ME/CFS patients and healthy controls reporting immune-related symptoms of at least moderate severity that occurred at least half of the time for the past 6 months.
NOTE: All patients fulfilled the Fukuda definition for CFS.
SOURCE: Jason et al., 2013b.

Although the prevalence of inflammatory symptoms reported in the literature ranges widely across studies that vary in time period, location, and case definition, it is evident that rates of this category of symptoms are elevated in ME/CFS patients: sore throat (19 to 84 percent), muscle pain (63 to 95 percent), joint pain (55 to 85 percent), tender/swollen axillary or cervical lymph nodes (23 to 76 percent), fever and/or chills (13 to 64 percent), flu-like feelings (56 to 81 percent), and new/worsened sensitivities (51 to 55 percent) (De Becker et al., 2001; Janal et al., 2006; Jason et al., 2013b; Kerr et al., 2010; Nacul et al., 2011; Naess et al., 2010; Solomon and Reeves, 2004). Jason and colleagues (2013b) showed that the presence of tender lymph nodes and sore throat was much greater in ME/CFS patients than in healthy controls (see Figure 5-2).

Assessment of Immune Impairment in ME/CFS

The evidence reviewed in this section pertains to the research setting because the usefulness of the tests employed in these studies has not yet been proved in the clinical setting. Alterations of natural killer (NK) cell count and function and perturbations in cytokine production have been the biomarkers studied most extensively because they have shown the most promising results.

NK cells are a part of the innate immune system and play an important role in preventing latent viruses from reactivating as well as in tumor surveillance. NK cell count is ascertained primarily by assay based on flow cytometry. Cytokine levels and function are most commonly measured through examination of plasma distribution via blood sample, but they may also be measured in cell supernatants following mitogenic stimulation of cells (Brenu et al., 2011, 2012b, 2014) or through various genomic methods (Carlo-Stella et al., 2006; Nakamura et al., 2013; Zhang et al., 2011). Most studies have not looked at cytokine function in the sense of measuring how well they function in their role as messengers (e.g., activation of the Janus kinase/signal transducer and activator of transcription [JAK-STAT] system). Other biomarkers with less consistent findings include humoral immunity and cellular cytotoxicity (Fischer et al., 2014). Overall, there is a large amount of variability across study protocols and laboratories in the methodology used for assessing biomarkers of immunology, which may contribute to inconsistency in the literature (Lyall et al., 2003).

Evidence for Immune Impairment in ME/CFS

The committee searched the literature for evidence with which to respond to one main question with respect to immunology: Is there a distinguishing feature of immune profile or function in ME/CFS? The methodology for the committee's review of the literature is described in Chapter 1.

Impaired Immune Function

One of the most consistent findings in ME/CFS subjects is poor NK cell function. Using K562 cells as target cells, 16 of 17 studies reviewed found poor function in subjects compared with healthy controls. However, this finding should be interpreted with caution as even the strongest of these studies are subject to methodological limitations discussed at the beginning of Chapter 4. Furthermore, it is unclear from the description of the methodology of some of the studies whether multiple studies included the same subjects. The largest study compared 176 ME/CFS subjects with 230 healthy controls and found a significant group effect of poorer NK cell function in the ME/CFS cohort (Fletcher et al., 2010). Curriu and colleagues (2013) showed that there were differences in mean cytotoxicity between ME/CFS subjects and healthy controls, but the range was the same. Brenu and colleagues (2012b) studied 65 ME/CFS patients and 21 matched controls in a longitudinal study of three time points over 12 months and found significant deficits in NK cytotoxic activity in the patient group at each time point using peripheral blood mononuclear cells (PBMCs) and a flow cytometric measure of killing. Caligiuri and colleagues (1987) demonstrated reduced cytotoxic activity of ME/CFS NK cells to K562 targets. On the other hand, one study with 26 ME/CFS patients and 50 controls failed to demonstrate impaired NK cell function in the ME/CFS patients using a K562 chromium (Cr) release assay of peripheral blood lymphocytes (PBLs) (Mawle et al., 1997). The authors of this study do not report NK cell counts or CD3-CD56+, but as described, NK numbers generally are not low in ME/CFS.

Low NK cytotoxicity is not specific to ME/CFS. It is also reported to be present in patients with rheumatoid arthritis, cancer, and endometriosis (Meeus et al., 2009; Oosterlynck et al., 1991; Richter et al., 2010). It is present as well in healthy individuals who are older, smokers, psychologically stressed, depressed, physically deconditioned, or sleep deprived (Fondell et al., 2011; Whiteside and Friberg, 1998; Zeidel et al., 2002).

A few studies found a correlation between the severity of NK cell functional impairment and the severity of disease in ME/CFS patients (Lutgendorf et al., 1995; Ojo-Amaize et al., 1994; Siegel et al., 2006). Others looked at mechanisms of cellular dysfunction in ME/CFS and identified abnormalities in early activation markers (Mihaylova et al., 2007) and perforin and granzyme concentration (Maher et al., 2005), as well as in the genes that regulate these cellular functions (Brenu et al., 2011, 2012a). However, no replication studies have been published.

There also are studies enumerating the numbers of NK cells in ME/CFS patients, sometimes employing different identifying markers. NK cell count shows substantial heterogeneity in these patients, and there are no consistent findings (Barker et al., 1994; Brenu et al., 2010, 2011, 2012b; Caligiuri et al., 1987; Curriu et al., 2013; Fletcher et al., 2010; Gupta and Vayuvegula, 1991; Henderson, 2014; Klimas et al., 1990; Levine et al., 1998; Maher et al., 2005; Mawle et al., 1997; Natelson et al., 1998; Peakman et al., 1997; Stewart et al., 2003; Straus et al., 1993; Tirelli et al., 1994).

Immune Activation

Immune activation has been studied using a variety of methods. The most consistent results are reported on pro-inflammatory cytokine production.

Cytokine abnormalities have been hypothesized to play a role in the pathogenesis of ME/CFS, although findings to support this idea are varied and inconsistent. Research to date has addressed levels of pro-inflammatory cytokines in ME/CFS patients compared with healthy controls.

The majority of studies yielded no significant findings (Jammes et al., 2009; Nakamura et al., 2010; Neu et al., 2014; White et al., 2010), including one study of monozygotic twins discordant for disease that showed no difference in pro-inflammatory cytokine levels between the affected and unaffected twins (Vollmer-Conna et al., 2007). However, several studies found elevated pro-inflammatory cytokine levels, particularly for TNF-α, in ME/CFS patients (Brenu et al., 2011, 2012b, 2014; Broderick et al., 2012; Maes et al., 2013; Neu et al., 2014).

Sample sizes of individual studies generally have been small, and only a few types of pro-inflammatory cytokines have been measured in multiple studies. Two studies used subgrouping to identify differences in cytokine levels between those with low and high prevalence, duration, or severity of PEM (Maes et al., 2012) or after physical exertion (White et al., 2010). In one study, postexercise increases in both pro-inflammatory and anti-inflammatory cytokines were associated with more severe symptom flares after exertion (White et al., 2010).

Fewer peer-reviewed papers report on functional studies of other aspects of immune function, and these studies yielded less consistent findings. There are reports of Immunoglobulin G (IgG) subclass deficiencies, diminished T and B cell response to mitogens, and abnormalities of neutrophil and macrophage functions. However, the subjects studied were limited to small series, and there are no replication studies (Fletcher et al., 2009; Lattie et al., 2012; Nakamura et al., 2013; Neu et al., 2014).

Emerging Areas

Autoimmunity ME/CFS has been reported to be associated with autoimmune disorders such as hypothyroidism and Sjogren's syndrome, raising the question of whether the disease may have an autoimmune component (Gaber and Oo, 2013; Nishikai et al., 1996; Sirois and Natelson, 2001). Antibodies frequently seen in other systemic autoimmune/rheumatic diseases are reported inconsistently in ME/CFS in the literature published to date. The prevalence of antinuclear antibodies in subjects varies widely (from 7 to 68 percent); antibody titers tend to be on the low side (less than 1:160); and no antigen (e.g., dsDNA, SS-A, Scl-70) has been identified as a unique marker (Buchwald and Komaroff, 1991; Konstantinov et al., 1996; Op De Beéck et al., 2012; Skowera et al., 2002; Tanaka et al., 2003; vonMikecz et al., 1997).

Three separate studies do point to one unusual antigen—the nuclear envelope protein lamin B, which has been associated with primary biliary cirrhosis. ME/CFS subjects with antibodies to this protein may be more likely to be affected by hypersomnia and cognitive difficulties (Konstantinov et al., 1996; Nishikai et al., 2001; vonMikecz et al., 1997); however, these observations have not been replicated in the ensuing years. Studies also found wide variation in autoantibodies to neural antigens (9 to 62 percent) (Klein and Berg, 1995; Ortega-Hernandez et al., 2009; Vernon and Reeves,

2005; vonMikecz et al., 1997) and cellular membranes (4 to 95 percent) (Hokama et al., 2009; Klein and Berg, 1995; Maes et al., 2006; Ortega-Hernandez et al., 2009). In other studies, ME/CFS or postviral fatigue syndrome patients showed antibodies to smooth muscle (36 percent) (Behan et al., 1985), heat shock protein 60 (24 percent) (Elfaitouri et al., 2013), and endothelial antigens (30 percent) (Ortega-Hernandez et al., 2009). The only clinical trial targeting antibodies found moderate to marked clinical improvements in 10 of 15 subjects treated with rituximab, a B cell depleting antibody, and 2 of 15 placebo arm subjects at a single time point (Fluge et al., 2011). This, however, was a post hoc analysis as the trial failed to meet its primary endpoint. Currently, researchers in the United Kingdom and Norway are conducting further studies addressing this question (Edwards, 2013; Mella and Fluge, 2014).

Systems biology Several groups are looking at the immune endocrine/ neuropeptide homeostatic balance in innovative ways that could lead to a better understanding of ME/CFS. Using genomic and proteomic techniques together with studies of immune function, immune activation, and chemokine/cytokine expression represents a "big picture" approach to a complex illness, although no significant risk alleles or disease signatures have yet been identified (Presson et al., 2009; Smylie et al., 2013).

Summary

The committee's literature review yielded data demonstrating poor NK cell cytotoxicity (NK cell function, not number) that correlates with illness severity in ME/CFS patients and could serve as a biomarker for the severity of the disease, although it is not specific to ME/CFS. More research is needed to address cytokine abnormalities and their potential use as biomarkers of possibly distinct subgroups of ME/CFS.

Conclusion: Sufficient evidence supports the finding of immune dysfunction in ME/CFS.

NEUROENDOCRINE MANIFESTATIONS

Description of Neuroendocrine Manifestations in ME/CFS

Linking a disease manifestation to a specific neuroendocrine abnormality is difficult. Neuroendocrine dysregulation or abnormalities may manifest with nonspecific signs and symptoms that present across multiple organ systems. Such manifestations as fatigue, achiness, weakness, sleep disturbances, and cognitive fog are nonspecific symptoms that may or may

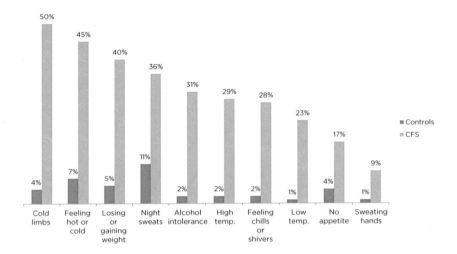

FIGURE 5-3 Percentage of ME/CFS patients and healthy controls reporting neuroendocrine manifestations of at least moderate severity that occurred at least half of the time for the past 6 months.
NOTE: All patients fulfilled the Fukuda definition for CFS.
SOURCE: Jason et al., 2013b.

not be caused by an underlying neuroendocrine abnormality. Further, if a neuroendocrine abnormality is contributing to these symptoms, it may be a secondary process.

The term and symptom category "neuroendocrine manifestations" appeared for the first time in the CCC. The Revised CCC retains the same group of symptoms, while the ME-ICC mentions only a few of these symptoms but classifies them under the "energy production/transportation impairments" category. According to Jason and colleagues (2013b), a greater percentage of ME/CFS patients compared to controls experience such symptoms as cold limbs, feeling hot or cold, losing or gaining weight, and night sweats compared with healthy controls (see Figure 5-3).

Assessment of Neuroendocrine Manifestations in ME/CFS

The complex multisystem nature of symptoms in ME/CFS patients has led researchers to explore central neural mechanisms such as dysregulation of the hypothalamic-pituitary-adrenal (HPA) and HP-growth hormone axes and the 5-hydroxytryptamine (5-HT) serotoninergic system (Fischer et al., 2014).

Numerous studies have focused on the HPA axis and measured cortisol concentrations in blood, saliva, and urine to assess the awakening, diurnal, and evening fluctuations in ME/CFS patients (Tomas et al., 2013). Researchers also have studied the role of the HP-growth hormone axis in ME/CFS and measured levels of growth hormone, insulin-like growth factor 1 (IGF-1), IGF-2, and IGF-binding protein 1 (IGFBP-1) (Allain et al., 1997). Various methods have been used to assess the HPA axis indirectly, including standardized stressors such as insulin-induced hypoglycemia; psychological duress or vigorous exercise; and administration of 5-HT (serotonin) precursors or receptor agonists, opioid antagonists, corticotropin-releasing hormone (CRH), or arginine vasopressin (AVP) (Tomas et al., 2013). For assessment of the 5-HT system, studies have measured plasma concentrations of 5-HT precursors (total and free tryptophan) in response to pharmacological challenge (i.e., d-fenfluramine) (Georgiades et al., 2003). A few other studies have examined both a serotonin transporter (5-HTT) gene promoter polymorphism and the density of serotonin transporters in the brain using positron emission tomography (PET) (Yamamoto et al., 2004).

Evidence for Neuroendocrine Manifestations in ME/CFS

Evaluation of the neuroendocrine literature was difficult for multiple reasons. First, there are myriad possible neuroendocrine abnormalities with different underlying pathophysiology. The physiology is sometimes complex, and knowledge about some of the physiology is evolving. For example, hormones of the neuroendocrine system generally are released in a pulsatile, cyclic, or feedback (negative and positive) responsive manner and in minutely detectable amounts. They may act on or be produced in several areas of the brain and be stored and released in others. Complex stimuli, including most of the "stressors" experienced by humans, are involved in their modulation and release, including peripheral and central signaling and sensory, autonomic, sleep, and emotional triggers, along with the positive and negative feedback of other endocrine signaling (Longo et al., 2012).

Second, studies addressing neuroendocrine manifestations have been heterogeneous and had multiple limitations, as described in Chapter 4. Most studies involved participants diagnosed with ME/CFS using the Fukuda definition, and they compared parameters in ME/CFS and healthy participants who were matched on age and gender. Few studies involved ME/CFS participants recruited from community samples or had comparison groups including patients with comorbidities. Studies evaluated multiple different stressors and used various measures to assess manifestations and outcomes. Some manifestations, such as fatigue severity and functional limitations, were rarely assessed. Cross-sectional comparisons that could not tease out cause-and-effect relationships were common. Some studies were small or exploratory and involved multiple statistical comparisons. Others failed to control for such important factors as time of day of measurement or sleep quality on the night before neuroendocrine evaluation.

The committee conducted a literature search with emphasis on the HPA axis to explore the following questions: (1) Are particular neuroendocrine abnormalities or manifestations pathognomonic for ME/CFS? and (2) How do neuroendocrine manifestations experienced by adults diagnosed with ME/CFS differ from those experienced by adults diagnosed with other chronic illnesses?

Hypothalamic-Pituitary-Adrenal Axis

The question of the contribution of low cortisol to ME/CFS was galvanized by a 1991 study demonstrating reduced 24-hour urinary cortisol in ME/CFS patients (Demitrack et al., 1991). Numerous studies found reduced overnight cortisol or 24-hour cortisol in patients compared with healthy controls (Cevik et al., 2004; Cleare et al., 2001; Crofford et al., 2004; Gur et al., 2004; Jerjes et al., 2007; Nater et al., 2008; Roberts et al., 2004), including three metanalyses (Powell et al., 2013; Rosmalen et al., 2010; Tak et al., 2011); however, many studies yielded contradictory or normal results (Di Giorgio et al., 2005; Jerjes et al., 2006; Markopoulou et al., 2010). Several studies found that participants with lower cortisol levels prior to treatment did not respond well to cognitive-behavioral therapy (Jason et al., 2007; Roberts et al., 2010). Lattie and colleagues (2013) reported that patients with worse PEM had lower awakening cortisol and a flatter diurnal curve. The committee could discern no single explanation for these findings.

There is some evidence of low CRH and AVP and blunted adrenocorticotropin hormone (ACTH) response in ME/CFS (Altemus et al., 2001; Bakheit et al., 1993; Di Giorgio et al., 2005; Gaab et al., 2002, 2005; Ottenweller et al., 2001; Parker et al., 2001; Racciatti et al., 2001; Scott et al., 1998a,b,c); however, there have been negative studies on this question as well (Gaab et al., 2003; Papadopoulos et al., 2009; Van Den Eede et al., 2008). CDC studied ME/CFS subjects extensively during a 3-day inpatient stay in a population-based study and found only decreased heart rate variability during sleep and low aldosterone levels (Boneva et al., 2007).

The results of physiological studies suggesting reduced HPA function and reduced blood volume producing orthostatic intolerance have led to several therapeutic studies using corticosteroids and mineralocorticoids. The committee reviewed two placebo-controlled studies using hydrocortisone (Cleare et al., 1999; McKenzie et al., 1998). The first used hydrocortisone 20-30 mg in the morning and 5 mg at 2 PM for 12 weeks. Of numerous outcome measures, only one showed small but significant improvement in the treated group. In addition, the authors found demonstrable evidence of adrenal cortical suppression in 12 of 33 hydrocortisone-treated participants and none in controls. They concluded that the risk of adrenal suppression negated the value of reported improvement (McKenzie et al., 1998). The second, much shorter study entailed administering hydrocortisone 5 or 10 mg daily for 1 month and placebo for 1 month in a crossover design. While on treatment, patients showed mild but statistically significant improvement in fatigue and disability compared with the placebo period without evidence of adrenal suppression (Cleare et al., 1999). Anecdotal discussion among clinicians during the open meetings held for this study indicated a lack of sustained effect using this treatment approach and concerns regarding the risks of long-term adrenal suppression. No further data on the effects of treating with hydrocortisone alone have appeared since 1999. A later study used both 5 mg of hydrocortisone and 50 mcg of fludrocortisone per day. These researchers found no effect on fatigue (Blockmans et al., 2003). Two studies that looked at treating with fludrocortisone alone also were negative (Peterson et al., 1998; Rowe et al., 2001).

Serotonin

Several studies found defective serotonergic signaling in the brain at or above the hypothalamus in ME/CFS patients (Bearn et al., 1995; Dinan et al., 1997; Sharpe et al., 1996). Higher prevalence of a 5-HTT gene promoter polymorphism (Narita et al., 2003) and reduced density of 5-HTT in the anterior cingulate (Yamamoto et al., 2004) were demonstrated in ME/CFS patients compared with healthy controls. Positive autoimmune activity was documented against 5-HT in a significant number of ME/CFS patients compared with chronic fatigue patients and healthy controls (Maes et al., 2013).

Growth Hormone

One study found normal levels of growth hormone or growth hormone responses in ME/CFS patients (Cleare et al., 2000), while others found reduced growth hormone (Allain et al., 1997; Bearn et al., 1995) and reduced nocturnal secretion of growth hormone (Berwaerts et al., 1998; Moorkens et al., 2000). Conflicting results were obtained in the growth hormone response to insulin-induced hypoglycemia, with responses being either reduced (Allain et al., 1997; Moorkens et al., 2000) or normal (Berwaerts et al., 1998). Various assessments of IGF-1 showed no consistent differences between ME/CFS patients and controls (Cleare et al., 2000; The et al., 2007).

Renin-aldosterone

Studies found low blood volume (orthostatic intolerance, small heart, and low cardiac index) and low aldosterone in ME/CFS patients (Miwa and Fujita, 2008, 2009, 2011, 2014). Renin is produced by the kidneys in response to low aldosterone and low blood volume. Abnormal function of the renin-angiotensin system, the autonomic nervous system, or the central nervous system could play a role (see the discussion of orthostatic intolerance and autonomic dysfunction in Chapter 4).

Summary

Patients with ME/CFS may have relatively reduced overnight cortisol, 24-hour urinary cortisol, CRH and/or AVP, and ACTH levels compared with healthy controls. The current preponderance of evidence points to normal adrenal function in such patients and suggests a secondary (central) rather than a primary (adrenal) cause of reduced but not absent cortisol production at the level of the pituitary, the hypothalamus, or higher. Patients with ME/CFS may have defective serotonergic signaling in the brain, localized to the level of the hypothalamus or higher, resulting in downstream dysregulation that may play a role in ME/CFS. The exact mechanism is not clear. Also, current evidence indicates that the growth hormone axis is intact in ME/CFS patients. If IGF-1 abnormalities are present, there may be many other causes (Brugts et al., 2009). ME/CFS patients may hyporeact to stressors, but that phenomenon may not be specific to a particular neurotransmitter or endocrine stimuli.

Conclusion: *Evidence is insufficient to conclude that any specific neuroendocrine abnormalities cause ME/CFS, or that any such abnormalities either uniformly differentiate those with ME/CFS from individuals with other illnesses or distinguish a subset of ME/CSF patients.*

INFECTION

Description of Infection in ME/CFS

Reports of several infectious disease outbreaks possibly leading to ME/CFS aroused early suspicion of an infectious etiology or an association of infection with the initiation of the illness (Acheson, 1955; Albrecht et al., 1964; Briggs and Levine, 1994; Buchwald et al., 1989; Clement et al., 1958; Daikos et al., 1959; Dillon et al., 1974; Klajman et al., 1960; Parish, 1978; Shelokov et al., 1957; Strickland et al., 2001). The observation that

ME/CFS cases commonly presented with an acute infection-like onset supported this belief (Komaroff, 1988), and an acute onset presentation was reported to be more common in ME/CFS patients than in those suffering from chronic fatigue only (Evengård et al., 2003). Yet while 25 to 80 percent of ME/CFS patients describe an infectious-like onset at the beginning of their illness (Ciccone and Natelson, 2003; Evengård et al., 2003; Naess et al., 2010), population-based studies using the Fukuda definition showed a predominance of gradual onset over an obvious acute infectious onset (Reyes et al., 2003). The variance in these rates likely is due to differences in recruitment of subjects, as well as varying interpretations of "acute," "infectious," and "gradual" onset.

While none of the case definitions discussed in Chapter 3 includes an infection-related onset as part of its main criteria, the CCC specifically uses this information to support the diagnosis of ME/CFS in patients who do not fulfill the sleep and pain criteria (Carruthers et al., 2003). Moreover, prospective studies of laboratory-documented acute Epstein-Barr virus (EBV)-associated glandular fever, non-EBV-associated glandular fever, Ross River virus, *Giardia duodenalis* enteritis, parvovirus B19, and Q fever infections demonstrated that 1 to 22 percent of patients go on to develop ME/CFS (Hickie et al., 2006; Kerr et al., 2002; Naess et al., 2012; Seishima et al., 2008; White et al., 1998). One of the few pediatric studies on infection and ME/CFS found a rate within this range after EBV-associated infectious mononucleosis: 13 percent after 6 months, 7 percent after 12 months, and 4 percent after 24 months (see the section on infection in Chapter 6) (Katz et al., 2009). Additionally, postviral onset differs from slow-onset illness, showing higher chronic immune activation markers years after onset (Porter et al., 2010).

Assessment of Infection in ME/CFS

Researchers have made numerous attempts to determine whether an infectious agent, particularly a virus, plays a role in the ongoing pathogenesis of ME/CFS. However, detecting active, pathological infections or differentiating an active infection or reactivation from a latent infection is highly challenging. Several studies tested patients with ME/CFS for the presence of serum antibody levels in response to viruses such as EBV, human herpes virus-6 (HHV-6), and cytomegalovirus (CMV) and found increased levels in a subset of patients (Ablashi et al., 2000; Gascon et al., 2006; Kawai and Kawai, 1992; Krueger et al., 1988; Lerner et al., 2002, 2004). However, these viruses are highly prevalent and associated with other diseases, and antibodies to them may be present even in asymptomatic people (Sumaya, 1991). An increase in such antibodies also may reflect a reactivation of the virus in people with an altered immune system. Moreover, the findings of increased serum antibody titers in ME/CFS patients have not been consistent, which may be due in part to the different serological tests used (Hellinger et al., 1988; Ilaria et al., 1995; Levine et al., 1992; Mawle et al., 1995; Reeves et al., 2000; Swanink et al., 1995; Whelton et al., 1992).

Prior studies also showed that peripheral blood samples may miss enterovirus, parvovirus, or herpes virus infections that continue to be present in, respectively, gut, brain, or heart tissues (Fotheringham et al., 2007; Halme et al., 2008; Kuhl et al., 2005; Yanai et al., 1997). Thus, ME/CFS researchers have looked for traces of infections elsewhere (Fremont et al., 2009; Ilaria et al., 1995). Enterovirus RNA assays have been performed on secretions, and immunohistochemistry has been used to look for enterovirus-specific antibodies or antigens in tissue (Chia and Chia, 2008; Chia et al., 2010). Newer techniques for detecting viruses, particularly when used in longitudinal therapeutic studies, may provide new insight into the etiology and treatment of some of these patients.

Because the immune system plays a vital role in the control of and response to pathogens, studies have been conducted to identify the presence of alterations to immune function in ME/CFS patients (Kerr and Tyrrell, 2003; Porter et al., 2010). The different markers tested to assess abnormalities in the immune function of ME/CFS patients were discussed earlier in the section of this chapter on immune impairment.

Evidence for Infection in ME/CFS

The committee searched the literature for evidence with which to address two main questions with respect to infection: (1) Is there an infectious agent that can precipitate ME/CFS? and (2) Is there evidence of an ongoing infection that plays a role in the disease? The description of the methodology used for the committee's literature search can be found in Chapter 1.

Viral Infections

Numerous studies have assessed the possible association between viral infections and ME/CFS. However, EBV is the only viral infection showing some consistent findings as a possible trigger of ME/CFS in these studies.

Herpes virus The possibility that EBV infection can be a trigger for ME/CFS is suggested by results of some prospective studies (Fark, 1991; Hickie et al., 2006; Jason et al., 2014a; White et al., 1998). Several studies also found high titers of certain antibodies to EBV in ME/CFS patients, including viral capsid antigen (VCA) IgG, persistent titers of VCA Immunoglobulin M (IgM), or the persistence of early antigen IgG, whereas healthy individuals who were previously infected with EBV had only VCA IgG and nuclear antigen IgG antibodies (Gascon et al., 2006; Kawai and Kawai, 1992; Lerner et al., 2004; Loebel et al., 2014; Manian, 1994; Natelson et al., 1990, 1994; Sairenji et al., 1995). Some studies, however, including a study of twins discordant for disease, were unable to find this difference (Buchwald et al., 1996; Fremont et al., 2009; Hellinger et al., 1988; Koelle et al., 2002; Levine et al., 1992; Mawle et al., 1995; Swanink et al., 1995). The severity of the acute illness may be a predictor of ME/CFS. Both a population-based study (Jason et al., 2014a) and a prospective study (Hickie et al., 2006) of ME/CFS patients after mononucleosis infection showed severity of illness, as measured by baseline autonomic symptoms and days spent in bed, to be a significant predictor of ME/CFS 6 months after the infection.

Evidence concerning the role of HHV-6 virus in ME/CFS is less consistent. Several studies found that ME/CFS patients have a significantly higher rate of HHV-6 antibodies (either IgG or IgM) compared with healthy controls (Ablashi et al., 2000; Patnaik et al., 1995; Sairenji et al., 1995; Yalcin et al., 1994). A few studies identified HHV-6 in human peripheral blood lymphocytes, recovered by culture and confirmed by immunofluorescence assay (IFA) and by polymerase chain reaction (PCR), more frequently in ME/CFS patients than in controls (Buchwald et al., 1992; Yalcin et al., 1994; Zorzenon, 1996). However, other research groups were unable to find any significant differences (Burbelo et al., 2012; Cameron et al., 2010; Enbom et al., 2000; Fremont et al., 2009).

A number of studies found release of early encoded viral proteins into the circulation of patients with ME/CFS, a phenomenon that some have suggested represents abortive lytic replication as whole virions are not present (Beqaj et al., 2008; Glaser et al., 2005, 2006; Jones et al., 1988; Lerner and Beqaj, 2011, 2012; Lerner et al., 2002, 2012; Loebel et al., 2014; Natelson et al., 1994; Patnaik et al., 1995). The clinical significance of unusual antibody profiles and incomplete viral replication in ME/CFS remains unclear.

Enterovirus A few studies focused on the role of persistent enterovirus infection in ME/CFS (Chia et al., 2010; Galbraith et al., 1995; Lane et al., 2003). Chia and Chia (2008) showed that in a subset of ME/CFS patients who reported significant gastrointestinal complaints, the prevalence of enterovirus infection as demonstrated in stomach biopsy samples was significantly higher compared with control subjects. Other investigators failed to reproduce an increased incidence of enterovirus infection in ME/CFS patients (Lindh et al., 1996).

Other viruses A few studies showed that ME/CFS may develop after an infection with parvovirus B19 (Fremont et al., 2009; Kerr et al., 2002; Seishima et al., 2008) and Ross River virus (Hickie et al., 2006). There is insufficient evidence for an association between ME/CFS and various other viral infections, such as bornavirus (Evengård et al., 1999; Kitani et al., 1996; Li et al., 2003), retrovirus (Heneine et al., 1994; Honda et al., 1993; Khan et al., 1993), and HHV-7 (Fremont et al., 2009; Levine et al., 2001).

Response to treatment Some have argued that antiviral medication helps a subset of ME/CFS patients (Watt et al., 2012). One double-blind, placebo-controlled trial showed symptom improvement after 6 months in patients with elevated IgG antibody titers against EBV and HHV-6 following treatment with valganciclovir. There were also statistically significant changes in monocyte and cytokine levels, suggesting that immunomodulation may have been a factor in their improvement. However, the number of patients studied was small (N = 30), there were no differences in viral antibody titers between the two arms, and the patients were followed for only 9 months (Montoya et al., 2013). A prospective review of 106 ME/CFS patients with elevated serum antibody titers to EBV, CMV, or HHV-6 showed that 75 percent responded to long-term treatment with valacyclovir and/or valganciclovir (mean duration = 2.4 years). A patient was categorized as a responder if the Energy Index Point Score effect was greater than or equal to 1 (Lerner et al., 2010). A single-blind, placebo-controlled trial found a significant increase in NK cell activity in ME/CFS patients following treatment with isoprinosine (Diaz-Mitoma et al., 2003). However, another double-blind, placebo-controlled trial of ME/CFS patients with elevated antibodies to EBV failed to show a difference in clinical improvement between acyclovir-treated participants and placebo controls at 37 days follow-up (Straus et al., 1988). This study included a small number of patients (N = 27) and did not assess immune parameters.

Other Infections

The evidence on bacterial infection as a possible trigger of ME/CFS is limited mainly to Q-fever and *Chlamydia pneumoniae* (Nicolson et al., 2003; Wildman et al., 2002). A case-control study in an endemic area found a higher rate of ME/CFS in Q-fever cases (5 years postinfection) than in healthy controls (42 versus 26 percent), and ME/CFS occurred more often in individuals with more severe symptoms (Ayres et al., 1998). Further evidence of Q-fever as a trigger for ME/CFS is limited to case reports (Ledina et al., 2007). A cross-sectional study showed no increased prevalence of ME/CFS in Q-fever patients compared with healthy controls (Strauss et al., 2012). These findings are in contrast to the results of a prospective study that found that some patients would develop ME/CFS after a laboratory-confirmed Q-fever infection (Hickie et al., 2006). Evidence is unconvincing regarding *Chlamydia pneumoniae* infection as a possible trigger for ME/

CFS (Chia and Chia, 1999). Large interventional trials have not been performed; thus, data on response to antibacterial therapy are retrospective or limited to case reports (Bottero, 2000; Frykholm, 2009; Iwakami et al., 2005; Jackson et al., 2013). The committee's literature review yielded no studies of posttreatment Lyme disease syndrome and ME/CFS; however, the two illnesses share some symptoms, and patients with Lyme disease often are identified as a subgroup among ME/CFS patients in specialty practices (Schutzer et al., 2011).

Literature on the association between ME/CFS and parasitic infection is limited to a few studies. Among a cohort of 1,262 laboratory-confirmed cases of *Giardia duodenalis*, 96 patients were diagnosed with long-lasting postinfectious fatigue; of those, 58 were diagnosed with ME/CFS (Naess et al., 2012). The data for a fungal etiology for ME/CFS are not convincing (Cater, 1995).

Summary

The literature indicates a possible relationship between EBV and ME/CFS. The evidence suggests that ME/CFS can be triggered by EBV infection, but there is insufficient evidence to conclude that all ME/CFS is caused by EBV or that ME/CFS is sustained by ongoing EBV infection. Improved diagnostic techniques may reveal as yet undetected associations. Further research in this area is warranted to determine whether patients in whom disease was triggered by EBV or patients with evidence of an ongoing abnormal response to EBV represent clinically significant subsets of ME/CFS.

There is insufficient evidence for an association between ME/CFS and bacterial, fungal, parasitic, and other viral infections. These infectious agents may, however, be comorbidities, and their presence may reflect the presence of problems with immune function in these patients. Future research may clarify the role of these infections in this illness.

Conclusion: There is sufficient evidence suggesting that ME/CFS follows infection with EBV and possibly other specific infections.

REFERENCES

Aaron, L. A., L. M. Arguelles, S. Ashton, M. Belcourt, R. Herrell, J. Goldberg, W. R. Smith, and D. Buchwald. 2002. Health and functional status of twins with chronic regional and widespread pain. *Journal of Rheumatology* 29(11):2426-2434.

Abbi, B., and B. H. Natelson. 2013. Is chronic fatigue syndrome the same illness as fibromyalgia: Evaluating the "single syndrome" hypothesis. *QJM: Monthly Journal of the Association of Physicians* 106(1):3-9.

Ablashi, D. V., H. B. Eastman, C. B. Owen, M. M. Roman, J. Friedman, J. B. Zabriskie, D. L. Peterson, G. R. Pearson, and J. E. Whitman. 2000. Frequent HHV-6 reactivation in multiple sclerosis (MS) and chronic fatigue syndrome (CFS) patients. *Journal of Clinical Virology* 16(3):179-191.

Acheson, E. D. 1955. Outbreak at the royal free. *Lancet* 266(6886):394-395.

Albrecht, R. M., V. L. Oliver, and D. C. Poskanzer. 1964. Epidemic neuromyasthenia. Outbreak in a convent in New York state. *Journal of the American Medical Association* 187:904-907.

Allain, T. J., J. A. Bearn, P. Coskeran, J. Jones, A. Checkley, J. Butler, S. Wessely, and J. P. Miell. 1997. Changes in growth hormone, insulin, insulinlike growth factors (IGFs), and IGF-binding protein-1 in chronic fatigue syndrome. *Biological Psychiatry* 41(5):567-573.

Altemus, M., J. K. Dale, D. Michelson, M. A. Demitrack, P. W. Gold, and S. E. Straus. 2001. Abnormalities in response to vasopressin infusion in chronic fatigue syndrome. *Psychoneuroendocrinology* 26(2):175-188.

Antepohl, W., L. Kiviloog, J. Andersson, and B. Gerdle. 2003. Cognitive impairment in patients with chronic whiplash-associated disorder—a matched control study. *Neuro-Rehabilitation* 18(4):307-315.

Ayres, J. G., N. Flint, E. G. Smith, W. S. Tunnicliffe, T. J. Fletcher, K. Hammond, D. Ward, and B. P. Marmion. 1998. Post-infection fatigue syndrome following Q fever. *QJM: Monthly Journal of the Association of Physicians* 91(2):105-123.

Bakheit, A. M., P. O. Behan, W. S. Watson, and J. J. Morton. 1993. Abnormal arginine-vasopressin secretion and water metabolism in patients with postviral fatigue syndrome. *Acta Neurologica Scandinavica* 87(3):234-238.

Barker, E., S. F. Fujimura, M. B. Fadem, A. L. Landay, and J. A. Levy. 1994. Immunologic abnormalities associated with chronic fatigue syndrome. *Clinical Infectious Diseases* 18(Suppl. 1):S136-S141.

Bearn, J., T. Allain, P. Coskeran, N. Munro, J. Butler, A. McGregor, and S. Wessely. 1995. Neuroendocrine responses to d-fenfluramine and insulin-induced hypoglycemia in chronic fatigue syndrome. *Biological Psychiatry* 37(4):245-252.

Behan, P. O., W. M. Behan, and E. J. Bell. 1985. The postviral fatigue syndrome—an analysis of the findings in 50 cases. *The Journal of Infection* 10(3):211-222.

Bennett, R. M., R. Friend, K. D. Jones, R. Ward, B. K. Han, and R. L. Ross. 2009. The Revised Fibromyalgia Impact Questionnaire (FIQR): Validation and psychometric properties. *Arthritis Research & Therapy* 11(4):R120.

Beqaj, S. H., A. M. Lerner, and J. T. Fitzgerald. 2008. Immunoassay with cytomegalovirus early antigens from gene products p52 and CM2 (UL44 and UL57) detects active infection in patients with chronic fatigue syndrome. *Journal of Clinical Pathology* 61(5):623-626.

Berwaerts, J., G. Moorkens, and R. Abs. 1998. Secretion of growth hormone in patients with chronic fatigue syndrome. *Growth Hormone & IGF Research* 8(Suppl. B):127-129.

Blockmans, D., P. Persoons, B. Van Houdenhove, M. Lejeune, and H. Bobbaers. 2003. Combination therapy with hydrocortisone and fludrocortisone does not improve symptoms in chronic fatigue syndrome: A randomized, placebo-controlled, double-blind, crossover study. *American Journal of Medicine* 114(9):736-741.

Boneva, R. S., M. J. Decker, E. M. Maloney, J. M. Lin, J. F. Jones, H. G. Helgason, C. M. Heim, D. B. Rye, and W. C. Reeves. 2007. Higher heart rate and reduced heart rate variability persist during sleep in chronic fatigue syndrome: A population-based study. *Autonomic Neuroscience: Basic and Clinical* 137(1-2):94-101.

Boomershine, C. S. 2012. A comprehensive evaluation of standardized assessment tools in the diagnosis of fibromyalgia and in the assessment of fibromyalgia severity. *Pain Research and Treatment* 2012:653714.

Bottero, P. 2000. Role of rickettsiae and chlamydiae in the psychopathology of chronic fatigue syndrome (CFS) patients: A diagnostic and therapeutic report. *Journal of Chronic Fatigue Syndrome* 6(3-4):147-161.

Brenu, E. W., D. R. Staines, O. K. Baskurt, K. J. Ashton, S. B. Ramos, R. M. Christy, and S. M. Marshall-Gradisnik. 2010. Immune and hemorheological changes in chronic fatigue syndrome. *Journal of Translational Medicine* 8.

Brenu, E. W., M. L. van Driel, D. R. Staines, K. J. Ashton, S. B. Ramos, J. Keane, N. G. Klimas, and S. M. Marshall-Gradisnik. 2011. Immunological abnormalities as potential biomarkers in chronic fatigue syndrome/myalgic encephalomyelitis. *Journal of Translational Medicine* 9:81.

Brenu, E. W., K. J. Ashton, M. van Driel, D. R. Staines, D. Peterson, G. M. Atkinson, and S. M. Marshall-Gradisnik. 2012a. Cytotoxic lymphocyte micrornas as prospective biomarkers for chronic fatigue syndrome/myalgic encephalomyelitis. *Journal of Affective Disorders* 141(2-3):261-269.

Brenu, E. W., M. L. van Driel, D. R. Staines, K. J. Ashton, S. L. Hardcastle, J. Keane, L. Tajouri, D. Peterson, S. B. Ramos, and S. M. Marshall-Gradisnik. 2012b. Longitudinal investigation of natural killer cells and cytokines in chronic fatigue syndrome/myalgic encephalomyelitis. *Journal of Translational Medicine* 10:88.

Brenu, E. W., T. K. Huth, S. L. Hardcastle, K. Fuller, M. Kaur, S. Johnston, S. B. Ramos, D. R. Staines, and S. M. Marshall-Gradisnik. 2014. Role of adaptive and innate immune cells in chronic fatigue syndrome/myalgic encephalomyelitis. *International Immunology* 26(4):233-242.

Briggs, N. C., and P. H. Levine. 1994. A comparative review of systemic and neurological symptomatology in 12 outbreaks collectively described as chronic fatigue syndrome, epidemic neuromyasthenia, and myalgic encephalomyelitis. *Clinical Infectious Diseases* 18(Suppl. 1):S32-S42.

Broderick, G., B. Z. Katz, H. Fernandes, M. A. Fletcher, N. Klimas, F. A. Smith, M. R. O'Gorman, S. D. Vernon, and R. Taylor. 2012. Cytokine expression profiles of immune imbalance in post-mononucleosis chronic fatigue. *Journal of Translational Medicine* 10:191.

Brown, A. A., L. A. Jason, M. A. Evans, and S. Flores. 2013. Contrasting case definitions: The ME international consensus criteria vs. the Fukuda et al. CFS criteria. *North American Journal of Psychology* 15(1):103-120.

Brugts, M. P., J. G. Luermans, E. G. Lentjes, N. J. van Trooyen-van Vrouwerff, F. A. van der Horst, P. H. Slee, S. W. Lamberts, and J. A. Janssen. 2009. Heterophilic antibodies may be a cause of falsely low total IGF1 levels. *European Journal of Endocrinology* 161(4):561-565.

Buchwald, D., and A. L. Komaroff. 1991. Review of laboratory findings for patients with chronic fatigue syndrome. *Reviews of Infectious Diseases* 13(Suppl. 1):S12-S18.

Buchwald, D. S., R. Biddle, F. Jolesz, R. Kikinis, P. R. Cheney, D. L. Peterson, and A. L. Komaroff. 1989. Central nervous-system (CNS) abnormalities on magnetic-resonance imaging (MRI) in an outbreak of chronic fatigue syndrome (CFS). *Clinical Research* 37(2):A309.

Buchwald, D., P. R. Cheney, D. L. Peterson, B. Henry, S. B. Wormsley, A. Geiger, D. V. Ablashi, S. Z. Salahuddin, C. Saxinger, R. Biddle, R. Kikinis, F. A, Jolesz, T. Folks, N. Balachandran, J. B. Peter, R. Gallo, and A. L. Komaroff. 1992. A chronic illness characterized by fatigue, neurologic and immunologic disorders, and active human herpesvirus type 6 infection. *Annals of Internal Medicine* 116(2):103-113.

Buchwald, D., R. L. Ashley, T. Pearlman, P. Kith, and A. L. Komaroff. 1996. Viral serologies in patients with chronic fatigue and chronic fatigue syndrome. *Journal of Medical Virology* 50(1):25-30.

Burbelo, P. D., A. Bayat, J. Wagner, T. B. Nutman, J. N. Baraniuk, and M. J. Iadarola. 2012. No serological evidence for a role of HHV-6 infection in chronic fatigue syndrome. *American Journal of Translational Research* 4(4):443-451.

Caligiuri, M., C. Murray, D. Buchwald, H. Levine, P. Cheney, D. Peterson, A. L. Komaroff, and J. Ritz. 1987. Phenotypic and functional deficiency of natural killer cells in patients with chronic fatigue syndrome. *Journal of Immunology* 139(10):3306-3313.

Cameron, B., L. Flamand, H. Juwana, J. Middeldorp, Z. Naing, W. Rawlinson, D. Ablashi, and A. Lloyd. 2010. Serological and virological investigation of the role of the herpesviruses EBV, CMV and HHV-6 in post-infective fatigue syndrome. *Journal of Medical Virology* 82(10):1684-1688.

Carlo-Stella, N., C. Badulli, A. De Silvestri, L. Bazzichi, M. Martinetti, L. Lorusso, S. Bombardieri, L Salvaneschi, and M. Cuccia. 2006. A first study of cytokine genomic polymorphisms in CFS: Positive association of TNF-857 and IFNgamma 874 rare alleles. *Clinical and Experimental Rheumatology* 24(2):179-182.

Carruthers, B. M., A. K. Jain, K. L. De Meirleir, D. L. Peterson, N. G. Klimas, A. M. Lemer, A. C. Bested, P. Flor-Henry, P. Joshi, A. C. P. Powles, J. A. Sherkey, and M. I. van de Sande. 2003. Myalgic encephalomyelitis/chronic fatigue syndrome: Clinical working case definition, diagnostic and treatment protocols (Canadian case definition). *Journal of Chronic Fatigue Syndrome* 11(1):7-115.

Carruthers, B. M., M. I. van de Sande, K. L. De Meirleir, N. G. Klimas, G. Broderick, T. Mitchell, D. Staines, A. C. P. Powles, N. Speight, R. Vallings, L. Bateman, B. Baumgarten-Austrheim, D. S. Bell, N. Carlo-Stella, J. Chia, A. Darragh, D. Jo, D. Lewis, A. R. Light, S. Marshall-Gradisbik, I. Mena, J. A. Mikovits, K. Miwa, M. Murovska, M. L. Pall, and S. Stevens. 2011. Myalgic encephalomyelitis: International consensus criteria. *Journal of Internal Medicine* 270(4):327-338.

Cater II, R. E. 1995. Chronic intestinal candidiasis as a possible etiological factor in the chronic fatigue syndrome. *Medical Hypotheses* 44(6):507-515.

Cevik, R., A. Gur, S. Acar, K. Nas, and A. J. Sarac. 2004. Hypothalamic-pituitary-gonadal axis hormones and cortisol in both menstrual phases of women with chronic fatigue syndrome and effect of depressive mood on these hormones. *BMC Musculoskeletal Disorders* 5:47.

Chia, J. K. S., and A. Y. Chia. 2008. Chronic fatigue syndrome is associated with chronic enterovirus infection of the stomach. *Journal of Clinical Pathology* 61(1):43-48.

Chia, J. K. S., and L. Y. Chia. 1999. Chronic chlamydia pneumoniae infection: A treatable cause of chronic fatigue syndrome. *Clinical Infectious Diseases* 29(2):452-453.

Chia, J., A. Chia, M. Voeller, T. Lee, and R. Chang. 2010. Acute enterovirus infection followed by myalgic encephalomyelitis/chronic fatigue syndrome (ME/CFS) and viral persistence. *Journal of Clinical Pathology* 63(2):165-168.

Ciccone, D. S., and B. H. Natelson. 2003. Comorbid illness in women with chronic fatigue syndrome: A test of the single syndrome hypothesis. *Psychosomatic Medicine* 65(2):268-275.

Clauw, D. J. 2014. Fibromyalgia: A clinical review. *Journal of the American Medical Association* 311(15):1547-1555.

Cleare, A. J., E. Heap, G. S. Malhi, S. Wessely, V. O'Keane, and J. Miell. 1999. Low-dose hydrocortisone in chronic fatigue syndrome: A randomised crossover trial. *Lancet* 353(9151):455-458.

Cleare, A. J., S. S. Sookdeo, J. Jones, V. O'Keane, and J. P. Miell. 2000. Integrity of the growth hormone/insulin-like growth factor system is maintained in patients with chronic fatigue syndrome. *Journal of Clinical Endocrinology & Metabolism* 85(4):1433-1439.

Cleare, A. J., D. Blair, S. Chambers, and S. Wessely. 2001. Urinary free cortisol in chronic fatigue syndrome. *American Journal of Psychiatry* 158(4):641-643.

Clement, W. B., P. Gorda, D. A. Henderson, J. W. Lawrence, and J. O. Bond. 1958. Epidemic neuromyasthenia, an outbreak in Punta Gorda, Florida; an illness resembling Iceland disease. *The Journal of the Florida Medical Association* 45(4):422-426.

Cook, D. B., P. R. Nagelkirk, A. Peckerman, A. Poluri, J. Mores, and B. H. Natelson. 2005. Exercise and cognitive performance in chronic fatigue syndrome. *Medicine & Science in Sports & Exercise* 37(9):1460-1467.

Cook, D. B., P. R. Nagelkirk, A. Poluri, J. Mores, and B. H. Natelson. 2006. The influence of aerobic fitness and fibromyalgia on cardiorespiratory and perceptual responses to exercise in patients with chronic fatigue syndrome. *Arthritis & Rheumatism* 54(10):3351-3362.

Crofford, L. J., E. A. Young, N. C. Engleberg, A. Korszun, C. B. Brucksch, L. A. McClure, M. B. Brown, and M. A. Demitrack. 2004. Basal circadian and pulsatile ACTH and cortisol secretion in patients with fibromyalgia and/or chronic fatigue syndrome. *Brain, Behavior & Immunity* 18(4):314-325.

Curriu, M., J. Carrillo, M. Massanella, J. Rigau, J. Alegre, J. Puig, A. M. Garcia-Quintana, J. Castro-Marrero, E. Negredo, B. Clotet, C. Cabrera, and J. Blanco. 2013. Screening NK-, B- and T-cell phenotype and function in patients suffering from chronic fatigue syndrome. *Journal of Translational Medicine* 11:68.

Daikos, G. K., S. Garzonis, A. Paleologue, G. A. Bousvaros, and N. Papadoyannakis. 1959. Benign myalgic encephalomyelitis. An outbreak in a nurses' school in Athens. *Lancet* 1(7075):693-696.

De Becker, P., N. McGregor, and K. De Meirleir. 2001. A definition-based analysis of symptoms in a large cohort of patients with chronic fatigue syndrome. *Journal of Internal Medicine* 250(3):234-240.

Demitrack, M. A., J. K. Dale, S. E. Straus, L. Laue, S. J. Listwak, M. J. Kruesi, G. P. Chrousos, and P. W. Gold. 1991. Evidence for impaired activation of the hypothalamic-pituitary-adrenal axis in patients with chronic fatigue syndrome. *Journal of Clinical Endocrinology and Metabolism* 73(6):1224-1234.

Di Giorgio, A., M. Hudson, W. Jerjes, and A. J. Cleare. 2005. 24-hour pituitary and adrenal hormone profiles in chronic fatigue syndrome. *Psychosomatic Medicine* 67(3):433-440.

Diaz-Mitoma, F., E. Turgonyi, A. Kumar, W. Lim, L. Larocque, and B. M. Hyde. 2003. Clinical improvement in chronic fatigue syndrome is associated with enhanced natural killer cell-mediated cytotoxicity: The results of a pilot study with isoprinosine®. *Journal of Chronic Fatigue Syndrome* 11(2):71-93.

Dillon, M. J., W. C. Marshall, J. A. Dudgeon, and A. J. Steigman. 1974. Epidemic neuromyasthenia: Outbreak among nurses at a children's hospital. *British Medical Journal* 1(5903):301-305.

Dinan, T. G., T. Majeed, E. Lavelle, L. V. Scott, C. Berti, and P. Behan. 1997. Blunted serotonin-mediated activation of the hypothalamic-pituitary-adrenal axis in chronic fatigue syndrome. *Psychoneuroendocrinology* 22(4):261-267.

Edwards, J. 2013. *UK rituximab trial—statements by professor Jonathan Edwards and invest in ME*. http://www.ukrituximabtrial.org/Rituximab%20news-July13%2001.htm (accessed May 14, 2014).

Elfaitouri, A., B. Herrmann, A. Bölin-Wiener, Y. Wang, C. G. Gottfries, O. Zachrisson, R. Pipkorn, L. Rönnblom, and J. Blomberg. 2013. Epitopes of microbial and human heat shock protein 60 and their recognition in myalgic encephalomyelitis. *PLoS ONE* 8(11):e81155.

Enbom, M., A. Linde, and B. Evengård. 2000. No evidence of active infection with human herpesvirus 6 (HHV-6) or HHV-8 in chronic fatigue syndrome. *Journal of Clinical Microbiology* 38(6):2457.

Evengård, B., C. G. Nilsson, G. Lindh, L. Lindquist, P. Eneroth, S. Fredrikson, L. Terenius, and K. G. Henriksson. 1998. Chronic fatigue syndrome differs from fibromyalgia. No evidence for elevated substance P levels in cerebrospinal fluid of patients with chronic fatigue syndrome. *Pain* 78(2):153-155.

Evengård, B., T. Briese, G. Lindh, S. Lee, and W. I. Lipkin. 1999. Absence of evidence of Borna disease virus infection in Swedish patients with chronic fatigue syndrome. *Journal of NeuroVirology* 5(5):495-499.

Evengård, B., E. Jonzon, A. Sandberg, T. Theorell, and G. Lindh. 2003. Differences between patients with chronic fatigue syndrome and with chronic fatigue at an infectious disease clinic in Stockholm, Sweden. *Psychiatry & Clinical Neurosciences* 57(4):361-368.

Fark, A. R. 1991. Infectious mononucleosis, Epstein-Barr virus, and chronic fatigue syndrome: A prospective case series. *Journal of Family Practice* 32(2):202, 205-206, 209.

FDA (Food and Drug Administration). 2013. *The voice of the patient: Chronic fatigue syndrome and myalgic encephalomyelitis.* Bethesda, MD: Center for Drug Evaluation and Research (CDER), FDA.

Fischer, D. B., A. H. William, A. C. Strauss, E. R. Unger, L. A. Jason, G. D. Marshall, Jr., and J. D. Dimitrakoff. 2014. Chronic fatigue syndrome: The current status and future potentials of emerging biomarkers. *Fatigue: Biomedicine, Health & Behavior* 2(2):93-109.

Fletcher, M. A., X. R. Zeng, Z. Barnes, S. Levis, and N. G. Klimas. 2009. Plasma cytokines in women with chronic fatigue syndrome. *Journal of Translational Medicine* 7:96.

Fletcher, M. A., X. R. Zeng, K. Maher, S. Levis, B. Hurwitz, M. Antoni, G. Broderick, and N. G. Klimas. 2010. Biomarkers in chronic fatigue syndrome: Evaluation of natural killer cell function and dipeptidyl peptidase IV/CD26. *PLoS ONE* 5(5):e10817.

Fluge, O., O. Bruland, K. Risa, A. Storstein, E. K. Kristoffersen, D. Sapkota, H. Naess, O. Dahl, H. Nyland, and O. Mella. 2011. Benefit from B-lymphocyte depletion using the anti-CD20 antibody rituximab in chronic fatigue syndrome. A double-blind and placebo-controlled study. *PLoS ONE* 6(10):e26358.

Fondell, E., J. Axelsson, K. Franck, A. Ploner, M. Lekander, K. Bälter, and H. Gaines. 2011. Short natural sleep is associated with higher T cell and lower NK cell activities. *Brain Behavior and Immunity* 25(7):1367-1375.

Fotheringham, J., N. Akhyani, A. Vortmeyer, D. Donati, E. Williams, U. Oh, M. Bishop, J. Barrett, J. Gea-Banacloche, and S. Jacobson. 2007. Detection of active human herpesvirus-6 infection in the brain: Correlation with polymerase chain reaction detection in cerebrospinal fluid. *The Journal of Infectious Diseases* 195(3):450-454.

Fremont, M., K. Metzger, H. Rady, J. Hulstaert, and K. De Meirleir. 2009. Detection of herpesviruses and parvovirus B19 in gastric and intestinal mucosa of chronic fatigue syndrome patients. *In Vivo* 23(2):209-213.

Frykholm, B. O. 2009. On the question of infectious aetiologies for multiple sclerosis, schizophrenia and the chronic fatigue syndrome and their treatment with antibiotics. *Medical Hypotheses* 72(6):736-739.

Fukuda, K., S. E. Straus, I. Hickie, M. C. Sharpe, J. G. Dobbins, A. Komaroff, A. Schluederberg, J. F. Jones, A. R. Lloyd, S. Wessely, N. M. Gantz, G. P. Holmes, D. Buchwald, S. Abbey, J. Rest, J. A. Levy, H. Jolson, D. L. Peterson, J. Vercoulen, U. Tirelli, B. Evengård, B. H. Natelson, L. Steele, M. Reyes, and W. C. Reeves. 1994. The chronic fatigue syndrome: A comprehensive approach to its definition and study. *Annals of Internal Medicine* 121(12):953-959.

Gaab, J., D. Hüster, R. Peisen, V. Engert, V. Heitz, T. Schad, T. H. Schürmeyer, and U. Ehlert. 2002. Hypothalalmic-pituitary-adrenal axis reactivity in chronic fatigue syndrome and health under psychological, physiological and pharmacological stimulation. *Psychosomatic Medicine* 64(6):951-962.

Gaab, J., D. Huster, R. Peisen, V. Engert, V. Heitz, T. Schad, T. Schurmeyer, and U. Ehlert. 2003. Assessment of cortisol response with low-dose and high-dose ACTH in patients with chronic fatigue syndrome and healthy comparison subjects. *Psychosomatics* 44(2): 113-119.

Gaab, J., N. Rohleder, V. Heitz, V. Engert, T. Schad, T. H. Schlümeyer, and U. Ehlert. 2005. Stress-induced changes in LPS-induced pro-inflammatory cytokine production in chronic fatigue syndrome. *Psychoneuroendocrinology* 30(2):188-198.

Gaber, T., and W. W. Oo. 2013. Prevalence of hypothyroidism in chronic fatigue syndrome patients (CFS/ME). *Journal of Neurology* 260:S98-S99.

Galbraith, D. N., C. Nairn, and G. B. Clements. 1995. Phylogenetic analysis of short enteroviral sequences from patients with chronic fatigue syndrome. *Journal of General Virology* 76(Pt. 7):1701-1707.

Gascon, J., T. Marcos, J. Vidal, A. G. Forcada, and M. Corachan. 2006. Cytomegalovirus and Epstein-Barr virus infection as a cause of chronic fatigue syndrome in travellers to tropical countries. *Journal of Travel Medicine* 2(1):41-44.

Georgiades, E., W. M. Behan, L. P. Kilduff, M. Hadjicharalambous, E. E. Mackie, J. Wilson, S. A. Ward, and Y. P. Pitsiladis. 2003. Chronic fatigue syndrome: New evidence for a central fatigue disorder. *Clinical Science* 105(2):213-218.

Glaser, R., D. A. Padgett, M. L. Litsky, R. A. Baiocchi, E. V. Yang, M. Chen, P. E. Yeh, N. G. Klimas, G. D. Marshall, T. Whiteside, R. Herberman, J. Kiecolt-Glaser, and M. V. Williams. 2005. Stress-associated changes in the steady-state expression of latent Epstein-Barr virus: Implications for chronic fatigue syndrome and cancer. *Brain, Behavior & Immunity* 19(2):91-103.

Glaser, R., M. L. Litsky, D. A. Padgett, R. A. Baiocchi, E. V. Yang, M. Chen, P. E. Yeh, K. B. Green-Church, M. A. Caligiuri, and M. V. Williams. 2006. EBV-encoded dutpase induces immune dysregulation: Implications for the pathophysiology of EBV-associated disease. *Virology* 346(1):205-218.

Gupta, S., and B. Vayuvegula. 1991. A comprehensive immunological analysis in chronic fatigue syndrome. *Scandinavian Journal of Immunology* 33(3):319-327.

Gur, A., R. Cevik, K. Nas, L. Colpan, and S. Sarac. 2004. Cortisol and hypothalamic-pituitary-gonadal axis hormones in follicular-phase women with fibromyalgia and chronic fatigue syndrome and effect of depressive symptoms on these hormones. *Arthritis Research & Therapy* 6(3):R232-R238.

Halme, L., J. Arola, K. Hockerstedt, and I. Lautenschlager. 2008. Human herpesvirus 6 infection of the gastroduodenal mucosa. *Clinical Infectious Diseases* 46(3):434-439.

Hellinger, W. C., T. F. Smith, R. E. Van Scoy, P. G. Spitzer, P. Forgacs, and R. S. Edson. 1988. Chronic fatigue syndrome and the diagnostic utility of antibody to Epstein-Barr virus early antigen. *Journal of the American Medical Association* 260(7):971-973.

Henderson, T. A. 2014. Valacyclovir treatment of chronic fatigue in adolescents. *Advances in Mind-Body Medicine* 28(1):4-14.

Heneine, W., T. C. Woods, S. D. Sinha, A. S. Khan, L. E. Chapman, L. B. Schonberger, and T. M. Folks. 1994. Lack of evidence for infection with known human and animal retroviruses in patients with chronic fatigue syndrome. *Clinical Infectious Diseases* 18(Suppl. 1):S121-S125.

Herr, K. A., and L. Garand. 2001. Assessment and measurement of pain in older adults. *Clinics in Geriatric Medicine* 17(3):vi, 457-478.

Hickie, I., T. Davenport, D. Wakefield, U. Vollmer-Conna, B. Cameron, S. D. Vernon, W. C. Reeves, A. Lloyd, and G. Dubbo Infection Outcomes Study. 2006. Post-infective and chronic fatigue syndromes precipitated by viral and non-viral pathogens: Prospective cohort study. *British Medical Journal* 333(7568):575.

Hokama, Y., C. E. Campora, C. Hara, T. Kuribayashi, D. Le Huynh, and K. Yabusaki. 2009. Anticardiolipin antibodies in the sera of patients with diagnosed chronic fatigue syndrome. *Journal of Clinical Laboratory Analysis* 23(4):210-212.

Honda, M., K. Kitamura, T. Nakasone, Y. Fukushima, S. Matsuda, K. Nishioka, J. Matsuda, N. Hashimoto, and S. Yamazaki. 1993. Japanese patients with chronic fatigue syndrome are negative for known retrovirus infections. *Microbiology and Immunology* 37(10):779-784.

Ickmans, K., M. Meeus, D. Kos, P. Clarys, G. Meersdom, L. Lambrecht, N. Pattyn, and J. Nijs. 2013. Cognitive performance is of clinical importance, but is unrelated to pain severity in women with chronic fatigue syndrome. *Clinical Rheumatology* 32(10):1475-1485.

Ilaria, Jr., R. L., A. L. Komaroff, L. R. Fagioli, W. C. Moloney, C. A. True, and S. J. Naides. 1995. Absence of parvovirus B19 infection in chronic fatigue syndrome. *Arthritis and Rheumatism* 38(5):638-641.

Iwakami, E., Y. Arashima, K. Kato, T. Komiya, Y. Matsukawa, T. Ikeda, Y. Arakawa, and S. Oshida. 2005. Treatment of chronic fatigue syndrome with antibiotics: Pilot study assessing the involvement of Coxiella burnetii infection. *Internal Medicine (Tokyo, Japan)* 44(12):1258-1263.

Jackson, M., H. Butt, M. Ball, D. Lewis, and D. Bruck. 2013. An association between changes in the intestinal microbial flora and the alteration of sleep in chronic fatigue syndrome: A pilot open label trial with use of the antibiotic erythromycin. *Sleep and Biological Rhythms* 11:55.

Jammes, Y., J. G. Steinberg, S. Delliaux, and F. Bregeon. 2009. Chronic fatigue syndrome combines increased exercise-induced oxidative stress and reduced cytokine and hsp responses. *Journal of Internal Medicine* 266(2):196-206.

Janal, M. N., D. S. Ciccone, and B. H. Natelson. 2006. Sub-typing CFS patients on the basis of "minor" symptoms. *Biological Psychology* 73(2):124-131.

Jason, L. A., J. A. Richman, A. W. Rademaker, K. M. Jordan, A. V. Plioplys, R. R. Taylor, W. McCready, C. F. Huang, and S. Plioplys. 1999. A community-based study of chronic fatigue syndrome. *Archives of Internal Medicine* 159(18):2129-2137.

Jason, L. A., S. R. Torres-Harding, A. Jurgens, and J. Helgerson. 2004. Comparing the Fukuda et al. criteria and the Canadian case definition for chronic fatigue syndrome. *Journal of Chronic Fatigue Syndrome* 12(1):37-52.

Jason, L. A., S. Torres-Harding, K. Maher, N. Reynolds, M. Brown, M. Sorenson, J. Donalek, K. Corradi, M. A. Fletcher, and T. Lu. 2007. Baseline cortisol levels predict treatment outcomes in chronic fatigue syndrome nonpharmacologic clinical trial. *Journal of Chronic Fatigue Syndrome* 14(4):39-59.

Jason, L. A., M. Evans, N. Porter, M. Brown, A. Brown, J. Hunnell, V. Anderson, A. Lerch, K. De Meirleir, and F. Friedberg. 2010. The development of a revised Canadian myalgic encephalomyelitis chronic fatigue syndrome case definition. *American Journal of Biochemistry and Biotechnology* 6(2):120-135.

Jason, L. A., A. Brown, E. Clyne, L. Bartgis, M. Evans, and M. Brown. 2012. Contrasting case definitions for chronic fatigue syndrome, myalgic encephalomyelitis/chronic fatigue syndrome and myalgic encephalomyelitis. *Evaluation and the Health Professions* 35(3):280-304.

Jason, L. A., A. Brown, M. Evans, M. Sunnquist, and J. L. Newton. 2013a. Contrasting chronic fatigue syndrome versus myalgic encephalomyelitis/chronic fatigue syndrome. *Fatigue* 1(3):168-183.

Jason, L. A., M. Sunnquist, A. Brown, M. Evans, S. Vernon, J. Furst, and V. Simonis. 2013b. Examining case definition criteria for chronic fatigue syndrome and myalgic encephalomyelitis. *Fatigue: Biomedicine, Health & Behavior* 2(1).

Jason, L. A., B. Z. Katz, Y. Shiraishi, C. Mears, Y. Im, and R. R. Taylor. 2014a. Predictors of post-infectious chronic fatigue syndrome in adolescents. *Health Psychology & Behavioural Medicine* 2(1):41-51.

Jason, L. A., M. Sunnquist, A. Brown, M. Evans, and J. L. Newton. 2014b. Are myalgic encephalomyelitis and chronic fatigue syndrome different illnesses? A preliminary analysis. *Journal of Health Psychology* [Epub ahead of print].

Jerjes, W. K., N. F. Taylor, T. J. Peters, S. Wessely, and A. J. Cleare. 2006. Urinary cortisol and cortisol metabolite excretion in chronic fatigue syndrome. *Psychosomatic Medicine* 68(4):578-582.

Jerjes, W. K., N. F. Taylor, P. J. Wood, and A. J. Cleare. 2007. Enhanced feedback sensitivity to prednisolone in chronic fatigue syndrome. *Psychoneuroendocrinology* 32(2):192-198.

Jones, J. F., M. Williams, R. T. Schooley, C. Robinson, and R. Glaser. 1988. Antibodies to Epstein-Barr virus-specific DNase and DNA polymerase in the chronic fatigue syndrome. *Archives of Internal Medicine* 148(9):1957-1960.

Katz, B. Z., Y. Shiraishi, C. J. Mears, H. J. Binns, and R. Taylor. 2009. Chronic fatigue syndrome following infectious mononucleosis in adolescents. *Pediatrics* 124(1):189-193.

Kawai, K., and A. Kawai. 1992. Studies on the relationship between chronic fatigue syndrome and Epstein-Barr virus in Japan. *Internal Medicine (Tokyo, Japan)* 31(3):313-318.

Kerr, J. R., and D. A. J. Tyrrell. 2003. Cytokines in parvovirus B19 infection as an aid to understanding chronic fatigue syndrome. *Current Pain and Headache Reports* 7(5):333-341.

Kerr, J. R., J. Bracewell, I. Laing, D. L. Mattey, R. M. Bernstein, I. N. Bruce, and D. A. Tyrrell. 2002. Chronic fatigue syndrome and arthralgia following parvovirus B19 infection. *Journal of Rheumatology* 29(3):595-602.

Kerr, J. R., J. Gough, S. C. Richards, J. Main, D. Enlander, M. McCreary, A. L. Komaroff, and J. K. Chia. 2010. Antibody to parvovirus B19 nonstructural protein is associated with chronic arthralgia in patients with chronic fatigue syndrome/myalgic encephalomyelitis. *Journal of General Virology* 91(Pt. 4):893-897.

Khan, A. S., W. M. Heneine, L. E. Chapman, H. E. Gary, Jr., T. C. Woods, T. M. Folks, and L. B. Schonberger. 1993. Assessment of a retrovirus sequence and other possible risk factors for the chronic fatigue syndrome in adults. *Annals of Internal Medicine* 118(4):241-245.

Kitani, T., H. Kuratsune, I. Fuke, Y. Nakamura, T. Nakaya, S. Asahi, M. Tobiume, K. Yamaguti, T. Machii, R. Inagi, K. Yamanishi, and K. Ikuta. 1996. Possible correlation between Borna disease virus infection and Japanese patients with chronic fatigue syndrome. *Microbiology and Immunology* 40(6):459-462.

Klajman, A., B. Pinkhas, and L. Rannon. 1960. An outbreak of an epidemic of benign myalgic encephalomyelitis. *Harefuah* 58:314-315.

Klein, R., and P. A. Berg. 1995. High incidence of antibodies to 5-hydroxytryptamine, gangliosides and phospholipids in patients with chronic fatigue and fibromyalgia syndrome and their relatives: Evidence for a clinical entity of both disorders. *European Journal of Medical Research* 1(1):21-26.

Klimas, N. G., F. R. Salvato, R. Morgan, and M. A. Fletcher. 1990. Immunologic abnormalities in chronic fatigue syndrome. *Journal of Clinical Microbiology* 28(6):1403-1410.

Koelle, D. M., S. Barcy, M. L. Huang, R. L. Ashley, L. Corey, J. Zeh, S. Ashton, and D. Buchwald. 2002. Markers of viral infection in monozygotic twins discordant for chronic fatigue syndrome. *Clinical Infectious Diseases* 35(5):518-525.

Komaroff, A. L. 1988. Chronic fatigue syndromes: Relationship to chronic viral infections. *Journal of Virological Methods* 21(1-4):3-10.

Komaroff, A. L., L. R. Fagioli, T. H. Doolittle, B. Gandek, M. A. Gleit, R. T. Guerriero, I. R. J. Kornish, N. C. Ware, J. E. Ware, Jr., and D. W. Bates. 1996. Health status in patients with chronic fatigue syndrome and in general population and disease comparison groups. *American Journal of Medicine* 101(3):281-290.

Konstantinov, K., A. von Mikecz, D. Buchwald, J. Jones, L. Gerace, and E. M. Tan. 1996. Autoantibodies to nuclear envelope antigens in chronic fatigue syndrome. *Journal of Clinical Investigation* 98(8):1888-1896.

Krueger, G. R., B. Koch, A. Ramon, D. V. Ablashi, S. Z. Salahuddin, S. F. Josephs, H. Z. Streicher, R. C. Gallo, and U. Habermann. 1988. Antibody prevalence to HBLV (human herpesvirus-6, HHV-6) and suggestive pathogenicity in the general population and in patients with immune deficiency syndromes. *Journal of Virological Methods* 21(1-4):125-131.

Kuhl, U., M. Pauschinger, B. Seeberg, D. Lassner, M. Noutsias, W. Poller, and H. P. Schultheiss. 2005. Viral persistence in the myocardium is associated with progressive cardiac dysfunction. *Circulation* 112(13):1965-1970.

Lane, R. J. M., B. A. Soteriou, H. Zhang, and L. C. Archard. 2003. Enterovirus related metabolic myopathy: A postviral fatigue syndrome. *Journal of Neurology, Neurosurgery & Psychiatry* 74(10):1382-1386.

Lattie, E. G., M. H. Antoni, M. A. Fletcher, F. Penedo, S. Czaja, C. Lopez, D. Perdomo, A. Sala, S. Nair, S. H. Fu, and N. Klimas. 2012. Stress management skills, neuroimmune processes and fatigue levels in persons with chronic fatigue syndrome. *Brain, Behavior & Immunity* 26(6):849-858.

Lattie, E. G., M. H. Antoni, S. Czaja, D. Perdomo, M. A. Fletcher, N. Klimas, and S. Nair. 2013. Post-exertional malaise symptoms, salivary cortisol, and coping self-efficacy in patients with ME/CFS. *Psychosomatic Medicine* 75(3):A66-A67.

Ledina, D., N. Bradaric, I. Milas, I. Ivic, N. Brncic, and N. Kuzmicic. 2007. Chronic fatigue syndrome after Q fever. *Medical Science Monitor* 13(7):CS88-CS92.

Lerner, A. M., and S. Beqaj. 2011. A paradigm linking herpesvirus immediate-early gene expression apoptosis and myalgic encephalomyelitis chronic fatigue syndrome. *Virus Adaptation and Treatment* 3(1):19-24.

Lerner, A. M., and S. Beqaj. 2012. Abortive lytic Epstein-Barr virus replication in tonsil-B lymphocytes in infectious mononucleosis and a subset of the chronic fatigue syndrome. *Virus Adaptation and Treatment* 4(1):85-91.

Lerner, A. M., S. H. Beqaj, R. G. Deeter, and J. T. Fitzgerald. 2002. IgM serum antibodies to human cytomegalovirus nonstructural gene products p52 and CM2(UL44 and UL57) are uniquely present in a subset of patients with chronic fatigue syndrome. *In Vivo* 16(3):153-159.

Lerner, A. M., S. H. Beqaj, R. G. Deeter, and J. T. Fitzgerald. 2004. IgM serum antibodies to Epstein-Barr virus are uniquely present in a subset of patients with the chronic fatigue syndrome. *In Vivo* 18(2):101-106.

Lerner, A. M., S. Beqaj, J. T. Fitzgerald, K. Gill, C. Gill, and J. Edington. 2010. Subset-directed antiviral treatment of 142 herpesvirus patients with chronic fatigue syndrome. *Virus Adaptation and Treatment* 2(1):47-57.

Lerner, A. M., M. E. Ariza, M. Williams, L. Jason, S. Beqaj, J. T. Fitzgerald, S. Lemeshow, and R. Glaser. 2012. Antibody to Epstein-Barr virus deoxyuridine triphosphate nucleotidohydrolase and deoxyribonucleotide polymerase in a chronic fatigue syndrome subset. *PLoS ONE* 7(11):e47891.

Levine, P. H., S. Jacobson, A. C. Pocinki, P. Cheney, D. Peterson, R. R. Connelly, R. Weil, S. M. Robinson, D. V. Ablashi, S. Z. Salahuddin, G. R. Pearson, and R. Hoover. 1992. Clinical, epidemiologic, and virologic studies in four clusters of the chronic fatigue syndrome. *Archives of Internal Medicine* 152(8):1611-1616.

Levine, P. H., T. L. Whiteside, D. Friberg, J. Bryant, G. Colclough, and R. B. Herberman. 1998. Dysfunction of natural killer activity in a family with chronic fatigue syndrome. *Clinical Immunology and Immunopathology* 88(1):96-104.

Levine, S., H. Eastman, and D. V. Ablashi. 2001. Prevalence of IgM and IgG antibody to HHV-6 and HHV-8 and results of plasma PCR to HHV-6 and HHV-7 in a group of CFS patients and healthy donors. *Journal of Chronic Fatigue Syndrome* 9(1-2):31-40.

Li, Y. J., D. X. Wang, F. M. Zhang, Z. D. Liu, A. Y. Yang, and K. Ykuta. 2003. Detection of antibody against Borna disease virus-p24 in the plasma of Chinese patients with chronic fatigue syndrome by western-blot analysis. *Chinese Journal of Experimental and Clinical Virology* 17(4):330-333.

Lindh, G., A. Samuelson, K. O. Hedlund, B. Evengård, L. Lindquist, and A. Ehrnst. 1996. No findings of enteroviruses in Swedish patients with chronic fatigue syndrome. *Scandinavian Journal of Infectious Diseases* 28(3):305-307.

Loebel, M., K. Strohschein, C. Giannini, U. Koelsch, S. Bauer, C. Doebis, S. Thomas, N. Unterwalder, V. von Baehr, P. Reinke, M. Knops, L. G. Hanitsch, C. Meisel, H. D. Volk, and C. Scheibenbogen. 2014. Deficient EBV-specific B- and T-cell response in patients with chronic fatigue syndrome. *PLoS ONE* 9(1):e85387.

Longo, D. L., A. S. Fauci, D. L. Kasper, S. L. Hauser, J. L. Jameson, and J. Loscalzo. 2012. *Harrison's principles of internal medicine:* 18th edition. New York: McGraw-Hill.

Lutgendorf, S., N. G. Klimas, M. Antoni, A. Brickman, and M. A. Fletcher. 1995. Relationships of cognitive difficulties to immune measures, depression and illness burden in chronic fatigue syndrome. *Journal of Chronic Fatigue Syndrome* 1(2):23-41.

Lyall, M., M. Peakman, and S. Wessely. 2003. A systematic review and critical evaluation of the immunology of chronic fatigue syndrome. *Journal of Psychosomatic Research* 55(2):79-90.

Maes, M., I. Mihaylova, and J.-C. Leunis. 2006. Chronic fatigue syndrome is accompanied by an IgM-related immune response directed against neoitopes formed by oxidative or nitrosative damage to lipids and proteins. *Neuroendocrinology Letters* 27(5):615-621.

Maes, M., F. N. M. Twisk, and C. Johnson. 2012. Myalgic encephalomyelitis (ME), chronic fatigue syndrome (CFS), and chronic fatigue (CF) are distinguished accurately: Results of supervised learning techniques applied on clinical and inflammatory data. *Psychiatry Research* 200(2-3):754-760.

Maes, M., K. Ringel, M. Kubera, G. Anderson, G. Morris, P. Galecki, and M. Geffard. 2013. In myalgic encephalomyelitis/chronic fatigue syndrome, increased autoimmune activity against 5-HT is associated with immuno-inflammatory pathways and bacterial translocation. *Journal of Affective Disorders* 150(2):223-230.

Maher, K. J., N. G. Klimas, and M. A. Fletcher. 2005. Chronic fatigue syndrome is associated with diminished intracellular perforin. *Clinical & Experimental Immunology* 142(3):505-511.

Manian, F. A. 1994. Simultaneous measurement of antibodies to Epstein-Barr virus, human herpesvirus 6, herpes simplex virus types 1 and 2, and 14 enteroviruses in chronic fatigue syndrome: Is there evidence of activation of a nonspecific polyclonal immune response? *Clinical Infectious Diseases* 19(3):448-453.

Markopoulou, K., A. Roberts, A. Papadopoulos, S. Wessely, T. Chalder, and A. Cleare. 2010. The ratio of cortisol/DHEA in chronic fatigue syndrome. *Journal of Affective Disorders* 122:S71.

Marshall, R., L. Paul, A. K. McFadyen, D. Rafferty, and L. Wood. 2010. Pain characteristics of people with chronic fatigue syndrome. *Journal of Musculoskeletal Pain* 18(2):127-137.

Maupin, C. 2014. *More than just "fatigue."* http://www.cfidsreport.com/Articles/CFS/Chronic_Fatigue_Syndrome-Fatigue.htm (accessed January 14, 2015).

Mawle, A. C., R. Nisenbaum, J. G. Dobbins, H. E. Gary, Jr., J. A. Stewart, M. Reyes, L. Steele, D. S. Schmid, and W. C. Reeves. 1995. Seroepidemiology of chronic fatigue syndrome: A case-control study. *Clinical Infectious Diseases* 21(6):1386-1389.

Mawle, A. C., R. Nisenbaum, J. G. Dobbins, H. E. Gary, Jr., J. A. Stewart, M. Reyes, L. Steele, D. S. Schmid, and W. C. Reeves. 1997. Immune responses associated with chronic fatigue syndrome: A case-control study. *Journal of Infectious Diseases* 175(1):136-141.

McCormack, H. M., D. J. Horne, and S. Sheather. 1988. Clinical applications of visual analogue scales: A critical review. *Psychological Medicine* 18(4):1007-1019.

McKenzie, R., A. O'Fallon, J. Dale, M. Demitrack, G. Sharma, M. Deloria, D. Garcia-Borreguero, W. Blackwelder, and S. E. Straus. 1998. Low-dose hydrocortisone for treatment of chronic fatigue syndrome: A randomized controlled trial. *Journal of the American Medical Association* 280(12):1061-1066.

Meeus, M., J. Nijs, and K. De Meirleir. 2007. Chronic musculoskeletal pain in patients with the chronic fatigue syndrome: A systematic review. *European Journal of Pain* 11(4):377-386.

Meeus, M., W. Mistiaen, L. Lambrecht, and J. Nijs. 2009. Immunological similarities between cancer and chronic fatigue syndrome: The common link to fatigue? *Anticancer Research* 29(11):4717-4726.

Meeus, M., L. Hermans, K. Ickmans, F. Struyf, D. Van Cauwenbergh, L. Bronckaerts, L. S. De Clerck, G. Moorken, G. Hans, S. Grosemans, and J. Nijs. 2014. Endogenous pain modulation in response to exercise in patients with rheumatoid arthritis, patients with chronic fatigue syndrome and comorbid fibromyalgia, and healthy controls: A double-blind randomized controlled trial. *Pain Practice* [Epub ahead of print].

Mella, O., and O. Fluge. 2014. *B-lymphocyte depletion using rituximab in chronic fatigue syndrome/myalgic encephalopathy (CFS/ME). A randomized phase-III study. (RituxME).* https://clinicaltrials.gov/ct2/show/NCT02229942 (accessed September 17, 2014).

Mihaylova, I., M. DeRuyter, J. L. Rummens, E. Bosmans, and M. Maes. 2007. Decreased expression of CD69 in chronic fatigue syndrome in relation to inflammatory markers: Evidence for a severe disorder in the early activation of T lymphocytes and natural killer cells. *Neuroendocrinology Letters* 28(4):477-483.

Miwa, K., and M. Fujita. 2008. Small heart syndrome in patients with chronic fatigue syndrome. *Clinical Cardiology* 31(7):328-333.

Miwa, K., and M. Fujita. 2009. Cardiac function fluctuates during exacerbation and remission in young adults with chronic fatigue syndrome and "small heart." *Journal of Cardiology* 54(1):29-35.

Miwa, K., and M. Fujita. 2011. Small heart with low cardiac output for orthostatic intolerance in patients with chronic fatigue syndrome. *Clinical Cardiology* 34(12):782-786.

Miwa, K., and M. Fujita. 2014. Renin-aldosterone paradox in patients with myalgic encephalomyelitis and orthostatic intolerance. *International Journal of Cardiology* 172(2):514-515.

Montoya, J. G., A. M. Kogelnik, M. Bhangoo, M. R. Lunn, L. Flamand, L. E. Merrihew, T. Watt, J. T. Kubo, J. Paik, and M. Desai. 2013. Randomized clinical trial to evaluate the efficacy and safety of valganciclovir in a subset of patients with chronic fatigue syndrome. *Journal of Medical Virology* 85(12):2101-2109.

Moorkens, G., J. Berwaerts, H. Wynants, and R. Abs. 2000. Characterization of pituitary function with emphasis on GH secretion in the chronic fatigue syndrome. *Clinical Endocrinology* 53(1):99-106.

Nacul, L. C., E. M. Lacerda, D. Pheby, P. Campion, M. Molokhia, S. Fayyaz, J. C. Leite, F. Poland, A. Howe, and M. L. Drachler. 2011. Prevalence of myalgic encephalomyelitis/chronic fatigue syndrome (ME/CFS) in three regions of England: A repeated cross-sectional study in primary care. *BMC Medicine* 9:91.

Naess, H., E. Sundal, K. M. Myhr, and H. I. Nyland. 2010. Postinfectious and chronic fatigue syndromes: Clinical experience from a tertiary-referral centre in Norway. *In Vivo* 24(2):185-188.

Naess, H., M. Nyland, T. Hausken, I. Follestad, and H. I. Nyland. 2012. Chronic fatigue syndrome after giardia enteritis: Clinical characteristics, disability and long-term sickness absence. *BMC Gastroenterology* 12:13.

Nakamura, T., S. K. Schwander, R. Donnelly, F. Ortega, F. Togo, G. Broderick, Y. Yamamoto, N. S. Cherniack, D. Rapoport, and B. H. Natelson. 2010. Cytokines across the night in chronic fatigue syndrome with and without fibromyalgia. *Clinical and Vaccine Immunology* 17(4):582-587.

Nakamura, T., S. Schwander, R. Donnelly, D. B. Cook, F. Ortega, F. Togo, Y. Yamamoto, N. S. Cherniack, M. Klapholz, D. Rapoport, and B. H. Natelson. 2013. Exercise and sleep deprivation do not change cytokine expression levels in patients with chronic fatigue syndrome. *Clinical and Vaccine Immunology* 20(11):1736-1742.

Narita, M., N. Nishigami, N. Narita, K. Yamaguti, N. Okado, Y. Watanabe, and H. Kuratsune. 2003. Association between serotonin transporter gene polymorphism and chronic fatigue syndrome. *Biochemical & Biophysical Research Communications* 311(2):264-266.

Naschitz, J. E., G. Slobodin, D. Sharif, M. Fields, H. Isseroff, E. Sabo, and I. Rosner. 2008. Electrocardiographic QT interval and cardiovascular reactivity in fibromyalgia differ from chronic fatigue syndrome. *European Journal of Internal Medicine* 19(3):187-191.

Natelson, B. H. 2010. Chronic fatigue syndrome and fibromyalgia: A status report in 2010. *MD Advisor* 3(3):18-25.

Natelson, B. H., N. Ye, and Y. C. Cheng. 1990. Evidence of actively replacing Epstein-Barr-virus in patients with the chronic fatigue syndrome. *Annals of Neurology* 28(2):252.

Natelson, B. H., N. Ye, D. E. Moul, F. J. Jenkins, D. A. Oren, W. N. Tapp, and Y. C. Cheng. 1994. High titers of anti-Epstein-Barr virus DNA polymerase are found in patients with severe fatiguing illness. *Journal of Medical Virology* 42(1):42-46.

Natelson, B. H., J. J. LaManca, T. N. Denny, A. Vladutiu, J. Oleske, N. Hill, M. T. Bergen, L. Korn, and J. Hay. 1998. Immunologic parameters in chronic fatigue syndrome, major depression, and multiple sclerosis. *American Journal of Medicine* 105(3A):43S-49S.

Nater, U. M., L. S. Youngblood, J. F. Jones, E. R. Unger, A. H. Miller, W. C. Reeves, and C. Heim. 2008. Alterations in diurnal salivary cortisol rhythm in a population-based sample of cases with chronic fatigue syndrome. *Psychosomatic Medicine* 70(3):298-305.

Neu, D., O. Mairesse, X. Montana, M. Gilson, F. Corazza, N. Lefevre, P. Linkowski, O. Le Bon, and P. Verbanck. 2014. Dimensions of pure chronic fatigue: Psychophysical, cognitive and biological correlates in the chronic fatigue syndrome. *European Journal of Applied Physiology* 114(9):1841-1851.

NICE (National Institute for Health and Clinical Excellence). 2007. *Chronic fatigue syndrome/myalgic encephalomyelitis (or encephalopathy): Diagnosis and management of CFS/ME in adults and children.* London, UK: NICE.

Nicolson, G. L., M. Y. Nasralla, K. De Meirleir, R. Gan, and J. Haier. 2003. Evidence for bacterial (mycoplasma, chlamydia) and viral (HHV-6) co-infections in chronic fatigue syndrome patients. *Journal of Chronic Fatigue Syndrome* 11(2):7-19.

Nishikai, M., K. Akiya, T. Tojo, N. Onoda, M. Tani, and K. Shimizu. 1996. "Seronegative" Sjögren's syndrome manifested as a subset of chronic fatigue syndrome. *British Journal of Rheumatology* 35(5):471-474.

Nishikai, M., S. Tomomatsu, R. W. Hankins, S. Takagi, K. Miyachi, S. Kosaka, and K. Akiya. 2001. Autoantibodies to a 68/48 kDa protein in chronic fatigue syndrome and primary fibromyalgia: A possible marker for hypersomnia and cognitive disorders. *Rheumatology* 40(7):806-810.

Ojo-Amaize, E. A., E. J. Conley, and J. B. Peter. 1994. Decreased natural killer cell activity is associated with severity of chronic fatigue immune dysfunction syndrome. *Clinical Infectious Diseases* 18(Suppl. 1):S157-S159.

Oosterlynck, D. J., F. J. Cornillie, M. Waer, M. Vandeputte, and P. R. Koninckx. 1991. Women with endometriosis show a defect in natural killer activity resulting in a decreased cytotoxicity to autologous endometrium. *Fertility and Sterility* 56(1):45-51.

Op De Beéck, K., P. Vermeersch, P. Verschueren, R. Westhovens, G. Mariën, D. Blockmans, and X. Bossuyt. 2012. Antinuclear antibody detection by automated multiplex immunoassay in untreated patients at the time of diagnosis. *Autoimmunity Reviews* 12(2):137-143.

Ortega-Hernandez, O.-D., M. Cuccia, S. Bozzini, N. Bassi, S. Moscavitch, L.-M. Diaz-Gallo, M. Blank, N. Agmon-Levin, and Y. Shoenfeld. 2009. Autoantibodies, polymorphisms in the serotonin pathway, and human leukocyte antigen class II alleles in chronic fatigue syndrome: Are they associated with age at onset and specific symptoms? In *Contemporary challenges in autoimmunity*, edited by Y. Shoenfeld and M. E. Gershwin. *Annals of the New York Academy of Sciences* 1173:589-599.

Ottenweller, J. E., S. A. Sisto, R. C. McCarty, and B. H. Natelson. 2001. Hormonal responses to exercise in chronic fatigue syndrome. *Neuropsychobiology* 43(1):34-41.

Papadopoulos, A., M. Ebrecht, A. D. L. Roberts, L. Poon, N. Rohleder, and A. J. Cleare. 2009. Glucocorticoid receptor mediated negative feedback in chronic fatigue syndrome using the low dose (0.5 mg) dexamethasone suppression test. *Journal of Affective Disorders* 112(1-3):289-294.

Parish, J. G. 1978. Early outbreaks of "epidemic neuromyasthenia." *Postgraduate Medical Journal* 54(637):711-717.

Park, D. C., J. M. Glass, M. Minear, and L. J. Crofford. 2001. Cognitive function in fibromyalgia patients. *Arthritis & Rheumatology* 44(9):2125-2133.

Parker, A. J. R., S. Wessely, and A. J. Cleare. 2001. The neuroendocrinology of chronic fatigue syndrome and fibromyalgia. *Psychological Medicine* 31(8):1331-1345.

Patnaik, M., A. L. Komaroff, E. Conley, E. A. Ojo-Amaize, and J. B. Peter. 1995. Prevalence of IgM antibodies to human herpesvirus 6 early antigen (p41/38) in patients with chronic fatigue syndrome. *Journal of Infectious Diseases* 172(5):1364-1367.

Peakman, M., A. Deale, R. Field, M. Mahalingam, and S. Wessely. 1997. Clinical improvement in chronic fatigue syndrome is not associated with lymphocyte subsets of function or activation. *Clinical Immunology and Immunopathology* 82(1):83-91.

Peterson, P. K., A. Pheley, J. Schroeppel, C. Schenck, P. Marshall, A. Kind, J. M. Haugland, L. J. Lambrecht, S. Swan, and S. Goldsmith. 1998. A preliminary placebo-controlled crossover trial of fludrocortisone for chronic fatigue syndrome. *Archives of Internal Medicine* 158(8):908-914.

Porter, N., A. Lerch, L. A. Jason, M. Sorenson, M. A. Fletcher, and J. Herrington. 2010. A comparison of immune functionality in viral versus non-viral CFS subtypes. *Journal of Behavioral and Neuroscience Research* 8(2):1-8.

Powell, D. J. H., C. Liossi, R. Moss-Morris, and W. Schlotz. 2013. Unstimulated cortisol secretory activity in everyday life and its relationship with fatigue and chronic fatigue syndrome: A systematic review and subset meta-analysis. *Psychoneuroendocrinology* 38(11):2405-2422.

Presson, A. P., E. M. Sobel, J. C. Papp, C. J. Suarez, T. Whistler, M. S. Rajeevan, S. D. Vernon, and S. Horvath. 2009. Integrated weighted gene co-expression network analysis with an application to chronic fatigue syndrome. *BMC Systems Biology* 2.

Racciatti, D., M. T. Guagnano, J. Vecchiet, P. L. De Remigis, E. Pizzigallo, R. Della Vecchia, T. Di Sciascio, D. Merlitti, and S. Sensi. 2001. Chronic fatigue syndrome: Circadian rhythm and hypothalamic-pituitary-adrenal (HPA) axis impairment. *International Journal of Immunopathology and Pharmacology* 14(1):11-15.

Reeves, W. C., F. R. Stamey, J. B. Black, A. C. Mawle, J. A. Stewart, and P. E. Pellett. 2000. Human herpesviruses 6 and 7 in chronic fatigue syndrome: A case-control study. *Clinical Infectious Diseases* 31(1):48-52.

Reeves, W. C., J. F. Jones, E. Maloney, C. Heim, D. C. Hoaglin, R. S. Boneva, M. Morrissey, and R. Devlin. 2007. Prevalence of chronic fatigue syndrome in metropolitan, urban, and rural Georgia. *Population Health Metrics* 5.

Reyes, M., R. Nisenbaum, D. C. Hoaglin, E. R. Unger, C. Emmons, B. Randall, J. A. Stewart, S. Abbey, J. F. Jones, N. Gantz, S. Minden, and W. C. Reeves. 2003. Prevalence and incidence of chronic fatigue syndrome in Wichita, Kansas. *Archives of Internal Medicine* 163(13):1530-1536.

Richter, J., V. Benson, V. Grobarova, J. Svoboda, J. Vencovsky, R. Svobodova, and A. Fiserova. 2010. CD161 receptor participates in both impairing NK cell cytotoxicity and the response to glycans and vimentin in patients with rheumatoid arthritis. *Clinical Immunology* 136(1):139-147.

Roberts, A. D. L., S. Wessely, T. Chalder, A. Papadopoulos, and A. J. Cleare. 2004. Salivary cortisol response to awakening in chronic fatigue syndrome. *British Journal of Psychiatry* 184:136-141.

Roberts, A. D. L., M. L. Charler, A. Papadopoulos, S. Wessely, T. Chalder, and A. J. Cleare. 2010. Does hypocortisolism predict a poor response to cognitive behavioural therapy in chronic fatigue syndrome? *Psychological Medicine* 40(3):515-522.

Rosmalen, J. G. M., L. M. Tak, J. Ormel, A. Manoharan, I. Kok, S. Wessely, and A. Cleare. 2010. Meta-analysis and meta-regression of hypothalamic-pituitary-adrenal axis activity in functional somatic disorders. *Journal of Psychosomatic Research* 68(6):659-660.

Rowe, P. C., H. Calkins, K. DeBusk, R. McKenzie, R. Anand, G. Sharma, B. A. Cuccherini, N. Soto, P. Hohman, S. Snader, K. E. Lucas, M. Wolff, and S. E. Straus. 2001. Fludrocortisone acetate to treat neurally mediated hypotension in chronic fatigue syndrome: A randomized controlled trial. *Journal of the American Medical Association* 285(1):52-59.

Russell, I. J., M. D. Orr, B. Littman, G. A. Vipraio, D. Alboukrek, J. E. Michalek, Y. Lopez, and F. MacKillip. 1994. Elevated cerebrospinal fluid levels of substance p in patients with the fibromyalgia syndrome. *Arthritis & Rheumatology* 37(11):1593-1601.

Sairenji, T., K. Yamanishi, Y. Tachibana, G. Bertoni, and T. Kurata. 1995. Antibody responses to Epstein-Barr virus, human herpesvirus 6 and human herpesvirus 7 in patients with chronic fatigue syndrome. *Intervirology* 38(5):269-273.

Schutzer, S. E., T. E. Angel, T. Liu, A. A. Schepmoes, T. R. Clauss, J. N. Adkins, D. G. Camp, B. K. Holland, J. Bergquist, P. K. Coyle, R. D. Smith, B. A. Fallon, and B. H. Natelson. 2011. Distinct cerebrospinal fluid proteomes differentiate post-treatment Lyme disease from chronic fatigue syndrome. *PLoS ONE* 6(2):e17287.

Scott, L. V., F. Burnett, S. Medbak, and T. G. Dinan. 1998a. Naloxone-mediated activation of the hypothalamic-pituitary-adrenal axis in chronic fatigue syndrome. *Psychological Medicine* 28(2):285-293.

Scott, L. V., S. Medbak, and T. G. Dinan. 1998b. Blunted adrenocorticotropin and cortisol responses to corticotropin-releasing hormone stimulation in chronic fatigue syndrome. *Acta Psychiatrica Scandinavica* 97(6):450-457.

Scott, L. V., S. Medbak, and T. G. Dinan. 1998c. The low dose ACTH test in chronic fatigue syndrome and in health. *Clinical Endocrinology* 48(6):733-737.

Seishima, M., Y. Mizutani, Y. Shibuya, and C. Arakawa. 2008. Chronic fatigue syndrome after human parvovirus B19 infection without persistent viremia. *Dermatology* 216(4):341-346.

Sharpe, M., A. Clements, K. Hawton, A. H. Young, P. Sargent, and P. J. Cowen. 1996. Increased prolactin response to buspirone in chronic fatigue syndrome. *Journal of Affective Disorders* 41(1):71-76.

Shelokov, A., K. Habel, E. Verder, and W. Welsh. 1957. Epidemic neuromyasthenia; an outbreak of poliomyelitislike illness in student nurses. *New England Journal of Medicine* 257(8):345-355.

Siegel, S. D., M. H. Antoni, M. A. Fletcher, K. Maher, M. C. Segota, and N. Klimas. 2006. Impaired natural immunity, cognitive dysfunction, and physical symptoms in patients with chronic fatigue syndrome: Preliminary evidence for a subgroup? *Journal of Psychosomatic Research* 60(6):559-566.

Sirois, D. A., and B. Natelson. 2001. Clinicopathological findings consistent with primary Sjögren's syndrome in a subset of patients diagnosed with chronic fatigue syndrome: Preliminary observations. *Journal of Rheumatology* 28(1):126-131.

Skowera, A., E. Stewart, E. T. Davis, A. J. Cleare, C. Unwin, L. Hull, K. Ismail, G. Hossain, S. C. Wessely, and M. Peakman. 2002. Antinuclear autoantibodies (ANA) in gulf war-related illness and chronic fatigue syndrome (CFS) patients. *Clinical & Experimental Immunology* 129(2):354-358.

Smylie, A. L., G. Broderick, H. Fernandes, S. Razdan, Z. Barnes, F. Collado, C. Sol, M. A. Fletcher, and N. Klimas. 2013. A comparison of sex-specific immune signatures in gulf war illness and chronic fatigue syndrome. *BMC Immunology* 14:29.

Solomon, L., and W. C. Reeves. 2004. Factors influencing the diagnosis of chronic fatigue syndrome. *Archives of Internal Medicine* 164(20):2241-2245.

Stewart, C. C., D. L. Cookfair, K. M. Hovey, K. E. Wende, D. S. Bell, and C. L. Warner. 2003. Predictive immunophenotypes: Disease-related profile in chronic fatigue syndrome. *Cytometry Part B, Clinical Cytometry* 53(1):26-33.

Straus, S. E., J. K. Dale, M. Tobi, T. Lawley, O. Preble, R. M. Blaese, C. Hallahan, and W. Henle. 1988. Acyclovir treatment of the chronic fatigue syndrome. Lack of efficacy in a placebo-controlled trial. *New England Journal of Medicine* 319(26):1692-1698.

Straus, S. E., S. Fritz, J. K. Dale, B. Gould, and W. Strober. 1993. Lymphocyte phenotype and function in the chronic fatigue syndrome. *Journal of Clinical Immunology* 13(1):30-40.

Strauss, B., M. Loschau, T. Seidel, A. Stallmach, and A. Thomas. 2012. Are fatigue symptoms and chronic fatigue syndrome following Q fever infection related to psychosocial variables? *Journal of Psychosomatic Research* 72(4):300-304.

Strickland, P. S., P. H. Levine, D. L. Peterson, K. O'Brien, and T. Fears. 2001. Neuromyasthenia and chronic fatigue syndrome (CFS) in northern Nevada/California: A ten-year follow-up of an outbreak. *Journal of Chronic Fatigue Syndrome* 9(3-4):3-14.

Sumaya, C. V. 1991. Serologic and virologic epidemiology of Epstein-Barr virus: Relevance to chronic fatigue syndrome. *Reviews of Infectious Diseases* 13(Suppl. 1):S19-S25.

Swanink, C. M., J. W. van der Meer, J. H. Vercoulen, G. Bleijenberg, J. F. Fennis, and J. M. Galama. 1995. Epstein-Barr virus (EBV) and the chronic fatigue syndrome: Normal virus load in blood and normal immunologic reactivity in the EBV regression assay. *Clinical Infectious Diseases* 20(5):1390-1392.

Tak, L. M., A. J. Cleare, J. Ormel, A. Manoharan, I. C. Kok, S. Wessely, and J. G. Rosmalen. 2011. Meta-analysis and meta-regression of hypothalamic-pituitary-adrenal axis activity in functional somatic disorders. *Biological Psychology* 87(2):183-194.

Tanaka, S., H. Kuratsune, Y. Hidaka, Y. Hakariya, K. I. Tatsumi, T. Takano, Y. Kanakura, and N. Amino. 2003. Autoantibodies against muscarinic cholinergic receptor in chronic fatigue syndrome. *International Journal of Molecular Medicine* 12(2):225-230.

The, G. K. H., G. Bleijenberg, and J. W. M. van der Meer. 2007. The effect of acclydine in chronic fatigue syndrome: A randomized controlled trial. *PLOS Clinical Trials* 2(5):e19.

Tirelli, U., G. Marotta, S. Improta, and A. Pinto. 1994. Immunological abnormalities in patients with chronic-fatigue-syndrome. *Scandinavian Journal of Immunology* 40(6):601-608.

Tomas, C., J. Newton, and S. Watson. 2013. A review of hypothalamic-pituitary-adrenal axis function in chronic fatigue syndrome. *ISRN Neuroscience* 2013:1-8.

Unger, E. 2013. Measures of CFS in a multi-site clinical study. Paper read at FDA Scientific Drug Development Workshop, April 26, 2013, Washington, DC.

Van Den Eede, F., G. Moorkens, W. Hulstijn, B. Van Houdenhove, P. Cosyns, B. G. C. Sabbe, and S. J. Claes. 2008. Combined dexamethasone/corticotropin-releasing factor test in chronic fatigue syndrome. *Psychological Medicine* 38(7):963-973.

Van Oosterwijck, J., J. Nijs, M. Meeus, I. Lefever, L. Huybrechts, L. Lambrecht, and L. Paul. 2010. Pain inhibition and postexertional malaise in myalgic encephalomyelitis/chronic fatigue syndrome: An experimental study. *Journal of Internal Medicine* 268(3):265-278.

Vernon, S. D., and W. C. Reeves. 2005. Evaluation of autoantibodies to common and neuronal cell antigens in chronic fatigue syndrome. *Journal of Autoimmune Diseases* 2(5).

Vollmer-Conna, U., B. Cameron, D. Hadzi-Pavlovic, K. Singletary, T. Davenport, S. Vernon, W. C. Reeves, I. Hickie, D. Wakefield, and A. R. Lloyd. 2007. Postinfective fatigue syndrome is not associated with altered cytokine production. *Clinical Infectious Diseases* 45(6):732-735.

vonMikecz, A., K. Konstantinov, D. S. Buchwald, L. Gerace, and E. M. Tan. 1997. High frequency of autoantibodies to insoluble cellular antigens in patients with chronic fatigue syndrome. *Arthritis and Rheumatism* 40(2):295-305.

Watt, T., S. Oberfoell, R. Balise, M. R. Lunn, A. K. Kar, L. Merrihew, M. S. Bhangoo, and J. G. Montoya. 2012. Response to valganciclovir in chronic fatigue syndrome patients with human herpesvirus 6 and Epstein-Barr virus IgG antibody titers. *Journal of Medical Virology* 84(12):1967-1974.

Weiner, D. K., T. E. Rudy, L. Morrow, J. Slaboda, and S. Lieber. 2006. The relationship between pain, neuropsychological performance, and physical function in community-dwelling older adults with chronic low back pain. *Pain Medicine* 7(1):60-70.

Whelton, C. L., I. Salit, and H. Moldofsky. 1992. Sleep, Epstein-Barr virus infection, musculoskeletal pain, and depressive symptoms in chronic fatigue syndrome. *Journal of Rheumatology* 19(6):939-943.

White, A. T., A. R. Light, R. W. Hughen, L. Bateman, T. B. Martins, H. R. Hill, and K. C. Light. 2010. Severity of symptom flare after moderate exercise is linked to cytokine activity in chronic fatigue syndrome. *Psychophysiology* 47(4):615-624.

White, K. P., M. Speechley, M. Harth, and T. Ostbye. 1999. The London fibromyalgia epidemiology study: The prevalence of fibromyalgia syndrome in London, Ontario. *Journal of Rheumatology* 26(7):1570-1576.

White, P. D., J. M. Thomas, J. Amess, D. H. Crawford, S. A. Grover, H. O. Kangro, and A. W. Clare. 1998. Incidence, risk and prognosis of acute and chronic fatigue syndromes and psychiatric disorders after glandular fever. *British Journal of Psychiatry* 173:475-481.

Whiteside, A., S. Hansen, and A. Chaudhuri. 2004. Exercise lowers pain threshold in chronic fatigue syndrome. *Pain* 109(3):497-499.

Whiteside, T. L., and D. Friberg. 1998. Natural killer cells and natural killer cell activity in chronic fatigue syndrome. *American Journal of Medicine* 105(3A):27S-34S.

Wildman, M. J., E. G. Smith, J. Groves, J. M. Beattie, E. O. Caul, and J. G. Ayres. 2002. Chronic fatigue following infection by Coxiella burnetii (Q fever): Ten-year follow-up of the 1989 UK outbreak cohort. *QJM: Monthly Journal of the Association of Physicians* 95(8):527-538.

Wolfe, F., K. Ross, J. Anderson, I. J. Russell, and L. Hebert. 1995. The prevalence and characteristics of fibromyalgia in the general population. *Arthritis & Rheumatology* 38(1):19-28.

Wolfe, F., D. J. Clauw, M. A. Fitzcharles, D. L. Goldenberg, R. S. Katz, P. Mease, A. S. Russell, I. J. Russell, J. B. Winfield, and M. B. Yunus. 2010. The American College of Rheumatology preliminary diagnostic criteria for fibromyalgia and measurement of symptom severity. *Arthritis Care & Research* 62(5):600-610.

Yalcin, S., H. Kuratsune, K. Yamaguchi, T. Kitani, and K. Yamanishi. 1994. Prevalence of human herpesvirus-6 variant-A and variant-B in patients with chronic-fatigue-syndrome. *Microbiology and Immunology* 38(7):587-590.

Yamamoto, S., Y. Ouchi, H. Onoe, E. Yoshikawa, H. Tsukada, H. Takahashi, M. Iwase, K. Yamaguti, H. Kuratsune, and Y. Watanabe. 2004. Reduction of serotonin transporters of patients with chronic fatigue syndrome. *NeuroReport: For Rapid Communication of Neuroscience Research* 15(17):2571-2574.

Yanai, H., K. Takada, N. Shimizu, Y. Mizugaki, M. Tada, and K. Okita. 1997. Epstein-Barr virus infection in non-carcinomatous gastric epithelium. *Journal of Pathology* 183(3):293-298.

Zeidel, A., B. Beilin, I. Yardeni, E. Mayburd, G. Smirnov, and H. Bessler. 2002. Immune response in asymptomatic smokers. *Acta Anaesthesiologica Scandinavica* 46(8):959-964.

Zhang, H. Y., Z. D. Liu, C. J. Hu, D. X. Wang, Y. B. Zhang, and Y. Z. Li. 2011. Up-regulation of TGF-β1 mRNA expression in peripheral blood mononuclear cells of patients with chronic fatigue syndrome. *Journal of the Formosan Medical Association* 110(11):701-704.

Zorzenon, M. 1996. Active HHV-6 infection in chronic fatigue syndrome patients from Italy: New data. *Journal of Chronic Fatigue Syndrome* 2(1):3-12.

6

Pediatric ME/CFS

Pediatric ME/CFS has been defined as a complex, multisystemic, and debilitating illness that is characterized by severe and medically unexplained fatigue and is usually accompanied by post-exertional malaise (PEM), orthostatic intolerance and other signs of autonomic dysfunction, and cognitive problems, as well as by unrefreshing sleep, headache, and other pain symptoms (Carruthers et al., 2003, 2011; Jason et al., 2006, 2010). Pediatric ME/CFS presents with either an acute (which can be infectious or noninfectious) or a gradual onset. Several studies showed that a gradual-onset pattern is more frequent (Bell et al., 2001; Nijhof et al., 2011), while others found an acute infectious onset to be more common, seen in 88 to 93 percent of young patients with ME/CFS (Kennedy et al., 2010b; Sankey et al., 2006). Patients often follow a prolonged and complex path before receiving a diagnosis of pediatric ME/CFS. Sankey and colleagues (2006) estimate that the median time from the start of symptoms to diagnosis is 8.5 months, while Nijhof and colleagues (2011) report 17 months. The challenges of diagnosis are described in Chapter 2.

The Royal College of Paediatrics and Child Health proposed pediatric criteria for ME/CFS in 2004 (Royal College, 2004). These authors considered whether a shorter time frame for diagnosis—3 months' duration rather than the 6 months for adults—is appropriate for children. In the absence of compelling epidemiological data, the authors concluded that the diagnosis of ME/CFS requires 6 months. They nonetheless suggest that pediatricians be "prepared to make a positive diagnosis of CFS/ME when a child or young person has characteristic symptoms supported by normal results and when the symptoms are causing significant functional impairment. This diagnosis does not depend on a specific time frame and a positive diagnosis of CFS/ME is not a prerequisite for the initiation of an appropriate management plan" (Royal College, 2004). The British National Institute for Health and Clinical Excellence (NICE) guidelines, published in 2007, recommend a duration of symptoms of 3 months for children and young people (NICE, 2007).

The International Association for Chronic Fatigue Syndrome/Myalgic Encephalomyelitis (IACFS/ME) developed a case definition for diagnosis of ME/CFS in children and adolescents using the DePaul Pediatric Health Questionnaire (DPHQ), a self-report measure for assessing ME/CFS symptoms in this population. This tool measures not only the presence of the symptoms but also their severity and frequency (Jason et al., 2006). The IACFS/ME Pediatric Case Definition incorporates elements of the Fukuda definition (see Chapter 3) and follows the structure of the 2003 Canadian Consensus Criteria (CCC). To make a diagnosis of ME/CFS, this definition requires the presence of symptoms more specific than those in the Fukuda definition, and it emphasizes the importance of such symptoms as dizziness, decreased endurance with symptoms, pain, and flu-like symptoms, which have frequently been reported by young ME/CFS patients (Jason et al., 2006). An important difference from the other case definitions is that the duration of symptoms required to make a diagnosis is 3 months rather than 6 months. However, subsequent work has shown that a large proportion of those with acute fatigue following infectious mononucleosis will take up to 6 months to improve (Jason et al., 2014; Katz et al., 2009). Most physicians and researchers still elect to apply the Fukuda definition when diagnosing these patients even though this definition was developed for use in research on the adult ME/CFS population (Knight et al., 2013b; Werker et al., 2013).

The prevalence of pediatric ME/CFS has been estimated in British, Dutch, and U.S. populations with numbers that vary widely, from 0.03 to 1.29 percent (Chalder et al., 2003; Crawley et al., 2011; Farmer et al., 2004; Jordan et al., 2006; Nijhof et al., 2011; Rimes et al., 2007). The differing estimates may be due to the different methodologies used in these studies, the application of different ME/CFS definitions, the use of self-reported data obtained from patients instead of physician diagnoses, and the use of community-based rather than tertiary care samples. Besides differences in methodology, underreporting of ME/CFS may occur if physicians make a diagnosis of postural orthostatic tachycardia syndrome (POTS) without assessing for ME/CFS, considering the large overlap in symptoms between these two entities in both children (Stewart et al., 1999b) and adults (Okamoto et al., 2012). ME/CFS has been reported less frequently in children younger than 10 years old than in older children (Bell et al., 2001; Davies and Crawley, 2008; Farmer et al., 2004). Some have argued that this may reflect a lesser ability of children at these younger ages to describe changes in their activity and the degree of fatigue they experience (Bell, 1995a). Regarding gender, most studies found a greater prevalence in girls, with a female-to-male ratio ranging from 2:1 to 6:1 (Farmer et al., 2004; Knight et al., 2013a; Nijhof et al., 2011).

Although the prognosis in this group often is described as being better than that in adults (Andersen et al., 2004; Cairns and Hotopf, 2005; Kennedy et al., 2010b), a very limited number of long-term follow-up studies reported recovery rates in the ME/CFS pediatric population. Several studies found that 20 to 48 percent of pediatric patients diagnosed using the Fukuda definition showed no improvement or actually had worse fatigue and physical impairment at follow-up times ranging from 2 to 13 years (Bell et al., 2001; Gill et al., 2004; Van Geelen et al., 2010).

There is clear evidence of the impact of ME/CFS on the education and social development of these young people (Kennedy et al., 2010b; Walford et al., 1993). The stigma and social effects of pediatric ME/CFS include the loss of normal childhood activities and, in some extreme instances, inappropriate forcible separation of children from their parents (Holder, 2010). Numerous studies found that school attendance is significantly reduced in a large percentage of patients (Crawley and Sterne, 2009; Smith et al., 1991; Van Geelen et al., 2010; Werker et al., 2013). For instance, Nijhof and colleagues (2011) found that approximately 90 percent of the patients they studied had "considerable" school absence (defined as missing 15 to 50 percent of all school days) during the previous 6 months. Further, a U.K. study showed that ME/CFS was the primary cause of long-term health-related school absence (Dowsett and Colby, 1997). Therefore, the use of such labels as "school refusal" or "school phobia" should be considered only after careful and thorough assessment of these patients. A consistent definition is required to make an accurate diagnosis and to allow physicians to provide adequate treatment for these patients as well as to prevent erroneously labeling them as having a psychiatric condition or as being malingerers (Jason et al., 2006).

When evaluating the available research to develop its findings, conclusions, and recommendations on pediatric ME/CFS, the committee was struck by the paucity of the research conducted to date in this population. For major ME/CFS symptoms such as PEM and sleep disturbances, no more than 10 papers were available on each of these topics. The methodology used to review the literature is described in Chapter 1. Moreover, to the limitations of the research base described in Chapter 4, it is important to add that numerous pediatric studies used a less restrictive ME/CFS definition than that used in other studies and classified children presenting with only "chronic fatigue" lasting for 3 months as ME/CFS cases, further complicating the understanding of this disease. With these caveats, the remainder of this chapter reviews the evidence for pediatric patients with respect to the symptoms of adult ME/CFS discussed in Chapters 4 and 5: PEM, orthostatic intolerance and autonomic dysfunction, neurocognitive manifestations, sleep-related symptoms, infection, immune impairment, neuroendocrine manifestations, and other symptoms (fatigue and pain). The potential for development of symptom constructs in pediatric ME/CFS also is discussed.

POST-EXERTIONAL MALAISE

PEM, as defined in Chapter 4, is the exacerbation of fatigue, cognitive problems, lightheadedness, pain, and a general sense of feeling sick after effort (see the section on PEM in adults in Chapter 4). It is widely considered to be a central feature of ME/CFS. The prevalence of PEM was found to be 71 percent in Australian children at the time of presentation of ME/CFS (Knight et al., 2013a), 80 percent in a cross-sectional study of Dutch adolescents (Nijhof et al., 2011), and 97 percent in a large referral population of British children with ME/CFS (Davies and Crawley, 2008).

Methodological differences account for some of the variability in PEM prevalence rates among studies. These differences may be related to the definition of the illness used, the duration of the illness at the time of the survey, the way the questions about PEM were posed, the types of effort (cognitive/physical activity or orthostatic stress) considered capable of provoking PEM symptoms, the duration of symptom provocation that qualified as PEM (hours versus more than 1 day), whether questions addressed symptom provocation for fatigue alone or for a wider range of posteffort symptoms, the numbers of questions asked to capture the desired information (the higher the number of questions asked, the higher the probability of detecting the phenomenon), the severity of the symptom provocation required to count as having PEM, and differences in the ongoing activity levels of the participants. As an example of the latter, after being evaluated and treated for ME/CFS, individuals might follow recommendations to modulate their activity to avoid triggering worse symptoms. The result would be a lower reported prevalence of PEM than these individuals might have reported if exposed to the same levels of physical, orthostatic, or cognitive stress (or combinations of these physiologic stressors) they experienced prior to the onset of illness.

Assessment of PEM in Pediatric ME/CFS

There is no standardized method of assessing PEM in children. Differences among studies in this regard may reflect in part the variability in the methods used to ask about the patients' symptoms.

Evidence for PEM in Pediatric ME/CFS

The committee examined the literature on the presentation of PEM in children and adolescents with ME/CFS and the differences compared with healthy or diseased controls. Data on PEM prevalence rates among active children or otherwise healthy sedentary controls typically have not been reported. No studies with concurrent controls investigated PEM symptoms in the days following formal exercise tests, and in contrast to the adult literature, no studies using a cardiopulmonary exercise test repeated the test the next day (Katz et al., 2010). Little work has been published on the prevalence of PEM in subsets of children or adolescents diagnosed with ME/CFS (e.g., those with gradual onset versus those with an apparent postinfectious onset).

All three studies involving an exercise stress test identified autonomic or circulatory differences between ME/CFS cases and controls during the exercise challenge (Katz et al., 2010; Takken et al., 2007; Wyller et al., 2008b). Katz and colleagues (2010) compared 21 adolescents who developed ME/CFS after infectious mononucleosis with 21 controls who had recovered from mononucleosis. The ME/CFS individuals exercised less efficiently than recovered controls, with a borderline significant 11 percent difference in predicted peak oxygen consumption ($p = 0.05$) and a significantly lower peak oxygen pulse (O_2 consumption per heartbeat) ($p = 0.03$). This study, however, did not find a significant difference in peak work capacity between ME/CFS patients and controls. Wyller and colleagues (2008b) compared 15 Norwegian adolescents with ME/CFS and 56 healthy adolescent controls. Those with ME/CFS had increased sympathetic activity at rest, with exaggerated cardiovascular responses to orthostatic stress, but attenuated cardiovascular responses to isometric exercise. Only one study assessed fatigue levels in pediatric ME/CFS patients and found that no child among the 20 who underwent exercise testing "reported excessive fatigue levels in the three days after the exercise test" (Takken et al., 2007, p. 582).

Overall, despite the limited research on the effect of exercise testing in pediatric ME/CFS, there is sufficient evidence that PEM is common in these patients.

ORTHOSTATIC INTOLERANCE AND AUTONOMIC DYSFUNCTION

The overlap in symptoms of pediatric orthostatic intolerance, most notably neurally mediated hypotension (NMH) and POTS, and pediatric ME/CFS was first emphasized in a small case series (Rowe et al., 1995) and a controlled study that included both adolescents and adults (Bou-Holaigah et al., 1995). (The definitions of NMH and POTS are discussed in the section on orthostatic intolerance and autonomic dysfunction in adults with ME/CFS in Chapter 4.) Stewart and colleagues (1999b) described in greater detail the differences among those with ME/CFS, those with POTS, and healthy controls. The prevalence of several symptoms was significantly higher in ME/CFS patients than in healthy controls: fatigue (100 versus 8 percent), lightheadedness (100 versus 15 percent), cognitive dysfunction (100 versus 0 percent), exercise intolerance (96 versus 23 percent), headache (92 versus 23 percent), sleep difficulties (80 versus 15 percent), and tender points (20 versus 0 percent). Those with POTS had an intermediate prevalence of the same symptoms. Of interest, frequent sore throat did not discriminate between ME/CFS patients and healthy children. The prevalence of orthostatic symptoms for adolescents with ME/CFS is above 90 percent (Stewart et al., 1999b; Wyller et al., 2008b).

Assessment of Orthostatic Intolerance and Autonomic Dysfunction in Pediatric ME/CFS

The methods used to assess for orthostatic intolerance are described in the section on orthostatic intolerance and autonomic dysfunction in adults with ME/CFS in Chapter 4.

Evidence for Orthostatic Intolerance and Autonomic Dysfunction in Pediatric ME/CFS

The committee examined the literature on the presentation of orthostatic intolerance and related autonomic abnormalities based on both patient report measures and objective testing in pediatric ME/CFS patients and the differences compared with healthy or diseased controls.

Orthostatic Testing in Pediatric ME/CFS

The committee reviewed five studies that compared rates of orthostatic intolerance between controls and those with ME/CFS. Bou-Holaigah and colleagues (1995) included some adolescents, but the mean age of participants was 34, so this paper is not included here.

Stewart and colleagues (1999a) describe NMH, POTS, or both in 96 percent (25/26) of adolescents with ME/CFS during the head-up tilt test. ME/CFS adolescents had a higher prevalence of circulatory abnormalities and clinical signs of acrocyanosis and cool extremities relative to those with recurrent syncope and healthy controls. Individuals with ME/CFS had a significantly higher mean heart rate and lower systolic blood pressure at rest and throughout the head-up tilt test compared with controls.

A study that assessed the impact of a 7-minute period of active standing in 28 Japanese adolescents with ME/CFS and 20 healthy adolescents showed that 57 percent of those with ME/CFS had orthostatic intolerance, compared with no healthy controls (p < 0.01), despite the brief duration of the orthostatic challenge. Among adolescents with ME/CFS, 18/28 experienced a prolonged reduction in oxy-hemoglobin during the 7 minutes of standing, compared with 4/20 controls (p < 0.01), a finding consistent with impaired cerebral hemodynamics (Tanaka et al., 2002).

Wyller and colleagues (2007a) in Norway examined the response to mild orthostatic stress (15 minutes of head-up tilt to just 20 degrees) in 27 adolescents with ME/CFS and 33 controls. At rest, those with ME/CFS had a higher total peripheral resistance index (TPRI), lower stroke index, and lower end-diastolic volume index than controls. With a 20-degree upright tilt, individuals with ME/CFS had greater increases in heart rate, diastolic blood pressure (both p < 0.001), mean blood pressure, and TPRI, as well as greater decreases in stroke index. Several other studies published by Stewart's and Wyller's groups substantiate the findings from their studies mentioned above. However, the independence of the participants from one study to the next is not always clear.

Galland and colleagues (2008) in New Zealand conducted a case-control study of 26 adolescents with ME/CFS and 26 controls. Participants underwent head-up tilt to 70 degrees for a maximum of 30 minutes, but could request that the test be stopped because of orthostatic symptoms before completion. Orthostatic intolerance was identified in 50 percent of ME/CFS patients versus 20 percent of controls (p = 0.04), with POTS being the most prominent problem in the ME/CFS patients. Adolescents with ME/CFS had a 3.2-fold increased risk of tachycardia during tilt.

Katz and colleagues (2012) conducted a nested case-control study comparing responses to 10 minutes of active standing in 36 adolescents with ME/CFS after infectious mononucleosis and 43 recovered controls. At the 6-month point after recovery from infectious mononucleosis, 25 percent of ME/CFS patients and 21 percent of controls met the study definition for orthostatic intolerance, a null finding that stands out from the rest of the literature.

Regardless of differences in methods of orthostatic testing, all studies with controls that examined adolescents with ME/CFS showed a numerically higher prevalence of circulatory disorders, most notably POTS and NMH, in ME/CFS patients. In most studies, the differences between ME/CFS patients and controls were statistically significant.

Heart Rate Variability

Six studies compared heart rate variability in pediatric ME/CFS patients and controls (Galland et al., 2008; Stewart, 2000; Stewart et al., 1998; Wyller et al., 2007c, 2008a, 2011). These studies showed that the R-R interval and measures of heart rate variability were reduced in those with ME/CFS. All of the studies revealed a sympathetic predominance of heart rate control and enhanced vagal withdrawal during either mild or moderate orthostatic stress or lower-body negative pressure (a method of simulating orthostatic stress). Traditional autonomic tests, such as the response to Valsalva maneuver, were found to be normal in pediatric ME/CFS patients (Stewart, 2000), although there are few studies on the topic.

Other Physiological Abnormalities Associated with Orthostatic Intolerance

Sommerfeldt and colleagues (2011) identified polymorphisms in adrenergic control genes (catechol-O-methyltransferase, beta 2 adrenergic receptor) that were associated with differential changes in sympathovagal balance in ME/CFS. Rowe and colleagues (1999) found an association of ME/CFS and orthostatic intolerance with Ehlers-Danlos syndrome (EDS). The association among EDS, joint hypermobility, chronic fatigue, and orthostatic intolerance has been confirmed by several other studies (De Wandele et al., 2014a,b; Gazit et al., 2003).

Treatment

One large randomized controlled trial compared the therapeutic and physiological responses to blocking of sympathetic tone with clonidine in 120 adolescents with ME/CFS. This study showed that successfully blocking sympathetic output with clonidine, as confirmed by a lower norepinephrine level in the treatment arm, led to worse ME/CFS symptoms, a lower number of steps per day, and lower C-reactive protein (Sulheim et al., 2014). The results were consistent with the hypothesis that systemic inflammation and sympathetic enhancement are mechanisms compensating for other physiological derangements in pediatric ME/CFS.

Open treatment of orthostatic intolerance has been described as being associated with improvement in ME/CFS symptoms in at least a subset of adolescents with ME/CFS (Bou-Holaigah et al., 1995; Rowe et al., 1995). Sulheim and colleagues (2012) report on a cohort study in which participants were seen at baseline and 3 to 17 months later. They confirm a correlation between improved hemodynamic variables on repeat 20-degree head-up tilt and improvement in fatigue, PEM, concentration problems, and overall function. The authors conclude that the concomitant improvement in symptoms, autonomic cardiovascular control, severity of ME/CFS-associated fatigue, and functional impairments is consistent with a possible causal relationship among these variables.

NEUROCOGNITIVE MANIFESTATIONS

Neurocognitive manifestations are among the most commonly reported symptoms in children and adolescents with ME/CFS, cited by 66 to 84 percent of patients in recent studies from Australia, Great Britain, and the Netherlands (Davies and Crawley, 2008; Knight et al., 2013a; Nijhof et al., 2011).

Assessment of Neurocognitive Manifestations in Pediatric ME/CFS

Other than a history that focuses on problems with concentration, short-term memory, and attention span, more formal methods used to assess neurocognitive symptoms in ME/CFS include neuropsychological testing at baseline and under conditions of cognitive or physiological stress. One such measure is the n-back test, which evaluates working memory, attention, concentration, and information processing (see the section on neurocognitive manifestations in adults with ME/CFS in Chapter 4). Questionnaires such as the Wood Mental Fatigue Inventory and elements from symptom surveys that address mental fatigue also are used to evaluate adolescents (Bentall et al., 1993; Wood et al., 1991).

Evidence for Neurocognitive Manifestations in Pediatric ME/CFS

The committee reviewed the literature to evaluate the neurocognitive symptoms experienced by pediatric ME/CFS patients and their differences from healthy and diseased controls. There are some broadly consistent themes. In study and clinic samples of those with pediatric ME/CFS not selected on the basis of greater difficulty with cognitive tasks, results of baseline neuropsychological testing are similar to those for healthy controls. Abnormalities emerge when participants are selected on the basis of increased difficulty with memory and concentration and when more complex challenges are employed, most notably those combining orthostatic and cognitive stresses (Haig-Ferguson et al., 2009; Kawatani et al., 2011; Ocon et al., 2012; Stewart et al., 2012; Tomoda et al., 2007; van de Putte et al., 2008).

Two studies conducted with adequate methodology, describing the same group of patients, assessed the effects of combined orthostatic stress and increasingly challenging neurocognitive tasks (Ocon et al., 2012; Stewart et al., 2012). The studies measured the response to n-back testing while supine and during progressive orthostatic stress (tilt table angles of 0, 15, 30, 45, 60, and 75 degrees). The authors conclude that orthostatic stress results in neurocognitive impairment in CFS/POTS but not in healthy controls. Stewart and colleagues (2012) also found that the expected increase in cerebral blood flow velocity during cognitive neuronal activation did not occur.

These findings are partially supported by Wyller and Helland (2013), who examined relationships among symptoms and autonomic cardiovascular control in 38 children with ME/CFS using the NICE guidelines. Cognitive symptoms were significantly and independently associated with a higher baseline heart rate, an enhanced heart rate response to orthostatic challenge, and older age within the adolescent age range (Wyller and Helland, 2013).

SLEEP-RELATED SYMPTOMS

Unrefreshing sleep and specific sleep disturbances—including insomnia, sleep cycle disturbances, and excessive sleeping—are among the most common symptoms reported in pediatric ME/CFS patients. The prevalence estimates for these sleep problems range from 84 to 96 percent (Davies and Crawley, 2008; Knight et al., 2013a; Nijhof et al., 2011).

Assessment of Sleep-Related Symptoms in Pediatric ME/CFS

Sleep problems usually are assessed by patient self-report during the clinical history. More formal studies are supplemented by sleep quality questionnaires, actigraphy, and polysomnography. (See the section on sleep-related symptoms in adults with ME/CFS in Chapter 4.)

Evidence for Sleep-Related Symptoms in Pediatric ME/CFS

The committee examined the literature on the presence of sleep-related symptoms in children/adolescents diagnosed with ME/CFS compared with other children/adolescents (healthy or otherwise). Taken together, these studies (Bell et al., 1994; Huang et al., 2010; Knook et al., 2000; Ohinata et al., 2008; Stores et al., 1998) suggest that children with ME/CFS have sleep disturbances, but they do not have a high prevalence of more severe sleep disorders such as obstructive sleep apnea or narcolepsy. The studies included in the committee's review used different case definitions and different measures with limited overlap in outcome variables, and there was little replication of results. Their findings therefore need to be interpreted with caution.

Two studies yielded higher-level data. Stores and colleagues (1998) performed home polysomnography in 18 British children with ME/CFS and 18 controls. Sleep efficiency was lower in those with ME/CFS (p < 0.001), in whom there were more awakenings of less than 2 minutes' duration, more awakenings of greater than 2 minutes, less non-rapid eye movement (NREM) stage 2 sleep, and less rapid eye movement (REM) sleep.

Hurum and colleagues (2011) compared ambulatory recordings of heart rate and blood pressure in 44 adolescents with ME/CFS and 52 healthy controls. This study used a relatively broad definition of ME/CFS, requiring at least 3 months of fatigue but no other somatic symptoms. Participants with ME/CFS were studied while staying overnight at an accommodation service, and controls were studied at home. During sleep, the ME/CFS patients had significantly higher heart rate, diastolic blood pressure, and mean arterial pressure. They also had higher heart rate during the waking hours.

INFECTION

The abrupt onset of illness for some adolescents with ME/CFS has stimulated investigation into infectious etiologies of the illness. Estimates of the proportion of pediatric ME/CFS patients with an abrupt infectious onset vary greatly across studies, from 22 to 93 percent. In a population-based study of 184 children from the Netherlands, Nijhof and colleagues (2011) found an overall rate of 32 percent with an acute onset, 22 percent of whom had an illness that began with an apparent infection. This study used the Fukuda definition. In a retrospective review of 59 Australian children attending an ME/CFS specialist clinic, 62 percent reported an infectious onset (Knight et al., 2013a). In a retrospective cohort study, Sankey and colleagues (2006) reported an acute onset in 93 percent of children diagnosed using the Oxford criteria (Sharpe et al., 1991) and evaluated in an English ME/CFS specialty service.

Assessment of Infection in Pediatric ME/CFS

Methods for assessing the association of ME/CFS with infection are described in the section on infection in adults with ME/CFS in Chapter 5.

Evidence for Infection in Pediatric ME/CFS

The committee identified and reviewed the two largest studies of the highest methodological quality on this topic. One prospective cohort study examined the rates of ME/CFS following acute infectious mononucleosis (Katz et al., 2009). To be eligible, participants had to have infectious mononucleosis, defined as a monospot-positive form of the illness. At 6, 12, and 24 months after infection, 13 percent, 7 percent, and 4 percent of adolescents, respectively, met criteria for ME/CFS, defined using the Jason pediatric criteria (Jason et al., 2006). There was a striking preponderance of females meeting ME/CFS criteria at all time points. At 6 months, 11.6 percent of females and 1.3 percent of males met criteria for ME/CFS, but only females continued to meet the criteria at 12 and 24 months (Katz et al., 2009). In a separate nested case-control study, stepwise logistic regression analysis identified (1) autonomic symptoms at baseline and (2) days spent in bed with the initial infection as the only significant risk factors for developing ME/CFS after infectious mononucleosis (Jason et al., 2014).

In a cross-sectional comparison of 120 Norwegian adolescents with established ME/CFS and 68 healthy controls, Sulheim and colleagues (2014)[1] examined serology for *B. burgdorferi*, Epstein-Barr virus (EBV), cytomegalovirus (CMV), and parvovirus B19. They also obtained results of polymerase chain reaction (PCR) tests for those organisms as well as for human herpes virus type 6 (HHV-6), enterovirus, and adenovirus. No adolescents with ME/CFS or controls were positive on PCR testing for *B. burgdorferi*, CMV, enterovirus, or adenovirus. PCR rates were low for the other infectious agents and did not differ between ME/CFS cases and healthy controls. Rates of seropositivity for immunoglobulin G (IgG) or immunoglobulin M (IgM) antibodies did not differ between ME/CFS patients and controls for any of the organisms for which testing was conducted (Sulheim et al., 2014).

In investigating a cluster of seven cases of ME/CFS in a rural community of northern New York state, Bell and colleagues (1991) found no evidence that the following organisms were a cause of the illness: *Brucella* species, *Coxiella*, CMV, EBV, human immunodeficiency virus, hepatitis B, parvovirus B19, *Toxoplasma gondii*, *B. burgdorferi*, and *Francisella tularensis*. A questionnaire distributed to the local school district identified 21 patients who met the criteria for ME/CFS, including 6 of the 7 index cases. These 21 were compared with 42 healthy controls, matching 2 controls to each case. Ingestion of raw milk, the presence of a second family member with ME/CFS symptoms, and a history of allergies or asthma emerged as risk factors for pediatric ME/CFS.

One study examined antibodies to human T-cell lymphotropic virus (HTLV)-I antigens by Western blot and HTLV-II gag sequences by PCR. The total pediatric sample is reported as 21, but results are given for only 18 pediatric ME/CFS patients. Of these, 11 (61 percent) had evidence of anti-HTLV-I antibodies, versus 3/17 (18 percent) controls (comprising

---

[1] This information can be found in the supplemental material of the Sulheim et al. (2014) paper.

7 healthy adults and 10 umbilical cord blood samples from newborns). PCR amplification of retroviral DNA was positive for the HTLV-II gag protein in 72 percent of the pediatric cases versus 12 percent of controls (DeFreitas et al., 1991). No age-matched pediatric controls were used in this study, and in the 23 years since publication of these results, they have not been independently confirmed.

A paper from Scotland describes coxsackie B virus antibody sero-positivity in 47 children ages 5 to 14 years with a diagnosis of ME/CFS. Using an enzyme-linked immunosorbent assay (ELISA) technique, 18/47 (38 percent) were positive, compared with a published rate in children ages ≤ 14 years of 5.5 percent with a positive coxsackie B virus IgM (Bell et al., 1988). Other studies, notably the Norwegian study of Sulheim and colleagues (2014), did not confirm such a high seroprevalence rate, and it is unclear why the IgM antibodies would remain positive long after the onset of ME/CFS.

A retrospective study of 53 children with ME/CFS in New Jersey found seropositivity for EBV and/or *B. burgdorferi* in 66 percent of patients. For those with less than 12 months' (n = 30), 12 to 24 months' (n = 17), or more than 24 months' (n = 6) duration of ME/CFS, seropositivity for EBV or *B. burgdorferi* or both was 63 percent, 82 percent, and 33 percent, respectively (Petrov et al., 2012).

Evidence of active infection has not been detected after the initial onset of ME/CFS. Pathogens for which the serological evidence argues against a causal role in a large proportion of pediatric ME/CFS cases are CMV, HHV-6, coxsackie viruses, and parvovirus B19.[2] There has been relatively little study of enteroviruses, however, and there is a relative paucity of data on *B. burgdorferi*.

IMMUNE IMPAIRMENT

Because ME/CFS often begins after an apparent infection, an important issue regarding the pathophysiology of the illness is whether its symptoms are due to a persistent infection or to the triggering infection acting as a "hit and run" phenomenon, initiating immune system or other physiologic dysfunctions that in turn cause chronic symptoms.

Assessment of Immune Impairment in Pediatric ME/CFS

Methods for assessing immune system dysfunction are described in the section on immune impairment in adults with ME/CFS in Chapter 5.

---

[2] Ibid.

Evidence for Immune Impairment in Pediatric ME/CFS

Among the five studies identified as relevant to this topic, one used the Jason pediatric definition of ME/CFS (Jason et al., 2006) and the remaining four used the Fukuda definition (CDC, 2012). These study results should be interpreted with caution. Several important methodological factors limit the strength of the results, including the relatively small sample size of four of the studies (Broderick et al., 2012; Itoh et al., 2012; Kavelaars et al., 2000; Kennedy et al., 2010a), which raises questions about the representativeness of the results. No study reporting an abnormality appears to have been replicated.

The studies varied widely in the types of immune dysfunction addressed. Abnormalities were examined in the following areas:

- both proliferative and inhibitory responses of T cells to specific agents (Kavelaars et al., 2000);
- elevations in interleukin (IL)-8 and reductions in IL-23 (Broderick et al., 2012);
- increased anti-Sa (a 62 kDa protein found in those with autoimmune fatigue syndrome) antibodies (Itoh et al., 2012);
- increased proportions of lymphocytes and neutrophils undergoing apoptosis (Kennedy et al., 2010a);
- rates of anergy (Rowe, 1997); and
- responses to intravenous immunoglobulin (IVIG) (Rowe, 1997).

Kavelaars and colleagues (2000) examined T cell proliferative responses to dexamethasone, as well as cytokine production by terbutaline, in 15 adolescents with ME/CFS and 14 controls. The peripheral blood cells of those with ME/CFS had higher proliferative responses of T cells to phytohemagglutinin (p = 0.044) and a lower inhibition of proliferation with dexamethasone (p = 0.001). The inhibitory effect of terbutaline on tumor necrosis factor (TNF)-alpha production was significantly lower in the ME/CFS patients, and terbutaline led to less enhancement of IL-10 production.

Broderick and colleagues (2012) used a 16-cytokine ELISA assay to compare 9 adolescents who met criteria for ME/CFS after infectious mononucleosis with 12 recovered controls at 24 months postinfection. There were significant differences in IL-8 and IL-23 between the two groups. IL-8 was significantly higher in the ME/CFS patients. IL-2 was also higher in the ME/CFS patients but less dramatically different from IL-2 levels in controls than was IL-8. IL-23 was significantly lower in the ME/CFS patients. IL-5 was lower as well, but less dramatically so. Katz and colleagues (2013) conducted a small case-control study in 9 adolescents who developed ME/CFS after infectious mononucleosis and 9 controls who had recovered uneventfully from the same illness. There were no differences between the groups in natural killer (NK) cell numbers or function.

Itoh and colleagues (2012) studied 15 Japanese children with fibromyalgia and 21 with ME/CFS over time. All had presented with fatigue. The authors measured antinuclear antibodies (ANAs), precipitin antibodies, T cells, B cells, and NK cells. Most fibromyalgia patients had low positive ANA titers in the 1:40 to 1:80 range; one had anti-Sa antibodies. ME/CFS participants had higher ANA titers, 11 of which had increased by the time ME/CFS was diagnosed. Among those with ME/CFS, 86 percent were positive for anti-Sa antibodies. The target antigen for anti-Sa antibodies is a lens epithelium-derived growth factor thought to confer resistance to stress-induced cell death (Itoh et al., 2012). These results have not been replicated in large samples. In contrast to data in adults with ME/CFS, lymphocyte subsets and NK cell activity were in the normal range in these ME/CFS patients.

Kennedy and colleagues (2010a) examined 25 children with ME/CFS from Great Britain and 23 healthy controls, focusing on markers of oxidative stress and measures of apoptosis. The ME/CFS participants had a significantly lower proportion of normal neutrophils (28 versus 46 percent) and a correspondingly higher proportion of neutrophils undergoing apoptosis relative to the healthy children (54 versus 36 percent). Similarly, those with ME/CFS had a significantly lower proportion of normal lymphocytes (44 versus 65 percent) and a correspondingly higher proportion of lymphocytes undergoing apoptosis (40 versus 25 percent).

Rowe (1997) conducted a randomized placebo-controlled trial of IVIG in 71 Australian adolescents with ME/CFS. There was a significant improvement in overall function at 6-month follow-up in those who had received IVIG in a dose of 1 gram/kg (max 60 grams) monthly for 3 months. Cell-mediated immunity was abnormal in 52 percent of ME/CFS participants at baseline. Given the scientific strength of the randomized controlled trial design, the larger sample size, and the reported benefit of IVIG for pediatric ME/CFS patients, further investigation of IVIG in the pediatric ME/CFS population is warranted.

NEUROENDOCRINE MANIFESTATIONS

The overlap of ME/CFS symptoms with those of adrenal insufficiency, together with inconsistent reports of lower cortisol values in adults with ME/CFS, has prompted several investigations into neuroendocrine abnormalities in pediatric ME/CFS. Similarly, reports of orthostatic intolerance have led to investigations of catecholamines and other hormones involved in the regulation of circulation in pediatric ME/CFS patients.

Assessment of Neuroendocrine Manifestations in Pediatric ME/CFS

Methods for assessing neuroendocrine abnormalities are described in the section on neuroendocrine manifestations in adults with ME/CFS in Chapter 5.

Evidence for Neuroendocrine Manifestations in Pediatric ME/CFS

The committee reviewed the available literature on neuroendocrine abnormalities in pediatric ME/CFS and the differences from those presented in healthy and diseased controls when available.

Adrenocortical Abnormalities

Several studies consistently found statistically lower mean cortisol levels in those with ME/CFS compared with controls (Nijhof et al., 2014; Segal et al., 2005; Sulheim et al., 2014; Tomoda et al., 2001). A study in the Netherlands compared a group of 108 adolescents with ME/CFS and 38 controls and found that those with ME/CFS had lower cortisol levels after awakening. The shape of the cortisol curves was similar for those with ME/CFS and controls, and it is unclear whether any adolescent with ME/CFS had clinically significantly low cortisol levels as opposed to statistically significant differences from controls. Cortisol levels at baseline did not predict recovery from ME/CFS during follow-up. The initial hypocortisolism was reversed after recovery from ME/CFS (Nijhof et al., 2014). In another cross-sectional study comparing 120 individuals with ME/CFS and 68 controls, performed in conjunction with a randomized trial of clonidine, those with ME/CFS showed lower urine cortisol-to-creatinine ratios (Sulheim et al., 2014). Tomoda and colleagues (2001) also found lower levels of cortisol and a 3-hour delay in the peak shift in cortisol in ME/CFS patients using 24-hour indwelling catheter measurements of cortisol every 4 hours.

Segal and colleagues (2005) used the low-dose synacthen test (LDST) to evaluate for subtle hypocortisolism in 23 children with ME/CFS and 17 controls of similar age and sex. The controls were retrospective, selected from among those with other endocrine disorders in whom an LDST had been performed with normal results. Studying a group suspected of having adrenal insufficiency would have been expected to bias against detection of a lower cortisol level in those with ME/CFS. Despite this limitation, children with ME/CFS had significantly lower mean cortisol levels than controls throughout the test. Their peak cortisol was lower, and the time to reach the peak level was longer. Girls had a more attenuated response to synacthen than boys.

One study examined the interaction between the neuroendocrine and immune systems by measuring cortisol, adrenocorticotropin hormone (ACTH), adrenaline, noradrenaline, and T cell proliferative responses to phytohemagluttinin and dexamethasone; cytokine production in response to terbutaline; and the response to corticotropin-releasing hormone (CRH) in a small sample of ME/CFS patients and controls. ACTH and cortisol responses were similar in response to CRH. Those with ME/CFS had higher proliferative responses of T cells to phytohemagluttinin but lower inhibition of proliferation with dexamethasone. The inhibitory effect of terbutaline on TNF-alpha production was lower in the ME/CFS patients, and there was less enhancement of IL-10 production (Kavelaars et al., 2000).

It is important to note, however, that even in studies reporting lower cortisol levels in adolescents with ME/CFS than in controls, the mean cortisol levels reported for those with ME/CFS remain within the normal range. Very little work has been done to determine whether the cortisol differences are related to sleep cycle abnormalities, as has been suggested in some adult studies, or are a secondary reflection of another aspect of being chronically ill.

Catecholamines

Two studies found elevations in supine epinephrine and norepinephrine in pediatric ME/CFS patients compared with controls (Sulheim et al., 2014; Wyller et al., 2008b). Kavelaars and colleagues (2000) also found higher epinephrine levels but no differences in supine norepinephrine levels in ME/CFS patients compared with controls. No differences were found between patients and controls for dopamine, normetanephrines, and metanephrines at rest (Wyller et al., 2007b).

Temperature Regulation

Tomoda and colleagues (2001) monitored deep body temperature in 41 Japanese children with ME/CFS and 9 controls. They found that the mean and nadir core body temperatures were higher in the ME/CFS patients than in the controls (both p < 0.0001).

Wyller and colleagues (2007b) studied thermoregulatory responses in 15 Norwegian ME/CFS adolescents and 57 controls. At baseline, ME/CFS patients had higher norepinephrine, epinephrine, and tympanic temperature than controls. During cooling of one hand, acral skin blood flow was reduced, vasoconstrictor events occurred at lower temperatures, and tympanic temperatures decreased more. However, catecholamines increased similarly in the two groups.

Other Neuroendocrine Findings

Knook and colleagues (2000) examined salivary melatonin levels in 13 adolescents with ME/CFS and 15 controls. Sleep onset and duration were the same in the two groups, but melatonin levels were higher in the ME/CFS patients, particularly after 10 PM. Wyller and colleagues (2010) examined 67 Norwegian adolescents with ME/CFS and 55 controls. Antidiuretic hormone (ADH) levels were lower in those with ME/CFS. Plasma renin and osmolality were increased; aldosterone, cortisol, and sex hormones did not differ. Segal and colleagues (2005) found that thyroid-stimulating hormone (TSH), free thyroxine, and prolactin were no different between ME/CFS and control groups. Levels of dehydroepiandrosterone (DHEA), androstenedione (A4), and 17-hydroxyprogesterone (17-OHP) for ME/CFS patients were similar to age and pubertal stage norms. These findings are relevant in light of the high incidence of orthostatic and circulatory dysfunction in pediatric ME/CFS.

A study suggesting a role for childhood trauma in ME/CFS used the broad empirical definition of ME/CFS, which resulted in a biased sample with overrepresentation of individuals with depression and posttraumatic stress disorder (PTSD) (Heim et al., 2009). The unusually high proportion of subjects with serious psychiatric problems likely explains the study finding of an association between ME/CFS and adverse childhood experiences. No other studies have suggested a higher rate of childhood trauma in those with confirmed ME/CFS as opposed to nonspecific chronic fatigue. In a study of 22 Norwegian adolescents with ME/CFS, no participant reported prior sexual abuse (Gjone and Wyller, 2009).

OTHER SYMPTOMS

Fatigue is universal in pediatric ME/CFS, usually to a degree that is sufficient in combination with other symptoms to lead to marked functional impairment (Davies and Crawley, 2008; Knight et al., 2013a; Nijhof et al., 2011). Kennedy and colleagues (2010b) showed that among 25 children with ME/CFS, recruited from support groups in the United Kingdom, only 1 attended regular classes. Compared with healthy controls, Child Health Questionnaire scores for the ME/CFS group were lowest on global health, physical function, and role/social limitations due to physical problems. Those with ME/CFS had lower physical function and greater general impairment than children with type 1 diabetes and asthma. Of 211 children with ME/CFS referred to a specialist clinic in England, 62 percent attended school 2 days per week or less. The factor most closely associated with school attendance was better physical function, whereas anxiety, gender, and age at assessment were not associated. Increasing fatigue was associated with worse physical function (Crawley and Sterne, 2009).

In pediatric ME/CFS studies, the prevalence of pain symptoms in the aggregate is relatively common at the time of presentation of ME/CFS, as demonstrated by a study of Australian children (Knight et al., 2013a), a cross-sectional study of Dutch adolescents (Nijhof et al., 2011), and a study of a large referral population of British children (Davies and Crawley, 2008). The most prevalent pain symptom is headaches, reported in 75 to 81 percent of patients in these studies. Reports of other specific pain symptoms are much more variable across studies and are less frequent than reports of headaches overall. Myalgia was observed in 52 to 73 percent, abdominal pain in 16 to 100 percent, arthralgia in 12 to 67 percent, sore throat in 25 to 62 percent, and tender glands in 12 to 50 percent of children (Bell, 1995b; Davies and Crawley, 2008; Knight et al., 2013a; Nijhof et al., 2011).

SYMPTOM CONSTRUCTS

Two pediatric studies used factor analysis to examine whether ME/CFS symptoms can be grouped in a way that defines separate phenotypes. Rowe and Rowe (2002) found that the pattern of symptoms in adolescents with ME/CFS was similar to the pattern in Australian adults, although nausea, abdominal pain, fevers, sweats, sore throat, and tender glands were more prevalent among the adolescents. Their sample included 189 adolescents ages 10 to 18 years who had noted a definite onset of ME/CFS over hours to several days, as well as 68 healthy adolescents. Among those with ME/CFS, more than 87 percent had experienced the following within the preceding month: prolonged fatigue following minor activity, headache, the need for excessive sleep, loss of ability to concentrate, disturbed sleep, excessive muscle fatigue, and myalgia following minor activity. In more than 60 percent, these symptoms were rated as moderately severe or severe. Interestingly, 14 of the symptoms had a low response frequency among both ME/CFS cases and controls and were grouped as somatic or involuntary muscle sensations. These factors were not a good fit to the data, accounting for less than 79 percent of the variance and covariance. Reports of symptoms unrelated to ME/CFS had low frequencies. The authors concluded that evidence for somatization disorder among those with ME/CFS was negligible. In contrast, factor analysis applied to the 24 symptoms judged to be salient on the basis of their frequency and severity scores identified five factors labeled muscle pain and fatigue, neurocognitive, abdominal/head/chest pain, neurophysiological, and immunological. This model accounted for 97 percent of the variance and covariance in the observed data. The immunological symptoms had significant direct and indirect effects on the other four key symptom factors and were thus judged to be primary (Rowe and Rowe, 2002).

May and colleagues (2010) performed exploratory factor analysis on 333 children and adolescents evaluated at the Bath specialist ME/CFS service. The median age of the participants was 14.9 years, with a range of 2 to 18 years. Three main phenotypes were identified. Based on the symptom clusters, these were labeled musculoskeletal, migraine, and sore throat. The musculoskeletal factor had the heaviest loading on muscle pain, joint pain, and hypersensitivity to touch, and it appears to be closest to the category for muscle pain and fatigue in the Australian model. The migraine factor had the heaviest loading on headaches, abdominal pain, nausea, hypersensitivity to light/noise/touch, and dizziness, and it appears to be similar to the abdominal, head, and chest pain factor in the Australian model. The sore throat phenotype loaded most heavily on sore throat and tender glands, thereby appearing to be similar to the immunological factor in the Australian model. The British factor analysis did not identify factors that corresponded to the neurocognitive and neurophysiological models in the Australian work. Among the three phenotypes, the musculoskeletal factor had the strongest association with fatigue, while the sore throat phenotype was the least severely affected group. The migraine group had the lowest physical function and had worse school attendance. None of the phenotypes was associated with depression; the migraine phenotype was associated with increased anxiety (May et al., 2010).

The two factor analyses thus achieved some qualitative similarity, although comparisons are limited by the different methods used to group and rate symptoms and by the types of symptoms collected. For example, the ascertainment of lightheadedness and other symptoms of orthostatic intolerance was incomplete. Whether the heterogeneous phenotypes reflect distinctive pathophysiologic factors is unknown.

SUMMARY

The data on orthostatic intolerance (notably POTS and NMH) and autonomic dysfunction in pediatric ME/CFS are strong and consistent across case definitions. While the available studies suggest the presence of only subtle neurocognitive problems at rest, children and adolescents with ME/CFS develop more robust and significant cognitive abnormalities under conditions of orthostatic stress or distraction. The evidence also indicates that PEM and unrefreshing sleep are common in pediatric ME/CFS, although studies are needed to better characterize the optimal method of assessing for these phenomena in children. Despite the evidence that these different pain symptoms are common in the aggregate, the high variability in the prevalence of these symptoms supports the committee's decision to not require pain for a diagnosis of ME/CFS. It is well documented that ME/CFS can follow EBV and non-EBV infectious mononucleosis. There is no evidence that other pathogens are consistently associated with the onset of pediatric ME/CFS. While there is no evidence of classic immunodeficiency or endocrine disorders in pediatric ME/CFS, the literature describes several discrete abnormalities in immune and endocrine system function in affected children and adolescents. These findings need to be interpreted with caution because of several important methodological issues and the lack of replications of these studies.

The committee adopted a 6-month duration of symptoms for the diagnosis of ME/CFS in children based on the literature described earlier in the chapter. Nonetheless, the committee emphasizes that this time criterion should not interfere with initiating appropriate symptom-based management long before 6 months has elapsed in children presenting with prolonged fatigue. Symptomatic treatment can begin at any point after the onset of fatigue as the diagnostic process continues to evaluate and exclude other potential causes for the patient's symptoms. Chapter 7 presents the committee's recommendations on diagnostic criteria for ME/CFS in children and adolescents.

Conclusion: There is sufficient evidence that orthostatic intolerance and autonomic dysfunction are common in pediatric ME/CFS; that neurocognitive abnormalities emerge when pediatric ME/CFS patients are tested under conditions of orthostatic stress or distraction; and that there is a high prevalence of profound fatigue, unrefreshing sleep, and post-exertional exacerbation of symptoms in these patients. There also is sufficient evidence that pediatric ME/CFS can follow acute infectious mononucleosis and EBV.

REFERENCES

Andersen, M. M., H. Permin, and F. Albrecht. 2004. Illness and disability in Danish chronic fatigue syndrome patients at diagnosis and 5-year follow-up. *Journal of Psychosomatic Research* 56(2):217-229.

Bell, D. S. 1995a. Chronic fatigue syndrome in children and adolescents: A review. *Focus & Opinion Pediatrics* 1(5):412-420.

Bell, D. S. 1995b. Chronic fatigue syndrome in children. *Journal of Chronic Fatigue Syndrome* 1(1):9-33.

Bell, D. S., K. M. Bell, and P. R. Cheney. 1994. Primary juvenile fibromyalgia syndrome and chronic fatigue syndrome in adolescents. *Clinical Infectious Diseases* 18(Suppl. 1):S21-S23.

Bell, D. S., K. Jordan, and M. Robinson. 2001. Thirteen-year follow-up of children and adolescents with chronic fatigue syndrome. *Pediatrics* 107(5):994-998.

Bell, E. J., R. A. McCartney, and M. H. Riding. 1988. Coxsackie B viruses and myalgic encephalomyelitis. *Journal of the Royal Society of Medicine* 81(6):329-331.

Bell, K. M., D. Cookfair, D. S. Bell, P. Reese, and L. Cooper. 1991. Risk factors associated with chronic fatigue syndrome in a cluster of pediatric cases. *Reviews of Infectious Diseases* 13(Suppl. 1):S32-S38.

Bentall, R. P., G. C. Wood, T. Marrinan, C. Deans, and R. H. T. Edwards. 1993. A brief mental fatigue questionnaire. *British Journal of Clinical Psychology* 32(3):375-377.

Bou-Holaigah, I., P. C. Rowe, J. Kan, and H. Calkins. 1995. The relationship between neurally mediated hypotension and the chronic fatigue syndrome. *Journal of the American Medical Association* 274(12):961-967.

Broderick, G., B. Z. Katz, H. Fernandes, M. A. Fletcher, N. Klimas, F. A. Smith, M. R. O'Gorman, S. D. Vernon, and R. Taylor. 2012. Cytokine expression profiles of immune imbalance in post-mononucleosis chronic fatigue. *Journal of Translational Medicine* 10:191.

Cairns, R., and M. Hotopf. 2005. A systematic review describing the prognosis of chronic fatigue syndrome. *Occupational Medicine (Oxford)* 55(1):20-31.

Carruthers, B. M., A. K. Jain, K. L. De Meirleir, D. L. Peterson, N. G. Klimas, A. M. Lerner, A. C. Bested, P. Flor-Henry, P. Joshi, A. C. P. Powles, J. A. Sherkey, and M. I. van de Sande. 2003. Myalgic encephalomyelitis/chronic fatigue syndrome: Clinical working case definition, diagnostic and treatment protocols (Canadian case definition). *Journal of Chronic Fatigue Syndrome* 11(1):7-115.

Carruthers, B. M., M. I. van de Sande, K. L. De Meirleir, N. G. Klimas, G. Broderick, T. Mitchell, D. Staines, A. C. P. Powles, N. Speight, R. Vallings, L. Bateman, B. Baumgarten-Austrheim, D. S. Bell, N. Carlo-Stella, J. Chia, A. Darragh, D. Jo, D. Lewis, A. R. Light, S. Marshall-Gradisbik, I. Mena, J. A. Mikovits, K. Miwa, M. Murovska, M. L. Pall, and S. Stevens. 2011. Myalgic encephalomyelitis: International consensus criteria. *Journal of Internal Medicine* 270(4):327-338.

CDC (Centers for Disease Control and Prevention). 2012. *Chronic fatigue syndrome: 1994 case definition.* http://www.cdc.gov/cfs/case-definition/1994.html (accessed December 16, 2013).

Chalder, T., R. Goodman, S. Wessely, M. Hotopf, and H. Meltzer. 2003. Epidemiology of chronic fatigue syndrome and self reported myalgic encephalomyelitis in 5-15 year olds: Cross sectional study. *British Medical Journal* 327(7416):654-655.

Crawley, E., and J. A. Sterne. 2009. Association between school absence and physical function in paediatric chronic fatigue syndrome/myalgic encephalopathy. *Archives of Disease in Childhood* 94(10):752-756.

Crawley, E. M., A. M. Emond, and J. A. C. Sterne. 2011. Unidentified chronic fatigue syndrome/myalgic encephalomyelitis (CFS/ME) is a major cause of school absence: Surveillance outcomes from school-based clinics. *BMJ Open* 1(2).

Davies, S., and E. Crawley. 2008. Chronic fatigue syndrome in children aged 11 years old and younger. *Archives of Disease in Childhood* 93(5):419-422.

De Wandele, I., P. Calders, W. Peersman, S. Rimbaut, T. De Backer, F. Malfait, A. De Paepe, and L. Rombaut. 2014a. Autonomic symptom burden in the hypermobility type of Ehlers-Danlos syndrome: A comparative study with two other EDS types, fibromyalgia, and healthy controls. *Seminars in Arthritis and Rheumatism* 44(3):353-361.

De Wandele, I., L. Rombaut, L. Leybaert, P. Van de Borne, T. De Backer, F. Malfait, A. De Paepe, and P. Calders. 2014b. Dysautonomia and its underlying mechanisms in the hypermobility type of Ehlers-Danlos syndrome. *Seminars in Arthritis and Rheumatism* 44(1):93-100.

DeFreitas, E., B. Hilliard, P. R. Cheney, D. S. Bell, E. Kiggundu, D. Sankey, Z. Wroblewska, M. Palladino, J. P. Woodward, and H. Koprowski. 1991. Retroviral sequences related to human T-lymphotropic virus type II in patients with chronic fatigue immune dysfunction syndrome. *Proceedings of the National Academy of Sciences of the United States of America* 88(7):2922-2926.

Dowsett, E. G., and J. Colby. 1997. Long-term sickness absence due to ME/CFS in UK schools: An epidemiological study with medical and educational implications. *Journal of Chronic Fatigue Syndrome* 3(2):29-42.

Farmer, A., T. Fowler, J. Scourfield, and A. Thapar. 2004. Prevalence of chronic disabling fatigue in children and adolescents. *British Journal of Psychiatry* 184:477-481.

Galland, B. C., P. M. Jackson, R. M. Sayers, and B. J. Taylor. 2008. A matched case control study of orthostatic intolerance in children/adolescents with chronic fatigue syndrome. *Pediatric Research* 63(2):196-202.

Gazit, Y., A. M. Nahir, R. Grahame, and G. Jacob. 2003. Dysautonomia in the joint hypermobility syndrome. *American Journal of Medicine* 115(1):33-40.

Gill, A. C., A. Dosen, and J. B. Ziegler. 2004. Chronic fatigue syndrome in adolescents: A follow-up study. *Archives of Pediatrics & Adolescent Medicine* 158(3):225-229.

Gjone, H., and V. B. Wyller. 2009. Chronic fatigue in adolescence—autonomic dysregulation and mental health: An exploratory study. *Acta Paediatrica, International Journal of Paediatrics* 98(8):1313-1318.

Haig-Ferguson, A., P. Tucker, N. Eaton, L. Hunt, and E. Crawley. 2009. Memory and attention problems in children with chronic fatigue syndrome or myalgic encephalopathy. *Archives of Disease in Childhood* 94(10):757-762.

Heim, C., U. M. Nater, E. Maloney, R. Boneva, J. F. Jones, and W. C. Reeves. 2009. Childhood trauma and risk for chronic fatigue syndrome association with neuroendocrine dysfunction. *Archives of General Psychiatry* 66(1):72-80.

Holder, N. 2010. Local family feels vindicated by breakthrough research. *Mountain Xpress.* September 14. http://mountainx.com/news/community-news/091510local-family-feels-vindicated-by-breakthrough-research (accessed April 15, 2014).

Huang, Y., B. Z. Katz, C. Mears, G. W. Kielhofner, and R. Taylor. 2010. Postinfectious fatigue in adolescents and physical activity. *Archives of Pediatrics and Adolescent Medicine* 164(9):803-809.

Hurum, H., D. Sulheim, E. Thaulow, and V. B. Wyller. 2011. Elevated nocturnal blood pressure and heart rate in adolescent chronic fatigue syndrome. *Acta Paediatrica, International Journal of Paediatrics* 100(2):289-292.

Itoh, Y., T. Shigemori, T. Igarashi, and Y. Fukunaga. 2012. Fibromyalgia and chronic fatigue syndrome in children. *Pediatrics International* 54(2):266-271.

Jason, L. A., D. S. Bell, K. Rowe, E. L. S. Van Hoof, K. Jordan, C. Lapp, A. Gurwitt, T. Miike, S. Torres-Harding, and K. De Meirleir. 2006. A pediatric case definition for myalgic encephalomyelitis and chronic fatigue syndrome. *Journal of Chronic Fatigue Syndrome* 13(2-3):1-44.

Jason, L. A., N. Porter, E. Shelleby, L. Till, D. Bell, C. Lapp, K. Rowe, and K. L. De Meirleir. 2010. Examining criteria to diagnose ME/CFS in pediatric samples. *Journal of Behavioral Health and Medicine* 3:186-195.

Jason, L. A., B. Z. Katz, Y. Shiraishi, C. Mears, Y. Im, and R. R. Taylor. 2014. Predictors of post-infectious chronic fatigue syndrome in adolescents. *Health Psychology & Behavioural Medicine* 2(1):41-51.

Jordan, K. M., L. A. Jason, C. J. Mears, B. Z. Katz, A. Rademaker, C. F. Huang, J. Richman, W. McCready, P. M. Ayers, and K. K. Taylor. 2006. Prevalence of pediatric chronic fatigue syndrome in a community-based sample. *Journal of Chronic Fatigue Syndrome* 13(2-3):75-78.

Katz, B. Z., Y. Shiraishi, C. J. Mears, H. J. Binns, and R. Taylor. 2009. Chronic fatigue syndrome following infectious mononucleosis in adolescents. *Pediatrics* 124(1):189-193.

Katz, B. Z., S. Boas, Y. Shiraishi, C. J. Mears, and R. Taylor. 2010. Exercise tolerance testing in a prospective cohort of adolescents with chronic fatigue syndrome and recovered controls following infectious mononucleosis. *Journal of Pediatrics* 157(3):468-472.

Katz, B. Z., J. M. Stewart, Y. Shiraishi, C. J. Mears, and R. Taylor. 2012. Orthostatic tolerance testing in a prospective cohort of adolescents with chronic fatigue syndrome and recovered controls following infectious mononucleosis. *Clinical Pediatrics* 51(9):835-839.

Katz, B. Z., D. Zimmerman, M. R. G. Gorman, C. J. Mears, Y. Shiraishi, and R. Taylor. 2013. Normal salivary cortisol and NK cell function in adolescents with chronic fatigue syndrome following infectious mononucleosis. *Archives of Pediatric Infectious Diseases* 2(4):211-216.

Kavelaars, A., W. Kuis, L. Knook, G. Sinnema, and C. J. Heijnen. 2000. Disturbed neuroendocrine-immune interactions in chronic fatigue syndrome. *Journal of Clinical Endocrinology & Metabolism* 85(2):692-696.

Kawatani, J., K. Mizuno, S. Shiraishi, M. Takao, T. Joudoi, S. Fukuda, Y. Watanabe, and A. Tomoda. 2011. Cognitive dysfunction and mental fatigue in childhood chronic fatigue syndrome—a 6-month follow-up study. *Brain & Development* 33(10):832-841.

Kennedy, G., F. Khan, A. Hill, C. Underwood, and J. J. F. Belch. 2010a. Biochemical and vascular aspects of pediatric chronic fatigue syndrome. *Archives of Pediatrics and Adolescent Medicine* 164(9):817-823.

Kennedy, G., C. Underwood, and J. J. Freda Belch. 2010b. Physical and functional impact of chronic fatigue syndrome/myalgic encephalomyelitis in childhood. *Pediatrics* 125(6):e1324-e1330.

Knight, S., A. Harvey, L. Lubitz, K. Rowe, C. Reveley, F. Veit, S. Hennel, and A. Scheinberg. 2013a. Paediatric chronic fatigue syndrome: Complex presentations and protracted time to diagnosis. *Journal of Paediatrics and Child Health* 49(11):919-924.

Knight, S. J., A. Scheinberg, and A. R. Harvey. 2013b. Interventions in pediatric chronic fatigue syndrome/myalgic encephalomyelitis: A systematic review. *Journal of Adolescent Health* 53(2):154-165.

Knook, L., A. Kavelaars, G. Sinnema, W. Kuis, and C. J. Heijnen. 2000. High nocturnal melatonin in adolescents with chronic fatigue syndrome. *Journal of Clinical Endocrinology & Metabolism* 85(10):3690-3692.

May, M., A. Emond, and E. Crawley. 2010. Phenotypes of chronic fatigue syndrome in children and young people. *Archives of Disease in Childhood* 95(4):245-249.

NICE (National Institute for Health and Clinical Excellence). 2007. *Chronic fatigue syndrome/myalgic encephalomyelitis (or encephalopathy): Diagnosis and management of CFS/ME in adults and children.* London, UK: NICE.

Nijhof, S. L., K. Maijer, G. Bleijenberg, C. Uiterwaal, J. L. L. Kimpen, and E. M. van de Putte. 2011. Adolescent chronic fatigue syndrome: Prevalence, incidence, and morbidity. *Pediatrics* 127(5):E1169-E1175.

Nijhof, S. L., J. M. Rutten, C. S. Uiterwaal, G. Bleijenberg, J. L. Kimpen, and E. M. Putte. 2014. The role of hypocortisolism in chronic fatigue syndrome. *Psychoneuroendocrinology* 42:199-206.

Ocon, A. J., Z. R. Messer, M. S. Medow, and J. M. Stewart. 2012. Increasing orthostatic stress impairs neurocognitive functioning in chronic fatigue syndrome with postural tachycardia syndrome. *Clinical Science* 122(5):227-238.

Ohinata, J., N. Suzuki, A. Araki, S. Takahashi, K. Fujieda, and H. Tanaka. 2008. Actigraphic assessment of sleep disorders in children with chronic fatigue syndrome. *Brain & Development* 30(5):329-333.

Okamoto, L. E., S. R. Raj, A. Peltier, A. Gamboa, C. Shibao, A. Diedrich, B. K. Black, D. Robertson, and I. Biaggioni. 2012. Neurohumoral and haemodynamic profile in postural tachycardia and chronic fatigue syndromes. *Clinical Science* 122(4):183-192.

Petrov, D., D. Marchalik, M. Sosin, and A. Bal. 2012. Factors affecting duration of chronic fatigue syndrome in pediatric patients. *Indian Journal of Pediatrics* 79(1):52-55.

Rimes, K. A., R. Goodman, M. Hotopf, S. Wessely, H. Meltzer, and T. Chalder. 2007. Incidence, prognosis, and risk factors for fatigue and chronic fatigue syndrome in adolescents: A prospective community study. *Pediatrics* 119(3):e603-e609.

Rowe, K. S. 1997. Double-blind randomized controlled trial to assess the efficacy of intravenous gammaglobulin for the management of chronic fatigue syndrome in adolescents. *Journal of Psychiatric Research* 31(1):133-147.

Rowe, K. S., and K. J. Rowe. 2002. Symptom patterns of children and adolescents with chronic fatigue syndrome. In *International perspectives on child and adolescent mental health*, Vol. 2, edited by N. N. Singh, T. H. Ollendick, and A. N. Singh. Oxford, UK: Elsevier. Pp. 395-421.

Rowe, P. C., I. Bou-Holaigah, J. S. Kan, and H. Calkins. 1995. Is neurally mediated hypotension an unrecognised cause of chronic fatigue? *Lancet* 345(8950):623-624.

Rowe, P. C., D. F. Barron, H. Calkins, I. H. Maumenee, P. Y. Tong, and M. T. Geraghty. 1999. Orthostatic intolerance and chronic fatigue syndrome associated with Ehlers-Danlos syndrome. *Journal of Pediatrics* 135(4):494-499.

Royal College. 2004. *Evidence based guideline for the management of CFS/ME in children and young people.* http://www.rcpch.ac.uk/system/files/protected/page/RCPCH%20CFS.pdf (accessed August 15, 2014).

Sankey, A., C. M. Hill, J. Brown, L. Quinn, and A. Fletcher. 2006. A follow-up study of chronic fatigue syndrome in children and adolescents: Symptom persistence and school absenteeism. *Clinical Child Psychology and Psychiatry* 11(1):126-138.

Segal, T. Y., P. C. Hindmarsh, and R. M. Viner. 2005. Disturbed adrenal function in adolescents with chronic fatigue syndrome. *Journal of Pediatric Endocrinology and Metabolism* 18(3):295-301.

Sharpe, M. C., L. C. Archard, J. E. Banatvala, L. K. Borysiewicz, A. W. Clare, A. David, R. H. Edwards, K. E. Hawton, H. P. Lambert, R. J. Lane, E. M. McDonald, J. F. Mowbray, D. J. Pearson, T. E. Peto, V. R. Preedy, A. P. Smith, D. G. Smith, D. J. Taylor, D. A. Tyrrell, S. Wessely, and P. D. White. 1991. A report-chronic fatigue syndrome—guidelines for research. *Journal of the Royal Society of Medicine* 84(2):118-121.

Smith, M. S., J. Mitchell, L. Corey, D. Gold, E. A. McCauley, D. Glover, and F. C. Tenover. 1991. Chronic fatigue in adolescents. *Pediatrics* 88(2):195-202.

Sommerfeldt, L., H. Portilla, L. Jacobsen, J. Gjerstad, and V. B. Wyller. 2011. Polymorphisms of adrenergic cardiovascular control genes are associated with adolescent chronic fatigue syndrome. *Acta Paediatrica* 100(2):293-298.

Stewart, J. M. 2000. Autonomic nervous system dysfunction in adolescents with postural orthostatic tachycardia syndrome and chronic fatigue syndrome is characterized by attenuated vagal baroreflex and potentiated sympathetic vasomotion. *Pediatric Research* 48(2):218-226.

Stewart, J., A. Weldon, N. Arlievsky, K. Li, and J. Munoz. 1998. Neurally mediated hypotension and autonomic dysfunction measured by heart rate variability during head-up tilt testing in children with chronic fatigue syndrome. *Clinical Autonomic Research* 8(4):221-230.

Stewart, J. M., M. H. Gewitz, A. Weldon, N. Arlievsky, K. Li, and J. Munoz. 1999a. Orthostatic intolerance in adolescent chronic fatigue syndrome. *Pediatrics* 103(1):116-121.

Stewart, J. M., M. H. Gewitz, A. Weldon, and J. Munoz. 1999b. Patterns of orthostatic intolerance: The orthostatic tachycardia syndrome and adolescent chronic fatigue. *Journal of Pediatrics* 135(2, Pt. 1):218-225.

Stewart, J. M., M. S. Medow, Z. R. Messer, I. L. Baugham, C. Terilli, and A. J. Ocon. 2012. Postural neurocognitive and neuronal activated cerebral blood flow deficits in young chronic fatigue syndrome patients with postural tachycardia syndrome. *American Journal of Physiology—Heart & Circulatory Physiology* 302(5):H1185-H1194.

Stores, G., A. Fry, and C. Crawford. 1998. Sleep abnormalities demonstrated by home polysomnography in teenagers with chronic fatigue syndrome. *Journal of Psychosomatic Research* 45(1):85-91.

Sulheim, D., H. Hurum, I. B. Helland, E. Thaulow, and V. B. Wyller. 2012. Adolescent chronic fatigue syndrome; a follow-up study displays concurrent improvement of circulatory abnormalities and clinical symptoms. *BioPsychoSocial Medicine* 6.

Sulheim, D., E. Fagermoen, A. Winger, A. M. Andersen, K. Godang, F. Muller, P. C. Rowe, J. P. Saul, E. Skovlund, M. G. Oie, and V. B. Wyller. 2014. Disease mechanisms and clonidine treatment in adolescent chronic fatigue syndrome: A combined cross-sectional and randomized clinical trial. *JAMA Pediatrics* 168(4):351-360.

Takken, T., T. Henneken, E. van de Putte, P. Helders, and R. Engelbert. 2007. Exercise testing in children and adolescents with chronic fatigue syndrome. *International Journal of Sports Medicine* 28(7):580-584.

Tanaka, H., R. Matsushima, H. Tamai, and Y. Kajimoto. 2002. Impaired postural cerebral hemodynamics in young patients with chronic fatigue with and without orthostatic intolerance. *Journal of Pediatrics* 140(4):412-417.

Tomoda, A., T. Jhodoi, and T. Miike. 2001. Chronic fatigue syndrome and abnormal biological rhythms in school children. *Journal of Chronic Fatigue Syndrome* 8(2):29-37.

Tomoda, A., K. Mizuno, N. Murayama, T. Joudoi, T. Igasaki, M. Miyazaki, and T. Miike. 2007. Event-related potentials in Japanese childhood chronic fatigue syndrome. *Journal of Pediatric Neurology* 5(3):199-208.

van de Putte, E. M., K. B. Bocker, J. Buitelaar, J. L. Kenemans, R. H. Engelbert, W. Kuis, J. L. Kimpen, and C. S. Uiterwaal. 2008. Deficits of interference control in adolescents with chronic fatigue syndrome. *Archives of Pediatrics and Adolescent Medicine* 162(12):1196-1197.

Van Geelen, S. M., R. J. Bakker, W. Kuis, and E. M. Van De Putte. 2010. Adolescent chronic fatigue syndrome: A follow-up study. *Archives of Pediatrics and Adolescent Medicine* 164(9):810-814.

Walford, G. A., W. M. Nelson, and D. R. McCluskey. 1993. Fatigue, depression, and social adjustment in chronic fatigue syndrome. *Archives of Disease in Childhood* 68(3):384-388.

Werker, C. L., S. L. Nijhof, and E. M. van de Putte. 2013. Clinical practice: Chronic fatigue syndrome. *European Journal of Pediatrics* 172(10):1293-1298.

Wood, G. C., R. P. Bentall, M. Gopfert, and R. H. T. Edwards. 1991. A comparative psychiatric-assessment of patients with chronic fatigue syndrome and muscle disease. *Psychological Medicine* 21(3):619-628.

Wyller, V. B., and I. B. Helland. 2013. Relationship between autonomic cardiovascular control, case definition, clinical symptoms, and functional disability in adolescent chronic fatigue syndrome: An exploratory study. *BioPsychoSocial Medicine* 7(5).

Wyller, V. B., R. Due, J. P. Saul, J. P. Amlie, and E. Thaulow. 2007a. Usefulness of an abnormal cardiovascular response during low-grade head-up tilt-test for discriminating adolescents with chronic fatigue from healthy controls. *American Journal of Cardiology* 99(7):997-1001.

Wyller, V. B., K. Godang, L. Mørkrid, J. P. Saul, E. Thaulow, and L. Walløe. 2007b. Abnormal thermoregulatory responses in adolescents with chronic fatigue syndrome: Relation to clinical symptoms. *Pediatrics* 120(1):e129-e137.

Wyller, V. B., J. P. Saul, J. P. Amlie, and E. Thaulow. 2007c. Sympathetic predominance of cardiovascular regulation during mild orthostatic stress in adolescents with chronic fatigue. *Clinical Physiology and Functional Imaging* 27(4):231-238.

Wyller, V. B., R. Barbieri, E. Thaulow, and J. P. Saul. 2008a. Enhanced vagal withdrawal during mild orthostatic stress in adolescents with chronic fatigue. *Annals of Noninvasive Electrocardiology* 13(1):67-73.

Wyller, V. B., J. P. Saul, L. Walloe, and E. Thaulow. 2008b. Sympathetic cardiovascular control during orthostatic stress and isometric exercise in adolescent chronic fatigue syndrome. *European Journal of Applied Physiology* 102(6):623-632.

Wyller, V. B., J. A. Evang, K. Godang, K. K. Solhjell, and J. Bollerslev. 2010. Hormonal alterations in adolescent chronic fatigue syndrome. *Acta Paediatrica, International Journal of Paediatrics* 99(5):770-773.

Wyller, V. B., R. Barbieri, and J. P. Saul. 2011. Blood pressure variability and closed-loop baroreflex assessment in adolescent chronic fatigue syndrome during supine rest and orthostatic stress. *European Journal of Applied Physiology* 111(3):497-507.

7

Recommendations

The committee's charge was to "develop evidence-based clinical diagnostic criteria for ME/CFS for use by clinicians, using a consensus-building methodology." To this end, the committee conducted a comprehensive review of the current literature pertinent to the diagnosis of ME/CFS—the results of which are reported in the preceding chapters—keeping in mind the views of clinicians, patients, and their families and caregivers, particularly as they shed light on the complex symptoms associated with this disorder. In the studies reviewed, detailed histories obtained using research questionnaires revealed that the majority of ME/CFS patients experienced post-exertional malaise (PEM) as well as intense fatigue, unrefreshing sleep, cognitive impairment, and autonomic dysfunction, regardless of the case definition or research tool used (findings that accord with those of the Centers for Disease Control and Prevention's [CDC's] Multi-Site Clinical Study).[1] Several signs and symptoms—PEM; orthostatic intolerance; and cognitive impairment, specifically slow information processing—have distinctive findings in ME/CFS patients.

> *Conclusion: It is clear from the evidence compiled by the committee that ME/CFS is a serious, chronic, complex, and multisystem disease that frequently and dramatically limits the activities of affected patients.*

---

[1] Personal communication from Elizabeth Unger, 2014. Preliminary analysis of CDC Multi-Site Clinical Study.

Relying on the findings reported in the literature reviewed, as well as stakeholder input, the committee refined diagnostic criteria that focus more on the central symptoms of this disease than many other definitions (see Box 7-1). The committee anticipates that use of these criteria will make it easier for clinicians to make appropriate and timely diagnoses of ME/CFS in both children and adults and to provide appropriate treatment and management while avoiding possibly harmful interventions. The proposed criteria are quite similar to the Canadian Consensus Criteria (CCC) (Carruthers et al., 2003). The committee recognizes that some patients diagnosed by other criteria, such as the Fukuda definition (Fukuda et al., 1994), will not fulfill all of the criteria proposed here, but it emphasizes that all patients should receive appropriate care.

The committee weighed several factors in reaching consensus on these diagnostic criteria: (1) the frequency and severity with which these symptoms were experienced by patients, (2) the strength of the scientific literature, and (3) the availability of objective measures supporting the association of particular symptoms with the diagnosis. Patient reports and

---

BOX 7-1
Proposed Diagnostic Criteria for ME/CFS

Diagnosis requires that the patient have the following three symptoms:

1. A substantial reduction or impairment in the ability to engage in pre-illness levels of occupational, educational, social, or personal activities that persists for more than 6 months and is accompanied by fatigue, which is often profound, is of new or definite onset (not lifelong), is not the result of ongoing excessive exertion, and is not substantially alleviated by rest,
2. Post-exertional malaise,* and
3. Unrefreshing sleep*

At least one of the two following manifestations is also required:

1. Cognitive impairment* or
2. Orthostatic intolerance

---

* Frequency and severity of symptoms should be assessed. The diagnosis of ME/CFS should be questioned if patients do not have these symptoms at least half of the time with moderate, substantial, or severe intensity.

symptom surveys as well as scientific evidence consistently showed that impaired function, PEM (an exacerbation of some or all of an individual's ME/CFS symptoms after physical or cognitive exertion, or orthostatic stress that leads to a reduction in functional ability), and unrefreshing sleep are characteristic symptoms almost universally present in ME/CFS; thus, the committee considered them to be core symptoms. The committee also found that cognitive impairment and orthostatic intolerance are frequently present in ME/CFS patients and have distinctive findings in these individuals that, particularly when viewed together with the core symptoms, distinguish ME/CFS from other fatiguing disorders. It is essential that clinicians assess the severity and duration of symptoms over an extended period of time because moderate or greater frequency and severity of symptoms are required to distinguish ME/CFS from other illnesses. Regarding the duration of the illness, the proposed criteria require 6 months to make a diagnosis in light of evidence that many other causes of similar fatigue do not last beyond 6 months (Jason et al., 2014; Nisenbaum et al., 1998). These criteria led the committee to create the diagnostic algorithm shown in Figure 7-1.

Other clinical features that may be seen in patients with this disorder are a history of certain infections known to act as triggers for ME/CFS that preceded the onset of symptoms and many types of pain, including headaches, arthralgia, and myalgia. Other complaints, such as gastrointestinal and genitourinary problems, sore throat, tender axillary/cervical lymph nodes, and sensitivity to external stimuli, are reported less frequently (Buchwald and Garrity, 1994; Jason et al., 2013; McGregor et al., 1996). These features, when present, can support the diagnosis of ME/CFS.

These criteria and the algorithm in Figure 7-1 can be used for pediatric patients as well. Although they experience the same symptoms as adult patients, current evidence suggests that children and adolescents with ME/CFS are more likely to have onset following infection with Epstein-Barr virus (EBV) and to have difficulty with orthostatic intolerance and autonomic dysfunction. Profound fatigue, unrefreshing sleep, PEM, and cognitive impairment under stress are common in pediatric patients.

The current evidence base is insufficient to determine whether the illness defined by existing ME/CFS criteria or by the new criteria proposed here has subtypes or is actually a collection of potentially distinguishable disorders. Fukuda and colleagues (1994, p. 956) urged that individuals with ME/CFS "be sub-grouped before analysis or stratified after analysis" by researcher-determined clinical characteristics (e.g., length of illness, infectious onset) or objective test results (e.g., treadmill testing, immunologic markers). Today, many clinicians and researchers agree that ME/CFS is a heterogeneous disease that may be composed of subgroups (Bassi et al., 2008; Carruthers et al., 2011; Jason et al., 2005; May et al., 2010). Yet in practice, large studies that include individuals with diverse symptoms and

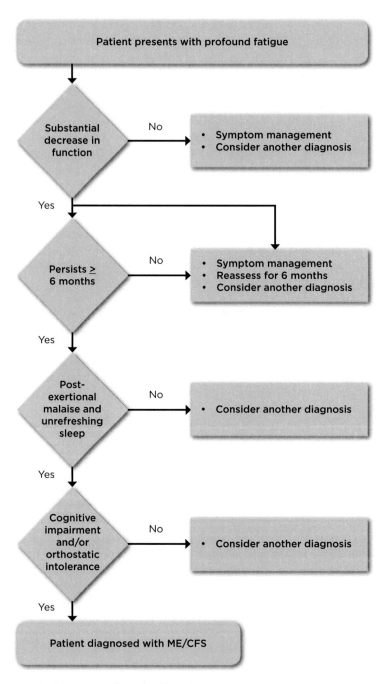

FIGURE 7-1 Diagnostic algorithm for ME/CFS.

yield diverse findings are needed to identify subgroups reliably, and few such studies have been conducted. Nor is there adequate evidence to enable comment on the manifestations of ME/CFS across the life course, except to the extent that orthostatic intolerance and postural orthostatic tachycardia syndrome (POTS) appear to be more prominent in children than in adults with the disorder (see the sections on orthostatic intolerance and autonomic dysfunction in adults and children with ME/CFS in Chapters 4 and 6, respectively). Notably, clinical impression suggests that a larger percentage of children and adolescents relative to adults recover from the disease, although this impression has not been confirmed by the few longitudinal studies conducted to date (Bell et al., 2001; Brown et al., 2012; Cairns and Hotopf, 2005). The committee notes, however, that many of these questions are under active investigation.

MAKING THE DIAGNOSIS

Conclusion: One of the committee's most important conclusions is that a thorough history, physical examination, and targeted work-up are necessary and often sufficient for diagnosis of ME/CFS.

Table 7-1 provides examples of (1) terms ME/CFS patients commonly use to describe their symptoms; (2) potential questions that can alert clinicians to the diagnosis; (3) in-office questionnaires, tools, or clinical observations that may aid diagnosis or indicate the need for further assessment or referral to a specialist (see also Appendix D); and (4) the objective tests that reveal distinctive findings in these patients. The information provided in this table can be used to operationalize the committee's proposed diagnostic criteria in the steps described below. Table 7-2 provides similar information for other symptoms/manifestations of ME/CFS that can support diagnosis.

Diagnostic Tools

First and foremost, listening to patients and taking a careful history are key diagnostic tools. Patients' symptoms and the words they frequently use in describing them should lead clinicians to consider the diagnosis of ME/CFS. Patients often use a variety of evocative words to describe particular symptoms. Histories of many of these symptoms are frequently and consistently elicited when any of an assortment of research questionnaires are used. Clinicians should ask a series of questions to elicit history consistent or inconsistent with ME/CFS. *It is essential that clinicians assess the severity and duration of symptoms over the past month or more. Chronic, frequent, and moderate or severe symptoms are required to distinguish ME/CFS from other illnesses.* Questionnaires and visual analog scales in

TABLE 7-1 Operationalizing the Proposed Criteria for Diagnosis of ME/CFS for Major Symptoms of the Illness

Major Symptom	Patient Descriptions	Potential Questions for Eliciting the Medical History (all questions should explore frequency and severity of symptoms)	Potential In-Office Questionnaires, Tools, or Clinical Observations	Abnormal Findings on Reliable Objective Tests That, When Considered in the Context of Other Symptoms, Support the Diagnosis of ME/CFS (these tests are not routinely required, nor do negative results preclude the diagnosis)
Fatigue	• "flu-like fatigue/exhaustion" • "wired but tired—I feel exhausted but I can't seem to relax or sleep" • "I feel like a battery that is never able to be recharged fully despite resting a lot and limiting my activities to only the bare essentials needed to get by" • "Thinking takes a lot more work than it used to" • "My arms, legs, body feel heavy and harder to move"	• How fatigued are you? • What helps your fatigue the most (resting, lying down, quiet situations, not exercising or avoiding exercise)?	History of this symptom can consistently be elicited using research questionnaires but without specificity. For information on tools or questionnaires for assessing fatigue in adults and children, see Appendix D. Observe for progressive fatigue, need for help or need to lie down during a prolonged exam.	

Substantial
decrease or
impairment in
function

- severe limitations in
  personal and household
  management
- loss of career
- being predominantly
  housebound
- decreased social
  interaction and increased
  isolation

Think back to what you
were able to do before you
became sick. How much has
this illness affected:

- your ability to work?
- your ability to take care
  of yourself/your family
  and to do chores?

What are you able to do
now? How does it compare
with what you were able to
do before?

Are you able to attend
school regularly? Are you
able to participate in any
extracurricular clubs or
sports activities?

- Work and Social
  Adjustment Scale
  (WSAS)
- Energy Index Point Score

For information on other
tools or questionnaires
for assessing decreased
or impaired function in
adults and children, see
Appendix D.

continued

TABLE 7-1 Continued

Major Symptom	Patient Descriptions	Potential Questions for Eliciting the Medical History (all questions should explore frequency and severity of symptoms)	Potential In-Office Questionnaires, Tools, or Clinical Observations	Abnormal Findings on Reliable Objective Tests That, When Considered in the Context of Other Symptoms, Support the Diagnosis of ME/CFS (these tests are not routinely required, nor do negative results preclude the diagnosis)
Post-exertional malaise (prolonged exacerbation of a patient's baseline symptoms after physical/cognitive/orthostatic stress; may be delayed relative to the trigger)	• "crash," "relapse," "collapse" • mentally tired after the slightest effort • physically drained or sick after mild activity • the more demanding or prolonged the activity, the more severe and prolonged the payback	• What happens to you after you engage in normal physical or mental exertion? • How long does it take you to feel bad? • How long does it take to recover from physical or mental effort? • If you go beyond your limits, what are the consequences? • What types of activities do you avoid because of what will happen if you do them? (Consider asking patients to keep a diary for a week or two, documenting activities and symptoms.)	History of this symptom can consistently be elicited using research questionnaires in adults and children (see Appendix D).	Two cardiopulmonary exercise tests (CPETs) separated by 24 hours that demonstrate marked inability to reproduce maximal or anaerobic threshold measures on the second day; values on the second CPET must be much lower than those on the first CPET (note that this test may induce severe exacerbation of symptoms in these patients); 2-day CPETs are not required for diagnosis, although they may be needed for other reasons, such as obtaining Social Security Disability.

Feeling unrefreshed despite sleeping many hours and other sleep disturbances	• "feeling like I never slept" • "cannot fall asleep or stay asleep" • "After long or normal hours of sleep, I still don't feel good in the morning"	• Do you have any problems getting to sleep or staying asleep? • How do you feel in the morning or after you've slept? • Do you need too much sleep? • Do you need to take more naps than other people? (there may be other sleep disruptors as well)	History of this symptom can be consistently elicited using research questionnaires (see Appendix D).	No evidence that currently available sleep studies contribute to the diagnosis of this disorder.
Cognitive impairments (problems with thinking exacerbated by exertion, effort, or stress or time pressure)	• "brain fog" • "confusion" • "disorientation" • "hard to concentrate, can't focus" • "inability to process information" • "can't find the right words" • "inability to multi-task" • "problems with decision making" • "absent-minded/forgetful"	• Do you have problems doing the following activities: driving, watching a movie, reading a book/magazine, completing complex tasks under time constraints, following/participating in conversation, doing more than one thing at a time? • Compared with before your illness, how is your performance at work or school now? • Do you have brain fog or cognitive problems?	• Wood Mental Fatigue Inventory While research questionnaires frequently elicit cognitive impairments (see Appendix D), they are less successful at eliciting issues with slow processing. Observe for difficulties with thinking during the clinic visit—unusual trouble remembering medications, relating details of history or understanding questions/recommendations, expressing self.	Formal neuropsychology testing is not required for diagnosis, although it may be needed for other reasons, such as obtaining Social Security Disability.

continued

TABLE 7-1 Continued

Major Symptom	Patient Descriptions	Potential Questions for Eliciting the Medical History (all questions should explore frequency and severity of symptoms)	Potential In-Office Questionnaires, Tools, or Clinical Observations	Abnormal Findings on Reliable Objective Tests That, When Considered in the Context of Other Symptoms, Support the Diagnosis of ME/CFS (these tests are not routinely required, nor do negative results preclude the diagnosis)
Orthostatic intolerance (Symptoms worsen upon assuming and maintaining upright posture and are ameliorated, though not necessarily abolished, by recumbency.)	• lightheadedness • dizziness • spatial disorientation • fainting • feeling unwell, dizzy, or lightheaded when sitting up or standing still for extended periods (Note "extended" can mean a few minutes for the severely affected.)	• How do you feel when you have been standing still for more than 1-2 minutes? • What happens to you after you get up rapidly after sitting for a long time? • How long can you stand before feeling ill? For example, can you do the dishes? Can you stand in line for a bus or movie? Are you able to grocery shop or be at a mall for more than a few minutes? Can you take a hot shower or hot bath without feeling tired and	This is an area that is not currently explored in depth in research questionnaires, but some suggestions are included in Appendix D. • These patients may need to lie down while they are being interviewed • Blood pressure and heart rate measurements taken lying, sitting, and standing for 10 minutes (Note that standard orthostatic vitals for 1-2 minutes will not be a long enough challenge to identify most forms of orthostatic intolerance.)	Standing test or tilt test to evaluate for postural tachycardia syndrome, neurally mediated hypotension, and orthostatic hypotension (See the section on orthostatic intolerance and autonomic dysfunction in Chapter 4.) Tilt testing is not required for diagnosis, although it may be needed for other reasons, such as obtaining Social Security Disability.

lightheaded? Do you have to sit down or lie down after a shower? Have you fainted or felt like you were going to faint while standing?

- Do these symptoms get worse in hot weather?
- Do you study in a reclining or prone position?
- Do you prefer to sit with knees to your chest or legs under you?

- Exam observations while standing; pallor, general discomfort, acrocyanosis, cold hands and feet, diminished peripheral pulses, sway, efforts to compensate by moving around

NOTES: The patient descriptions included in this table were obtained from the Food and Drug Administration's *Voice of the Patient* report (FDA, 2013), the public comments submitted for the study, and the ME/CFS experts on the committee.

TABLE 7-2 Assessing Other Symptoms/Manifestations of ME/CFS That May Support Diagnosis

Other Symptoms/ Manifestations	Patient Descriptions	Potential Questions for Eliciting the Medical History (all questions should explore frequency and severity of symptoms)	Potential In-Office Questionnaires, Tools, or Clinical Observations	Abnormal Findings on Reliable Objective Tests That, When Considered in the Context of Other Symptoms, Support the Diagnosis of ME/CFS (these tests are not routinely required, nor do negative results preclude the diagnosis)
Pain	• vague achiness all over • muscle pain ("my muscles constantly burn") • joint pain • headaches ("my brain was going to explode")	• Do you have any pain? • Where does it hurt? • How does it feel (e.g., burning, tingling, aching)? • How often do you have pain? How severe is it? How long does it last? What makes it better? What makes it worse?	For information on tools or questionnaires for assessing decreased or impaired function, see Appendix D.	
History of prior triggering infection from which patient never recovered	Patients report coming down with a viral-like, respiratory, or gastrointestinal infection from which they never recovered entirely.	• How did your illness begin? • Were there any events or exposures you consider significant?		Laboratory evidence of prior infection is not required to diagnose this disorder, although it may be needed for other reasons, such as obtaining Social Security Disability; the presence of virus-specific immunoglobulin M (IgM), if documented near the onset of illness, may support diagnosis.

| Abnormal immune function | Patients may report that they are more or less susceptible to infections. | • Are you more susceptible to infection than others or than before your other symptoms began?
• Does it take you longer to recover? | Decreased function of natural killer cells in those with severe disease (Note that this is not unique to this disorder and that commercially available tests may not give accurate results.) |

NOTES: The patient descriptions included in this table were obtained from the Food and Drug Administration's *Voice of the Patient* report (FDA, 2013), the public comments submitted for the study, and the ME/CFS experts on the committee.

which patients rate the frequency and severity of symptoms may be helpful in making these assessments (see Appendix D).

Second, there are several in-office tests and clinical observations that may aid in making the diagnosis or indicate a need for further evaluation or referral. The clinical utility of these tests and observations, however, needs more thorough evaluation. There are objective measures of function that can be helpful in making or confirming the diagnosis. The committee notes that these tests are not required in every case; indeed, they should be performed for purposes of diagnosis *only* when the initial assessment is not definitive. The tests are neither pathognomonic nor diagnostic of ME/CFS on their own, nor does every patient have to have abnormal results on any particular test. Indeed, some tests should be undertaken with caution as they may seriously exacerbate the patient's symptoms. Rather, the results of these tests, when performed in cases of uncertainty, should be considered in the context of the patient's overall clinical picture. The committee recognizes that objective tests also may be useful for patient management but notes that evaluating such uses is beyond its charge.

Conclusion: The central point is that ME/CFS is a diagnosis to be made.

The clinician who suspects this disorder should obtain a detailed history, perform a comprehensive physical examination, and consider conducting an appropriate symptom-focused diagnostic work-up to determine a differential diagnosis and, where clinically indicated, to exclude other disorders that could cause the patient's symptoms as well as to identify any comorbid conditions. As noted previously, the objective functional tests listed in Table 7-1 and Appendix D frequently are not required to make the diagnosis of ME/CFS. If these tests are performed, however, abnormal results can support the diagnosis.

Evidence shows that some tests are not helpful in making the diagnosis of ME/CFS. The committee found tests of neuroendocrine function to be an example, warranted only if disorders in those systems are suspected on other clinical grounds. Similarly, currently available sleep studies are not useful for identifying the presence or absence of unrefreshing sleep.

Recommendation 1: Physicians should diagnose myalgic encephalomyelitis/chronic fatigue syndrome if diagnostic criteria are met following an appropriate history, physical examination, and medical work-up. A new code should be assigned to this disorder in the *International Classification of Diseases*, Tenth Revision (ICD-10), that is not linked to "chronic fatigue" or "neurasthenia."

Even if patients do not meet the criteria for this disorder, clinicians should address their symptoms and concerns. Patients who have not yet been symptomatic for 6 months should be followed over time to see whether they meet the criteria for ME/CFS at a later time.

> **Recommendation 2: The Department of Health and Human Services should develop a toolkit appropriate for screening and diagnosing patients with myalgic encephalomyelitis/chronic fatigue syndrome in a wide array of clinical settings that commonly encounter these patients, including primary care practices, emergency departments, mental/behavioral health clinics, physical/occupational therapy units, and medical subspecialty services (e.g., rheumatology, infectious diseases, neurology).**

CDC's *CFS Toolkit* (CDC, 2014) and the International Association for CFS/ME's *ME/CFS: Primer for Clinical Practitioners* (IACFS/ME, 2014) may be potential places to start, but both need updating in a number of areas in light of the findings presented in this report. The development of clinical questionnaire or history tools that are valid across populations of patients should be an urgent priority. The DePaul Symptom Questionnaire, which has been used extensively in research (DePaul Research Team, 2010), as well as the CDC Symptom Inventory (Wagner et al., 2005), may provide a solid base from which to begin developing questionnaires and interview guides that can be validated for clinical use. Also critical is the development of brief in-office tests for detecting PEM and orthostatic intolerance, for which there are known distinctive findings on more complex clinical tests. For example, evaluation of the extent to which results of the 10-minute lean test correlate with abnormalities on tilt table testing would be useful. It would also be helpful to develop a brief set of neuropsychology tests targeting the information processing problems that affect patients with ME/CFS. This is a particular need as current neuropsychology tests require many hours to complete, frequently precipitating symptoms that patients may find intolerable, and often are impractical for patients because they are quite expensive and not covered by many insurance plans (Lange, 2010). Identification of a set of distinctive biomarkers for this disorder should also be a priority. Finally, all of the above tools should be evaluated to determine how well they distinguish ME/CFS from other complex, multisystem, and fatiguing disorders.

Comorbidities

Over the years, case definitions of ME/CFS have differed significantly in their classification of exclusionary conditions and comorbidities. As a result, a number of disorders, such as morbid obesity and an array of psychiatric disorders, are listed as exclusionary in one definition and as comorbid in another, despite the lack of scientific evidence that being affected by such disorders precludes having ME/CFS. Indeed, it has become increasingly clear that many patients with ME/CFS have other disorders as well, some of which—including fibromyalgia, irritable bowel syndrome, metabolic syndrome, sleep disorders, and depression—may have symptoms that overlap with those of ME/CFS (Buchwald and Garrity, 1994; Johnson et al., 1996; Maloney et al., 2010). Some of these other disorders may develop as part of the spectrum of ME/CFS or in response to the burdens of this disorder.

The committee decided against developing a comprehensive list of potential comorbid conditions, but it points to conditions that clinicians may wish to consider that have been identified by the International Consensus Criteria for ME (ME-ICC) and CCC, including fibromyalgia, myofascial pain syndrome, temporomandibular joint syndrome, irritable bowel syndrome, interstitial cystitis, irritable bladder syndrome, Raynaud's phenomenon, prolapsed mitral valve, depression, migraine, allergies, multiple chemical sensitivities, Sicca syndrome, obstructive or central sleep apnea, and reactive depression or anxiety.

In the section on pain in Chapter 5, the committee discusses the presence of fibromyalgia in patients with ME/CFS. The lack of rigorous studies assessing how ME/CFS patients with fibromyalgia differ from those without fibromyalgia and from patients with fibromyalgia who do not meet criteria for ME/CFS prevents a complete understanding of how these two entities differ. However, the available literature shows that differences between them exist. In addition to the evidence presented in Chapter 5, Cook and colleagues (2012) found that patients with ME/CFS + fibromyalgia showed cardiopulmonary changes during submaximal exercise that differentiated them from controls; the ME/CFS-only group did not show these effects. Also, an analysis of sleep records showed very different results for the two study groups: those with ME/CFS alone had a significantly higher probability of transitioning from rapid eye movement (REM) sleep to wakefulness relative to the ME/CFS + fibromyalgia group; the latter group, on the other hand, showed both sleep pressure and sleep disruption—increased transitions from wakefulness to light sleep and increased transitions from deep to lighter sleep or wakefulness, respectively (Kishi et al., 2011). More research in this area is clearly needed.

The committee recognizes that diagnosis and treatment of comorbid conditions are necessary when caring for patients. For example, a patient with ME/CFS with a prominent history of snoring and sleep apnea may have polysomnography diagnostic of sleep apnea. Treatment with continuous positive airway pressure could improve the patient's overall condition but not resolve all the symptoms of ME/CFS, signifying that in this individual, obstructive sleep apnea is a comorbid condition rather than the cause of the patient's ME/CFS symptoms.

Areas Deserving Further Study

While there was sufficient evidence with which to carry out the first steps of its task, the committee was struck by the relative paucity of research on ME/CFS conducted to date in many areas related to this disorder. Remarkably little research funding has been made available to study the etiology, pathophysiology, and effective treatment of this disease, especially given the number of people afflicted. Thus, the committee was unable to define subgroups of patients or even to clearly define the natural history of the disease. More research is essential.

Future diagnostic research will be most instructive when protocols include patients identified using the committee's proposed diagnostic criteria for ME/CFS as well as patients with other complex fatiguing disorders. Almost all of the studies conducted to date have compared patients with ME/CFS with healthy controls rather than with patients with these other fatiguing disorders. As a result, there is a paucity of data to guide clinicians in distinguishing among these disorders, a gap that urgently needs to be filled.

Finding the cause of and cure for ME/CFS may require research that enlists a homogeneous sample of patients from which important subsets can be identified in terms of disease symptomatology, responses to physical and cognitive stressors, brain imaging, the microbiome, virology, immune function, and gene expression. Integrative approaches using systems biology may be useful in unraveling illness triggers. Studies aimed at assessing the natural history of the disease and its temporal characteristics (onset, duration, severity, recovery, and functional deficits) are essential for a better understanding of ME/CFS and also are important to further refine the diagnostic criteria proposed in this report.

DISSEMINATING THE DIAGNOSTIC CRITERIA

The criteria proposed here will not improve the diagnosis and care of patients unless health care providers use them. Accordingly, the committee developed an outreach strategy for disseminating the clinical diagnostic criteria resulting from this study nationwide to health care professionals so patients will receive this diagnosis in an accurate and timely manner (see Chapter 8). The committee believes that focusing dissemination efforts on reaching primary care and other providers who encounter these patients will increase awareness of and familiarity with the new criteria in a manner that will be most beneficial to patients with ME/CFS.

UPDATING THE DIAGNOSTIC CRITERIA

The committee recognizes that new and accumulating evidence will likely enable refinement of the diagnostic criteria proposed in this report and possibly define subtypes of the disease or even distinct entities. Ideally, diagnostic criteria should be updated when evidence supports a change in order to improve the identification and care of affected individuals (IOM, 2011). The need for reexamination could arise for a number of reasons. Evidence providing greater understanding of the etiology and pathophysiology of ME/CFS might facilitate more discriminating, efficient, or precise diagnostic approaches. Evidence validating either screening or diagnostic tools that are practical for widespread use by generalists might lead to improved identification of affected individuals and so warrant inclusion. And a demonstration of subtypes or even discrete disease entities within the current case definition might enable better prognostication and help target treatment approaches.

Given the current pace of scientific research, the committee expects that the criteria proposed here may warrant reassessment in the not too distant future. Therefore, the committee recommends continuing surveillance of the evidence and revisiting of the criteria in no more than 5 years. Efforts to update the criteria should comply with the process recommendations set forth in the Institute of Medicine (IOM) report *Clinical Practice Guidelines We Can Trust*, which were developed for clinical practice guidelines but are also pertinent to the development of trustworthy diagnostic criteria (IOM, 2011). Regardless of who convenes the update effort, the process for updating should be transparent and open to the views of all stakeholders to ensure that all relevant perspectives are considered. An evidence review that is guided by well-formulated questions informed by stakeholders' views and is conducted by individuals with methodological expertise should underpin any update effort. Ideally, experienced individuals without significant conflicts of interest should conduct a systematic literature review to address the key questions. A multidisciplinary group that includes individuals with clinical expertise should identify those questions and rely heavily on the findings derived from the literature review when making recommendations about modifications of the diagnostic criteria. Members of this group should clearly disclose their potential conflicts of interest, and the conveners of the group should try to limit the number of members with significant conflicts, who should in no case represent a majority of the group's membership. It is critical that support for these activities come from nonconflicted sources such as the Agency for Healthcare Research and Quality (AHRQ) or foundations.

Recommendation 3: A multidisciplinary group should reexamine the diagnostic criteria set forth in this report when firm evidence supports modification to improve the identification or care of affected individuals. Such a group should consider, in no more than 5 years, whether modification of the criteria is necessary. Funding for this update effort should be provided by nonconflicted sources, such as the Agency for Healthcare Research and Quality through its Evidence-based Practice Centers process, and foundations.

NAMING THE DISORDER

As noted in Chapter 3, many concerns have been raised about the term "chronic fatigue syndrome" by clinicians and particularly by patients, their families, and their caregivers.

Conclusion: The committee agrees that the term "chronic fatigue syndrome" can result in stigmatization and trivialization and should no longer be used as the name of this illness.

In response to its directive to "recommend whether new terminology for ME/CFS should be adopted" (see Box 1-1 in Chapter 1), the committee considered the variety of case definitions and diagnostic criteria that have been proposed for ME/CFS as well as the public comments submitted for this study (see Box 3-2 in Chapter 3). In considering what name would be most appropriate, the committee turned first to "myalgic encephalomyelitis" or "encephalopathy" (ME), which was the name most commonly supported in the public comments. The committee, however, was concerned that the term "encephalomyelitis" is not well supported by the evidence and that there is substantial controversy surrounding the two versions of this name. Neither version conveys the full complexity of this disorder. The committee notes that many of the other names that have been proposed focus on particular organ systems. Others suggest particular etiologies, such as immune or infectious, for this disorder that are not yet proven.

The committee was convinced of the value of creating a name that conveys the central elements of this disease, a practice for which there is much precedent in medicine for disorders whose etiology or pathophysiology is not yet well understood. After extensive consideration, and being mindful of the concerns expressed by patients and their advocates, the committee recommends that the disorder described in this report be named "systemic exertion intolerance disease" (SEID). "Systemic exertion intolerance" captures the fact that exertion of any sort—physical, cognitive, emotional—can adversely affect these patients in many organ systems and in many aspects of their lives. The committee intends for this name to convey the complexity and severity of this disorder.

> **Recommendation 4: The committee recommends that this disorder be renamed "systemic exertion intolerance disease" (SEID). SEID should replace myalgic encephalomyelitis/chronic fatigue syndrome for patients who meet the criteria set forth in this report.**

CLOSING THOUGHTS

The committee's careful review of the literature, together with the input of patients and clinicians, revealed that ME/CFS is a complex disorder characterized by a prolonged, significant decrease in function; fatigue; post-exertional malaise; unrefreshing sleep; difficulties with information processing, especially under time pressure; and orthostatic intolerance. ME/CFS frequently is accompanied by pain and a variety of other symptoms. It often is triggered by specific infections. Although research using complex investigative testing is yielding some unique findings, there is an urgent need to develop a series of questionnaires and objective tests that can easily be used to diagnose these patients in a variety of clinical settings. Current evidence does provide a path forward now, which is outlined in this report, but it is the committee's hope that new developments in research, particularly in the creation of clinical diagnostic tools, will warrant revisiting these guidelines in the near future. To that end, the committee has proposed a process that should be used in updating its proposed diagnostic criteria.

In what will likely be its most controversial recommendation, the committee has proposed that the name "chronic fatigue syndrome" no longer be used to describe this disorder. The committee repeatedly heard from patients that this term was stigmatizing and too often precluded their receiving appropriate care. The committee instead determined that the name "systemic exertion intolerance disease" (SEID) better characterizes the disorder for which its proposed diagnostic criteria were developed.

REFERENCES

Bassi, N., D. Amital, H. Amital, A. Doria, and Y. Shoenfeld. 2008. Chronic fatigue syndrome: Characteristics and possible causes for its pathogenesis. *Israel Medical Association Journal* 10(1):79-82.

Bell, D. S., K. Jordan, and M. Robinson. 2001. Thirteen-year follow-up of children and adolescents with chronic fatigue syndrome. *Pediatrics* 107(5):994-998.

Brown, M. M., D. S. Bell, L. A. Jason, C. Christos, and D. E. Bell. 2012. Understanding long-term outcomes of chronic fatigue syndrome. *Journal of Clinical Psychology* 68(9):1028-1035.

Buchwald, D., and D. Garrity. 1994. Comparison of patients with chronic fatigue syndrome, fibromyalgia, and multiple chemical sensitivities. *Archives of Internal Medicine* 154(18):2049-2053.

Cairns, R., and M. Hotopf. 2005. A systematic review describing the prognosis of chronic fatigue syndrome. *Occupational Medicine (Oxford)* 55(1):20-31.

Carruthers, B. M., A. K. Jain, K. L. De Meirleir, D. L. Peterson, N. G. Klimas, A. M. Lemer, A. C. Bested, P. Flor-Henry, P. Joshi, A. C. P. Powles, J. A. Sherkey, and M. I. van de Sande. 2003. Myalgic encephalomyelitis/chronic fatigue syndrome: Clinical working case definition, diagnostic and treatment protocols (Canadian case definition). *Journal of Chronic Fatigue Syndrome* 11(1):7-115.

Carruthers, B. M., M. I. van de Sande, K. L. De Meirleir, N. G. Klimas, G. Broderick, T. Mitchell, D. Staines, A. C. P. Powles, N. Speight, R. Vallings, L. Bateman, B. Baumgarten-Austrheim, D. S. Bell, N. Carlo-Stella, J. Chia, A. Darragh, D. Jo, D. Lewis, A. R. Light, S. Marshall-Gradisbik, I. Mena, J. A. Mikovits, K. Miwa, M. Murovska, M. L. Pall, and S. Stevens. 2011. Myalgic encephalomyelitis: International consensus criteria. *Journal of Internal Medicine* 270(4):327-338.

CDC (Centers for Disease Control and Prevention). 2014. *CDC CFS toolkit.* http://www.cdc.gov/cfs/toolkit (accessed July 22, 2014).

Cook, D. B., A. J. Stegner, P. R. Nagelkirk, J. D. Meyer, F. Togo, and B. H. Natelson. 2012. Responses to exercise differ for chronic fatigue syndrome patients with fibromyalgia. *Medicine & Science in Sports & Exercise* 44(6):1186-1193.

DePaul Research Team. 2010. *DePaul symptom questionnaire.* http://condor.depaul.edu/ljason/cfs/measures.html (accessed August 20, 2014).

FDA (Food and Drug Administration). 2013. *The voice of the patient: Chronic fatigue syndrome and myalgic encephalomyelitis.* Bethesda, MD: Center for Drug Evaluation and Research (CDER), FDA.

Fukuda, K., S. E. Straus, I. Hickie, M. C. Sharpe, J. G. Dobbins, and A. Komaroff. 1994. The chronic fatigue syndrome: A comprehensive approach to its definition and study. *Annals of Internal Medicine* 121(12):953-959.

IACFS/ME (International Association for Chronic Fatigue Syndrome/Myalgic Encephalomyelitis). 2014. *ME/CFS: Primer for clinical practitioners.* Chicago, IL: IACFS/ME.

IOM (Institute of Medicine). 2011. *Clinical practice guidelines we can trust.* Washington, DC: The National Academies Press.

Jason, L. A., K. Corradi, S. Torres-Harding, R. R. Taylor, and C. King. 2005. Chronic fatigue syndrome: The need for subtypes. *Neuropsychology Review* 15(1):29-58.

Jason, L. A., M. Sunnquist, A. Brown, M. Evans, S. Vernon, J. Furst, and V. Simonis. 2013. Examining case definition criteria for chronic fatigue syndrome and myalgic encephalomyelitis. *Fatigue: Biomedicine, Health & Behavior Fatigue: Biomedicine, Health & Behavior* 2(1).

Jason, L. A., B. Z. Katz, Y. Shiraishi, C. Mears, Y. Im, and R. R. Taylor. 2014. Predictors of post-infectious chronic fatigue syndrome in adolescents. *Health Psychology & Behavioural Medicine* 2(1):41-51.

Johnson, S. K., J. DeLuca, and B. H. Natelson. 1996. Depression in fatiguing illness: Comparing patients with chronic fatigue syndrome, multiple sclerosis and depression. *Journal of Affective Disorders* 39(1):21-30.

Kishi, A., B. H. Natelson, F. Togo, Z. R. Struzik, D. M. Rapoport, and Y. Yamamoto. 2011. Sleep-stage dynamics in patients with chronic fatigue syndrome with or without fibromyalgia. *Sleep* 34(11):1551-1560.

Lange, G. 2010. *Cognitive function in CFS: A measure of disability?* http://www.hhs.gov/advcomcfs/meetings/presentations/presentation_10132010_gudrunlannge.pdf (accessed August 5, 2014).

Maloney, E. M., R. S. Boneva, J. M. Lin, and W. C. Reeves. 2010. Chronic fatigue syndrome is associated with metabolic syndrome: Results from a case-control study in Georgia. *Metabolism: Clinical & Experimental* 59(9):1351-1357.

May, M., A. Emond, and E. Crawley. 2010. Phenotypes of chronic fatigue syndrome in children and young people. *Archives of Disease in Childhood* 95(4):245-249.

McGregor, N. R., R. H. Dunstan, M. Zerbes, H. L. Butt, T. K. Roberts, and I. J. Klineberg. 1996. Preliminary determination of the association between symptom expression and urinary metabolites in subjects with chronic fatigue syndrome. *Biochemical and Molecular Medicine* 58(1):85-92.

Nisenbaum, R., M. Reyes, A. C. Mawle, and W. C. Reeves. 1998. Factor analysis of unexplained severe fatigue and interrelated symptoms: Overlap with criteria for chronic fatigue syndrome. *American Journal of Epidemiology* 148(1):72-77.

Wagner, D., R. Nisenbaum, C. Heim, J. F. Jones, E. R. Unger, and W. C. Reeves. 2005. Psychometric properties of the CDC symptom inventory for assessment of chronic fatigue syndrome. *Population Health Metrics* 3(8).

8

Dissemination Strategy

A fter evaluating the evidence, recommending new clinical diagnostic criteria for ME/CFS that address the needs of health care providers and patients and their caregivers, and suggesting a new name for ME/CFS ("systemic exertion intolerance disease" [SEID]), the committee's final task was to develop an outreach strategy for disseminating its diagnostic criteria nationwide to health care professionals.

OBJECTIVE

The adoption of new clinical information can be a slow process, sometimes taking many years before new evidence-based findings make their way into clinical practice (Balas and Boren, 2000). With a constant flow of new information about the practice of medicine and patient care, it is difficult for health care providers to remain up to date. In addition, a provider may be aware of new information but not familiar with or able to accept or apply it. The objective of the committee's dissemination strategy is to provide recommendations for dissemination of the new diagnostic criteria for SEID that will result in patients receiving this diagnosis in an accurate and timely manner.

CONTEXT

Prior to the implementation of any dissemination strategy, it is important to examine the internal and external environments that can influence the strategy—both positively and negatively. The internal environment

231

refers to the strengths, weaknesses, capacities, and resources of the Department of Health and Human Services (HHS) and its affiliated agencies. The external environment comprises those factors that are not controlled by HHS or its agencies but that need to be considered in designing and implementing the dissemination strategy.

Internal Environment

HHS and its affiliated agencies generally are well positioned to increase awareness of and familiarity with the new diagnostic criteria:

- The Centers for Disease Control and Prevention (CDC) provided the initial case definition of CFS in 1988 and helped launch one of the first national programs to educate the American public and health care providers about the illness.
- Surveys of the American public have found a relatively high level of trust of HHS—and an even greater trust of CDC—as agencies that provide factual information. A national survey conducted by the Pew Research Center during October 9-13, 2013, among 1,504 adults in the United States found that 75 percent had a favorable opinion of CDC—the highest level of approval among the 13 agencies included in the survey (Pew Research Center for the People & the Press, 2013).
- Many studies point to a rise in use of the Internet by health care providers and the public to seek health information (Dolan, 2010; Fox and Duggan, 2013). A search of "chronic fatigue syndrome" on major search engines such as Google and Yahoo generated many federally managed websites among the top results. Information on websites controlled by CDC, the National Institutes of Health (NIH), and the Office on Women's Health are ranked highly on search engine returns, which results in large numbers of annual visitors (CDC, 2014b). In contrast, a search of "myalgic encephalomyelitis" returns primarily nongovernmental or non-U.S. websites because of the relatively rare use of this term until 2011, when U.S. federal agencies began using the term "ME/CFS."
- HHS also has existing ties to many ME/CFS opinion leaders and advocates through its Chronic Fatigue Syndrome Advisory Committee and CDC's Chronic Fatigue Syndrome (CFS) Patient-Centered Outreach and Communication Activity (PCOCA) Conference Calls. These could be excellent venues for disseminating the committee's diagnostic criteria and recommendations.
- As the single largest payer for health care services in the United States (through Medicare and Medicaid), HHS has a great deal

of influence over and ability to communicate with nearly all physicians.

While generally trusted by the American public, HHS and its affiliated agencies have faced strong criticism in previous years from patients with ME/CFS and their care providers and advocates. A Government Accountability Office (GAO) report released in June 2000 was highly critical of CDC's appropriation of a significant proportion of CFS funds for programs and activities that were not related to CFS (GAO, 2000). HHS needs to be prepared to address possible questions or concerns regarding this issue and to share information about the positive changes that have been made since the GAO report was issued.

HHS also has faced some criticism for requesting that this committee be convened to develop new diagnostic criteria for ME/CFS. As noted in Chapter 1, a number of researchers and clinicians with strong ties to the ME/CFS community formally called for HHS to abandon this Institute of Medicine (IOM) effort and instead use the funds to support further ME/CFS research (An Open Letter, 2013).

External Environment

Several positive external environmental factors may support HHS in its efforts to disseminate the committee's new diagnostic criteria. The following are examples:

- Designated awareness efforts, such as International Chronic Fatigue Syndrome [and Fibromyalgia] Awareness Day, held on May 12, and National Chronic Fatigue Syndrome Awareness Month, held in March, have helped somewhat to raise general awareness of ME/CFS. These observances also have traditionally served as times to share information about ME/CFS, especially with the public.
- A number of independent ME/CFS organizations exist both in the United States and internationally (e.g., the Solve ME/CFS Initiative and the ME Association in the United Kingdom) to support and share information with patients with ME/CFS and their care providers.

As dissemination activities are planned, however, it is also important to recognize the various external environmental factors that may present challenges to dissemination efforts. One of the more concerning of these external factors is the lack of awareness and continuing skepticism among many health care providers of ME/CFS as a legitimate physical illness.

Indeed, the main barriers to appropriate and timely diagnosis of

ME/CFS appear to be primarily attitudinal rather than knowledge based. A study published in 2010 by CDC found that 96 percent of health care providers were aware of ME/CFS and were able to recall accurately some symptoms associated with the 1994 Fukuda definition (Brimmer et al., 2010). Yet the same study also found that a significant portion of providers had doubts and misconceptions about the illness. Some providers still were expressing the belief that "people with [ME/CFS] are just depressed" and 30 to 43 percent link the illness to high socioeconomic status or pre-illness "competitive/compulsive" personality traits. These findings led the authors of the study to recommend that future education efforts for providers address diagnosis and be delivered through venues used by providers as their primary sources of reliable and accurate information. As part of the CDC study, physicians reported that professional journals, the Internet, and continuing education programs were their top three sources for information on ME/CFS. Similarly, a 2011 study found that 85 percent of health care providers still believed the illness was wholly or partially a psychiatric rather than a medical one (Unger, 2011). Numerous studies also have documented skepticism among clinicians about ME/CFS being a distinct clinical entity (Bayliss et al., 2014).

Other attitudinal barriers include physicians' low self-efficacy and lack of positive outcome expectancy with respect to ME/CFS. A recent CDC-sponsored Medscape continuing medical education program found that a high percentage of the more than 2,000 respondents were "not at all confident" or only "somewhat confident" about making a diagnosis of ME/CFS (Harmon et al., 2014). In a separate study, almost 70 percent of clinicians who had previously diagnosed patients with ME/CFS still believed the illness to be more difficult to diagnose than other illnesses (Brimmer et al., 2010). Finally, some physicians, despite being somewhat knowledgeable about and believing in the legitimacy of the condition, may not share those thoughts with their patients because of the mistaken belief that giving them a diagnosis of ME/CFS will "inhibit a patient's motivation to get better" as it prevents them from engaging fully with the existential conditions of their life, which is what they cannot cope with (Brimmer et al., 2010, p. 10). Consequently, successful dissemination of the committee's new clinical diagnostic criteria will entail not only educating clinicians about the content of the criteria but also addressing the attitudes and beliefs that could hinder the criteria's acceptance.

It is also important to note that, as discussed in Chapter 7, the diagnostic label "chronic fatigue syndrome" is viewed negatively by the majority of patients (Jason et al., 2004). Many patient groups argue that the label trivializes the illness and creates unnecessary stigma (Jason et al., 2007). In addition, a study found that physicians may even perceive the condition as being less serious as a result of this name (Jason et al., 2002).

Finally, despite the above barriers to the accurate diagnosis of ME/CFS among health care providers, it is important for the dissemination of the new diagnostic criteria to build on previous efforts that have helped increase awareness of ME/CFS among health care providers and the public. Key to doing so will be the continued positioning of SEID as a legitimate disease that occurs in children and adults and should be properly diagnosed and treated. Another key is emphasizing that the diagnosis of SEID should be made if a patient fits the diagnostic criteria, instead of a diagnosis of exclusion being made after no medical explanation can be found for the patient's symptoms. Many patients already diagnosed with ME/CFS will also qualify for the diagnosis of SEID and should receive the latter diagnosis and be cared for accordingly. Others who do not meet the new criteria should continue to be diagnosed by other criteria as their symptoms and evaluations dictate. In addition, it is essential that patients who do not qualify for a diagnosis of SEID receive appropriate care.

STRATEGIC CHOICES

Strategic choices that will inform the dissemination strategy relate to both audiences and messaging.

Audiences

To accomplish the task of disseminating the new diagnostic criteria for SEID nationwide to health care providers, multiple audiences will need to be included in the dissemination effort. The audiences identified include not only the key decision makers (i.e., primary care providers [PCPs]) but also other health care providers traditionally associated with the diagnosis and care of patients with ME/CFS. Audiences that can be engaged by HHS to help influence PCPs and other health care providers also have been identified.

Primary Care Providers

While it is important for a variety of health care providers to have knowledge of the new diagnostic criteria, the need to educate and influence PCPs is paramount. These professionals usually are the first providers seen by patients with SEID, and as with other chronic illnesses, they frequently continue to care for these patients over the long term. As noted by patients currently diagnosed with ME/CFS, their PCP's lack of knowledge of the disorder or unwillingness to provide a diagnosis often has resulted in the need to see multiple physicians and unnecessary delays in diagnosis. An estimated 84 percent of Americans afflicted with what is currently known as ME/CFS have yet to be diagnosed (Solomon and Reeves, 2004), and in one patient survey, many of those who had been diagnosed reported seeing more than five doctors across a period of 6 years or more before receiving their diagnosis (ProHealth, 2008). The committee believes that focusing dissemination efforts on reaching PCPs will increase awareness of and familiarity with the new clinical diagnostic criteria for SEID in a manner that will be most beneficial to patients.

According to the Agency for Healthcare Research and Quality, there are an estimated 300,000 PCPs in the United States. Potential PCPs for patients with SEID include

- internists (American College of Physicians: www.acponline.org; American Medical Association: www.ama-assn.org/ama),
- family physicians (American Academy of Family Physicians: www.aafp.org; American Medical Association: www.ama-assn.org/ama),
- general practitioners (American Academy of General Physicians: www.aagp.org),
- pediatricians (American Academy of Pediatrics: www.aap.org; American Medical Association: www.ama-assn.org/ama),
- nurse practitioners (American Association of Nurse Practitioners: www.aanp.org), and
- physician assistants (American Academy of Physician Assistants: www.aapa.org).

Additional Care Providers

While PCPs should be the primary target audience of the dissemination strategy, PCPs frequently will consult with specialists when making a diagnosis of SEID. In addition, many other health care providers often diagnose and/or care for patients with SEID (IACFS/ME, 2013). These secondary audiences include the following health care providers:

- obstetricians/gynecologists (Montefiore Medical Center, 2013) (American College of Obstetricians and Gynecologists: www.acog.org),
- emergency medicine practitioners (American Academy of Emergency Medicine: www.aaem.org),
- psychologists (American Psychological Association: www.apa.org),
- psychiatrists (American Psychiatric Association: www.psychiatry.org),
- neurologists (FM/CFS/ME Resources, 2014) (American Academy of Neurology: www.aan.com),

- rheumatologists (American College of Rheumatology: www.rheumatology.org),
- gastroenterologists (American College of Gastroenterology: www.gi.org),
- sports medicine practitioners (American Medical Society for Sports Medicine: www.amssm.org),
- sleep medicine practitioners (Jackson and Bruck, 2012) (American Academy of Sleep Medicine: www.aasmnet.org),
- infectious disease practitioners (Infectious Diseases Society of America: www.idsociety.org),
- cardiologists (DeNoon, 2003) (American College of Cardiology: www.cardiosource.org),
- physical therapists (American Physical Therapy Association: www.apta.org),
- occupational therapists (American Occupational Therapy Association: www.aota.org),
- chiropractors (American Chiropractic Association: www.acatoday.org),
- osteopathic practitioners (American Osteopathic Association: www.osteopathic.org), and
- fitness instructors (American Council on Exercise: www.acefitness.org).

School-Based Professionals

Given that SEID has been shown to be among the top medical causes of long-term absence from school for the K-12 population (Crawley et al., 2011), outreach efforts also should target school nurses (National Association of School Nurses: www.nasn.org), school psychologists (National Association of School Psychologists: www.nasponline.org), and other professionals who have contact with children who have problems attending school because of health issues. Currently, some students with SEID and their families struggle to obtain accommodations for their education because school personnel do not understand the clinical impact of the illness.

Professional Societies

Studies have found that professional societies rank among health care providers' top sources for new information. As such, they are an important audience for HHS's efforts to reach out to and educate and influence health care providers. A sampling of potential societies was noted above; however, the committee recognizes that HHS should potentially consider many other societies as well.

Independent ME/CFS Organizations

In addition to professional societies, health care providers recognize patients as sources of new information. For this reason, it is important for HHS to engage organizations with strong connections to patients as well as other important audiences. Potential targets include

- International Association for CFS/ME (www.iacfsme.org),
- Massachusetts CFIDS/ME & FM [Fibromyalgia] Association (www.masscfids.org),
- ME/CFS Forums (www.mecfsforums.com),
- New Jersey Chronic Fatigue Syndrome Association, Inc. (www. njcfsa.org),
- Organization for Fatigue & Fibromyalgia Education & Research (OFFER) (www.offerutah.org),
- Patient Alliance for Neuro-endocrine-immune Disorders Organization for Research and Advocacy (PANDORA) (www.pandoraorg. net),
- Phoenix Rising (www.phoenixrising.me),
- Rocky Mountain CFS/ME & FM Association (www.rmcfa.org),
- Solve ME/CFS Initiative (www.solvecfs.org), and
- Wisconsin ME/CFS Association, Inc. (www.wicfs-me.org).

As discussed in earlier chapters, patients with SEID often have other comorbidities and thus seek help from organizations that focus on those conditions. Similarly, members of professional organizations that address these other conditions may encounter SEID. Some examples of such organizations are

- Dysautonomia International (www.dysautonomiainternational. org),
- Dysautonomic Youth Network of America (www.dynainc.org),
- National Fibromyalgia and Chronic Pain Association (www. fmcpaware.org), and
- National Fibromyalgia Association (www.fmaware.org).

Messaging

The messaging that is part of the dissemination strategy needs to support the objective of increasing awareness that SEID is a serious, chronic, complex, and multisystem medical condition, and that knowledge and use of the new diagnostic criteria will enable patients with SEID to receive an accurate diagnosis in a timely manner. Effective messaging informs, persuades, and moves a target audience to action. The following suggested messages are designed to serve as a framework for use in conjunction with all dissemination activities:

- Patients deserve to receive an accurate diagnosis of their illness as quickly as possible.
- SEID is a disease that occurs in both children and adults and needs to be properly diagnosed and managed.
- The IOM's new diagnostic criteria should be used to diagnose SEID quickly and accurately.
- By using the new diagnostic criteria, health care providers will enable patients with SEID to receive the diagnosis of their illness and appropriate care.

With regard to the committee's new term for ME/CFS, HHS's messaging should communicate that the diagnostic label "systemic exertion intolerance disease" (SEID) more accurately reflects the disease's characteristics than "ME/CFS." It is also important to stress that adoption of the new name will help remove some of the stigma associated with the "ME/CFS" label.

In addition, as noted earlier, some patients diagnosed by other criteria, such as the Fukuda definition, may or may not fulfill all criteria for a diagnosis of SEID. HHS will need to communicate that all of these patients should still receive appropriate care.

DISSEMINATION ACTIVITIES

Strategic dissemination is vital for developing awareness of and familiarity with the new diagnostic criteria. Whenever possible, it is important to use the most direct tactics possible to reach the targeted audiences. It is also important to note that no single tactic is effective in all circumstances for all people. Successful dissemination will require the use of multiple tactics. The following tactics have been shown to be effective as means of sharing information with health care providers and influencing their behaviors.

Educational Material

HHS should explore options for producing and directly distributing (via traditional mail, email, or other means) an educational summary of this report and the new diagnostic criteria directly to PCPs. Information on how to obtain a copy of the full report should also be provided.

In addition, an audit should be conducted to identify any existing materials regarding ME/CFS that are already available from HHS and its affiliated agencies (e.g., CDC's *Recognition and Management of CFS: A Resource Guide for Health Care Professionals*) (CDC, 2014a). These materials should then be reviewed and updated as needed to reflect the committee's new diagnostic criteria and terminology. HHS also should strive for consistent information and messaging across all of its agencies' materials.

Presentations/Exhibits at Major Medical Meetings

Sharing information about the new diagnostic criteria and terminology at major medical meetings is an excellent way to reach large numbers of attending PCPs. In addition to having information about the new diagnostic criteria available to share as part of educational exhibits at these meetings, HHS should seek opportunities for opinion leaders (discussed later in this section) to be included as part of the formal program to allow for an in-depth presentation of the new diagnostic criteria and terminology. Examples of possible meetings to target include

- American Academy of Family Physicians Scientific Assembly, September 29-October 3, 2015 (http://www.aafp.org/events/assembly/about/past-future.html);
- American College of Physicians Internal Medicine Meeting, April 30-May 2, 2015 (http://im2015.acponline.org);
- American Academy of Pediatrics National Conference, October 24-27, 2015 (http://www.aapexperience.org);
- American Association of Nurse Practitioners National Conference, June 9-14, 2015 (http://www.aanp.org/conferences/national-conference); and
- American Academy of Physician Assistants, May 23-27, 2015 (http://www.aapaconference.org/?utm_source=aapa.org&utm_medium=events&utm_campaign=aapa15).

As resources allow, HHS should pursue sharing information at additional medical meetings that reach not just PCPs but also the additional health care providers previously identified.

Online Outreach

Studies have found that physicians are increasingly using the Internet to locate information to assist in the treatment of patients and keep up to date on health topics (Google/Hall & Partners, 2009; Hornby, 2004; Wolters Kluwer Health, 2011). HHS should make information about the new diagnostic criteria and terminology available online, including both on websites operated by HHS and its affiliated agencies and on leading third-party websites. Websites of HHS and its affiliated agencies include

- Agency for Healthcare Research and Quality (National Guideline Clearinghouse) (http://www.guideline.gov),
- CDC (http://www.cdc.gov/cfs; http://www.cdc.gov/cfs/es/index.html),
- HHS (healthfinder.gov) (http://www.healthfinder.gov/FindServices/SearchContext.aspx?topic=171),
- National Library of Medicine (MedlinePlus) (http://www.nlm.nih.gov/medlineplus/chronicfatiguesyndrome.html), and
- Office on Women's Health (http://www.womenshealth.gov/publications/our-publications/fact-sheet/chronic-fatigue-syndrome.html).

HHS should undertake a thorough audit of all of its online resources to ensure that the information presented reflects the new criteria and terminology.

Examples of third-party websites that have been cited by health care providers as leading sources for new information include (De Leo et al., 2006; Glenn, 2013)

- Epocrates (www.epocrates.com),
- Mayo Clinic (MayoClinic.com),
- Mdconsult (www.mdconsult.com),
- Medscape (www.medscape.com),
- Skyscape (www.skyscape.com),
- Uptodate (www.uptodate.com),
- WebMD (www.webmd.com), and
- Wikipedia (www.wikipedia.com).

Collaboration with Professional Societies

PCPs and other health care providers trust their professional societies and use them as a resource for keeping up to date on health information. In addition to the aforementioned national meetings, large professional societies typically have available multiple channels of communication, such as websites, newsletters, and educational programming, to allow for the sharing of information with their members. HHS should seek opportunities to collaborate with these professional societies in the distribution of the new diagnostic criteria and terminology.

One of the most effective channels of communication available to professional societies is their journals, which, as noted earlier, rank among the main resources used by health care providers to obtain information to aid in diagnosing patients. For example, the *Journal of the American Medical Association* has a regular column, "Medical News and Perspectives," featuring news from various government agencies, while the *New England Journal of Medicine* has "Clinical Crossroads," where an individual patient with a common medical problem is presented, followed by discussion of existing guidelines and recommendations. HHS should actively seek to have information about the new diagnostic criteria and terminology included in these journals.

As appropriate, HHS also should request that the societies express official support for this report. Any positive support for the new diagnostic criteria should then be shared and incorporated into any future communication activities.

Collaboration with Large Health Care Systems/Medical Groups, Managed Care Organizations, and Insurance Providers

Many PCPs and other health care providers are employed by large and highly organized health care systems/medical groups or managed care organizations (e.g., Ascension Health, Permanente Medical Groups). HHS should reach out to the largest of these systems to seek their assistance and ideas for educating their member physicians (SK&A, 2015). These organizations often have committees that review recent recommendations/guidelines and work to implement them within their own standards of care. HHS also should share the new diagnostic criteria with large insurance providers that issue diagnostic guides and manuals to participating physicians (Heilbrunn, 2014). In addition to private-sector organizations, HHS should reach out to federally supported provider networks, such as

- National Association of Community Health Clinics,
- Society of Federal Health Professionals, and
- U.S. Public Health Service.

Media Outreach

PCPs and other health care providers are consumers of mass media, and they report that the media—particularly news outlets—play a significant role in their awareness of new health information (van Bekkum and Hilton, 2013). Targeted mass media outlets, including but not limited to broadcast, print, and online outlets, should be the focus of HHS efforts to share information about and obtain positive coverage of the new diagnostic criteria.

Given that SEID is more common among women than among men (Jason et al., 1999), HHS should make a special effort to secure coverage with media outlets that reach women. However, approximately 25 percent of affected patients are men, and there is evidence suggesting that a similar condition, fibromyalgia, is underdiagnosed to a much greater extent in men than in women (Vincent et al., 2013). Therefore, efforts to educate professionals and the public via media sources that target men (e.g., the magazines *Men's Health* and *Men's Fitness*) also are needed. In addition, some studies suggest that ethnic minorities with SEID are diagnosed less frequently and may have a higher prevalence of and more severe illness (Jason et al., 1999, 2003), so it is important also to try to place stories with media outlets that reach these populations.

The submission of editorials by opinion leaders (see below) about the new diagnostic criteria and the need for physicians to overcome barriers to diagnosing patients with SEID would also be useful. This outreach should include traditional media outlets such as *The New York Times* and *The Washington Post*, as well as newer media outlets such as The Health Care Blog and KevinMD.com.

Social Media Outreach

Research has shown that social media applications may be an efficient and effective way for health care providers to keep up to date and to share newly acquired medical knowledge with other providers, thereby improving the quality of patient care (McGowan et al., 2012). As with its websites, HHS should employ the social media applications (Facebook, Twitter, blogs, etc.) used by the department and its affiliated agencies to help disseminate the new diagnostic criteria and terminology. Examples of possible activities include

- an announcement about the new diagnostic criteria on the Office on Women's Health's Facebook page (www.facebook.com/HHSOWH),
- a Twitter chat hosted by HHS (twitter.com/hhsgov), and
- a YouTube video with various opinion leaders discussing the new diagnostic criteria and terminology (www.youtube.com/user/usgovhhs).

Outreach to Opinion Leaders

Highly regarded individuals within the health care community influence the practice of their peers (Flodgren et al., 2011; Lomas et al., 1991; Valente and Davis, 1999). Thus, it is important for HHS to identify and educate opinion leaders within the existing ME/CFS professional and patient communities about the new criteria and terminology. These leaders should then be enlisted to address barriers and promote the new criteria and terminology at every opportunity, both formally and informally. Members of this IOM committee, the HHS Chronic Fatigue Syndrome Advisory Committee, and the NIH Trans-NIH Myalgic Encephalomyelitis/Chronic Fatigue Syndrome Research Working Group could provide a good base of opinion leaders, as well as insight into other possible opinion leaders. It is important that the identified opinion leaders be thoroughly briefed on the new diagnostic criteria and terminology and be provided with approved talking points to help ensure consistent messaging.

Patient-Directed Interventions

Patients are increasingly seeking out health information, especially from the Internet, in addition to seeking help from health care providers (Diaz et al., 2002). They often share the information they discover directly with their providers or use the information to shape communication with their providers. As HHS seeks to include information for professionals on websites operated by the department and its affiliated agencies, it should include information for patients as well. In addition, any media outreach should include professional and general outlets to help inform both providers and patients.

To help increase awareness among possible patients with SEID, HHS also should work with ME/CFS organizations (identified previously) that serve as a resource for health care providers and patients. It is also recommended that CDC host a special CFS PCOCA Conference Call to discuss the new diagnostic criteria and terminology.

Educational Awareness Campaign

HHS should consider launching a public awareness campaign similar to that launched by CDC in 2006. This campaign should be a collaboration that includes appropriate federal agencies and participation by ME/CFS organizations and professional medical societies. The campaign should place a heavy emphasis on directly addressing barriers to PCPs' adequately diagnosing SEID and explain the benefits of the new diagnostic criteria and terminology.

Collaboration with Training and Examination Organizations

Studies have found that younger and less experienced physicians may be more open to adopting new practices relative to older physicians (Francke et al., 2008). Therefore, efforts aimed at introducing the new diagnostic criteria to medical students and trainees should be considered. HHS should share the new diagnostic criteria and terminology with the Association of American Medical Colleges (AAMC) and explore working with that organization to incorporate the new information into the curricula for medical students.

Furthermore, curricula of training programs often are dictated by topics that will be covered in various training examinations, so outreach to groups that develop and administer those examinations can be valuable. HHS should share the new diagnostic criteria and terminology with the American Council for Graduate Medical Education and National Board of Medical Examiners and work to have the new information accurately reflected in the examinations they administer.

Collaboration with Licensure and Certification Organizations

As with training and examination organizations, HHS should share information about the new diagnostic criteria and terminology with state medical licensing and certification boards. Opportunities to have the new information incorporated into the processes of these organizations should be explored.

Continuing Medical Education Opportunities

PCPs and other health care providers use continuing medical education as an opportunity to learn new information. In addition, continuing medical education points can be an incentive for providers to seek out specific information. HHS should work to update CDC's current continuing medical education course Diagnosis and Management of Chronic Fatigue Syndrome (http://www.cdc.gov/cfs/education/diagnosis/index.html [accessed January 14, 2015]) to include information about the new diagnostic criteria.

Designation of an HHS Point Person

HHS should consider appointing an individual to oversee the dissemination of the new diagnostic criteria nationwide to health care professionals (i.e., a "SEID czar" within the department). This person should have access to the necessary resources and the authority to implement the dissemination plans for the new criteria and address any questions or concerns that arise. Having such an individual in place will also help demonstrate HHS's responsiveness to this issue.

EVALUATION

As the dissemination strategy is implemented, it will be important for HHS to include an evaluation component in order to monitor progress. The evaluation should include both quantitative and qualitative measures. These measures should be established prior to the start of the implementation effort and reviewed periodically throughout its course to identify any issues and refine the strategy accordingly.

Examples of possible quantitative measures that HHS could use include tracking the number of visits to government websites containing SEID information and the number of health care providers reached at conferences/meetings where the new diagnostic criteria and terminology are presented. A possible qualitative evaluation measure is a study similar to the 2010 study "U.S. Healthcare Providers' Knowledge, Attitudes, Beliefs, and Perceptions Concerning Chronic Fatigue Syndrome" (Brimmer et al., 2010). This study could serve as a baseline for the tracking of any changes in knowledge, attitudes, and behaviors among providers as a result of the new diagnostic criteria and terminology.

REFERENCES

An Open Letter. 2013. *An open letter to the honorable Kathleen Sebelius, U.S. Secretary of Health and Human Services*, September 23, 2013. https://dl.dropboxusercontent.com/u/89158245/Case%20Definition%20Letter%20Sept%2023%202013.pdf (accessed July 17, 2014).

Balas, E. A., and S. A. Boren. 2000. Managing clinical knowledge for health care improvement. In *Yearbook of medical informatics 2000: Patient-centered systems*, edited by J. Bemmel and A. McCray. Stuttgart, Germany: Schattinauer. Pp. 65-70.

Bayliss, K., M. Goodall, A. Chisholm, B. Fordham, C. Chew-Graham, L. Riste, L. Fisher, K. Lovell, S. Peters, and A. Wearden. 2014. Overcoming the barriers to the diagnosis and management of chronic fatigue syndrome/ME in primary care: A meta synthesis of qualitative studies. *BMC Family Practice* 15(1):44.

Brimmer, D. J., F. Fridinger, J. M. Lin, and W. C. Reeves. 2010. U.S. healthcare providers' knowledge, attitudes, beliefs, and perceptions concerning chronic fatigue syndrome. *BMC Family Practice* 11:28.

CDC (Centers for Disease Control and Prevention). 2014a. *Recognition and management of chronic fatigue syndrome: A resource guide for health care professionals.* http://www.cdc.gov/cfs/pdf/cfs-resource-guide.pdf (accessed July 23, 2014).

CDC. 2014b. *Top referrers (inbound links) to CDC.gov.* http://www.cdc.gov/metrics/cdcgov/referrers.html (accessed July 23, 2014).

Crawley, E. M., A. M. Emond, and J. A. C. Sterne. 2011. Unidentified chronic fatigue syndrome/myalgic encephalomyelitis (CFS/ME) is a major cause of school absence: Surveillance outcomes from school-based clinics. *BMJ Open* 1(2).

De Leo, G., C. LeRouge, C. Ceriani, and F. Niederman. 2006. Websites most frequently used by physician for gathering medical information. *AMIA Annual Symposium Proceedings Archive* 902.

DeNoon, D. 2003. *Tricky heart may cause chronic fatigue.* http://www.webmd.com/chronic-fatigue-syndrome/news/20030414/tricky-heart-may-cause-chronic-fatigue?lastselected guid=%7B5FE84E90-BC77-4056-A91C-9531713CA348 (accessed August 4, 2014).

Diaz, J. A., R. A. Griffith, J. J. Ng, S. E. Reinert, P. D. Friedman, and A. W. Moulton. 2002. Patients' use of the Internet for medical information. *Journal of General Internal Medicine* 17(3):180-185.

Dolan, P. L. 2010. *86% of physicians use internet to access health information.* http://www.amednews.com/article/20100104/business/301049966/7 (accessed August 15, 2014).

Flodgren, G., E. Parmelli, G. Doumit, M. Gattellari, M. A. O'Brien, J. Grimshaw, and M. P. Eccles. 2011. Local opinion leaders: Effects on professional practice and health care outcomes. *Cochrane Database of Systematic Reviews* (8):Cd000125.

FM/CFS/ME (Fibromyalgia/Chronic Fatigue Syndrome/Myalgic Encephalomyelitis) Resources. 2014.http://fmcfsme.com (accessed August 21, 2014).

Fox, S., and M. Duggan. 2013. *Health online 2013.* http://www.pewinternet.org/2013/01/15/health-online-2013 (accessed September 29, 2014).

Francke A. L., M. C. Smit, A. J. E. de Veer, and P. Mistiaen. 2008. Factors influencing the implementation of clinical guidelines for health care professionals: A systematic meta-review. *BMC Medical Informatics and Decision Making* 8.

GAO (Government Accountability Office). 2000. *Chronic fatigue syndrome: CDC and NIH research activities are diverse, but agency coordination is limited.* Washington, DC: GAO.

Glenn, B. 2013. Physicians' top 5 most-used medical apps for smartphones and tablets. *Medical Economics Online.* http://medicaleconomics.modernmedicine.com/medical-economics/content/tags/american-ehr-partners/physicians-top-5-most-used-medical-apps-smartph (accessed January 14, 2015).

Google/Hall & Partners. 2009. *Connecting with physicians online.* http://www.gstatic.com/ads/research/en/2009_ConnectingwithPhysiciansOnline.pdf (accessed August 4, 2014).

Harmon, M., C. Bateman, C. Lapp, and K. McCleary. 2014. *Chronic fatigue syndrome: Diagnosis to management.* http://www.medscape.org/viewarticle/581527_10 (accessed August 20, 2014).

Heilbrunn, E. 2014. *Top health insurance companies: Best? Not necessarily. But these health insurers have the biggest market share.* http://health.usnews.com/health-news/health-insurance/articles/2013/12/16/top-health-insurance-companies (accessed December 12, 2014).

Hornby, K. 2004. The Internet as an evidence-based medicine tool. *British Columbia Medical Journal* 46:282-284.

IACFS/ME (International Association for Chronic Fatigue Syndrome/Myalgic Encephalomyelitis). 2013. *ME/CFS management an approach to finding physician care.* http://www.iacfsme.org/MECFSManagementAnApproachtoFindingPhysician/tabid/313/Default.aspx (accessed August 20, 2014).

Jackson, M. L., and D. Bruck. 2012. Sleep abnormalities in chronic fatigue syndrome/myalgic encephalomyelitis: A review. *Journal of Clinical Sleep Medicine* 8(6):719-728.

Jason, L. A., J. A. Richman, A. W. Rademaker, K. M. Jordan, A. V. Plioplys, R. R. Taylor, W. McCready, C. F. Huang, and S. Plioplys. 1999. A community-based study of chronic fatigue syndrome. *Archives of Internal Medicine* 159(18):2129-2137.

Jason, L. A., R. R. Taylor, S. Plioplys, Z. Stepanek, and J. Shlaes. 2002. Evaluating attributions for an illness based upon the name: Chronic fatigue syndrome, myalgic encephalopathy and Florence Nightingale disease. *American Journal of Community Psychology* 30(1):133-148.

Jason, L. A., A. V. Plioplys, S. Torres-Harding, and K. Corradi. 2003. Comparing symptoms of chronic fatigue syndrome in a community-based versus tertiary care sample. *Journal of Health Psychology* 8(4):459-464.

Jason, L. A., C. Holbert, S. Torres-Harding, and R. Taylor. 2004. Stigma and the term chronic fatigue syndrome. *Journal of Disability Policy Studies* 14(4):222-228.

Jason, L. A., J. Richman, N. Porter, and M. Benton. 2007. Why the name of an illness is of importance. Paper read at 8th International IACFS Conference, Florida.

Lomas, J., M. Enkin, G. M. Anderson, W. J. Hannah, E. Vayda, and J. Singer. 1991. Opinion leaders vs audit and feedback to implement practice guidelines. Delivery after previous cesarean section. *Journal of the American Medical Association* 265(17):2202-2207.

McGowan, B. S., M. Wasko, B. S. Vartabedian, R. S. Miller, D. D. Freiherr, and M. Abdolra-sulnia. 2012. Understanding the factors that influence the adoption and meaningful use of social media by physicians to share medical information. *Journal of Medical Internet Research* 14(5):e117.

Montefiore Medical Center. 2013. *Study finds young, minority women most likely to visit Ob/Gyn as primary care provider*. News release. http://www.montefiore.org/body.cfm?id=1738&action=detail&ref=1031 (accessed September 2, 2014).

Pew Research Center for the People & the Press. 2013. *Trust in government nears record low, but most federal agencies are viewed favorably*. http://www.people-press.org/2013/10/18/trust-in-government-nears-record-low-but-most-federal-agencies-are-viewed-favorably (accessed September 29, 2014).

ProHealth. 2008. *A profile of ME/CFS patients: How many years and how many doctors?* http://www.prohealth.com/library/showarticle.cfm?libid=13672 (accessed August 28, 2104).

SK&A. 2015. *SK&A's 50 largest medical groups*. http://www.skainfo.com/health_care_market_reports/largest_medical_groups.pdf (accessed January 12, 2015).

Solomon, L., and W. C. Reeves. 2004. Factors influencing the diagnosis of chronic fatigue syndrome. *Archives of Internal Medicine* 164(20):2241-2245.

Unger, A. 2011. CFS knowledge and illness management behavior among U.S. healthcare providers and the public. Paper read at IACFS/ME Biennial International Conference Ottawa, Ontario, Canada.

Valente, T., and R. Davis. 1999. Accelerating the diffusion of innovations using opinion leaders. *The Annals of the American Academy* 566.

van Bekkum, J., and S. Hilton. 2013. Primary care nurses' experiences of how the mass media influence frontline healthcare in the UK. *BMC Family Practice* 14:178.

Vincent, A., B. D. Lahr, F. Wolfe, D. J. Clauw, M. O. Whipple, T. H. Oh, D. L. Barton, and J. St. Sauver. 2013. Prevalence of fibromyalgia: A population-based study in Olmsted County, Minnesota, utilizing the Rochester Epidemiology Project. *Arthritis Care and Research* 65(5):786-792.

Wolters Kluwer Health. 2011. *Wolters Kluwer Health 2011: Point-of-care survey*. http://www.wolterskluwerhealth.com/news/documents/white%20papers/wolters%20kluwer%20health%20survey%20executive%20summary-media.pdf (accessed September 2, 2014).

A

Public Session Agendas[1]

January 27, 2014
Keck Center of The National Academies
500 Fifth Street, NW, Room 100
Washington, DC

1:00-1:15 PM **Introduction to Public Session**
Ellen Wright Clayton, Committee Chair

1:15-2:00 PM **Background and Charge to the Committee**
Nancy C. Lee, M.D., Designated Federal Officer for
the Chronic Fatigue Syndrome Advisory Committee
(CFSAC), Deputy Assistant Secretary for Health-
Women's Health and Director of the Office on Women's
Health (OWH) in the Office of the Secretary, Department
of Health and Human Services

Q and A from Committee

2:00-2:30 PM **Methodology for the CDC Multi-Site Clinical Study**
Elizabeth Unger, Chief of the Chronic Viral Diseases
Branch (CVDB), Centers for Disease Control and
Prevention

---

[1] Presentation materials available by request through the National Academies Public Access
Records Office, (202) 334-3543 or paro@nas.edu.

2:30-3:00 PM   NIH/Office of Disease Prevention (ODP) Pathways
to Prevention Workshop: Myalgic Encephalomyelitis/
Chronic Fatigue Syndrome (ME/CFS)
Susan Maier, Deputy Director, Office of Research on
Women's Health (ORWH), Department of Health and
Human Services

3:00-3:15 PM   Break

3:15-3:45 PM   The Voice of the Patient Report
Sara Eggers, Office of Program and Strategic Analysis/
Office of Strategic Programs, Center for Drug Evaluation
and Research, Food and Drug Administration

3:45-4:45 PM   Remarks from ME/CFS Advocates and Associations
Adin Burroughs, Phoenix Rising
Lori Chapo-Kroger, PANDORA
Carol Head, CFIDS Association of America
Pat LaRosa, New Jersey Chronic Fatigue Syndrome
Association, Inc.
Charmian Proskauer, Massachusetts CFIDS/ME & FM
Association
Mary Schweitzer, Wisconsin ME/CFS Association, Inc.
Jennie Spotila, OccupyCFS

4:45-5:30 PM   Public Comment Session (15 slots of 3 minutes each)

5:30 PM   Adjournment of Public Session
Ellen Wright Clayton, Committee Chair

May 5, 2014
National Academy of Sciences Building
2101 Constitution Avenue, NW, Room 120
Washington, DC

1:00-1:15 PM   Introduction to Public Session
Ellen Wright Clayton, Committee Chair

1:15-2:45 PM   Patient and Advocate Panel: Challenges Faced by
ME/CFS Patients When Interacting with the
Health Care System
Joseph Landson
Denise and Matthew Lopez-Majano
Robert Miller
Annette Whittemore

2:45-3:15 PM   Q and A from Committee

3:15-3:30 PM   Break

3:30-4:00 PM   Diagnostic Criteria Issues for ME/CFS
Leonard A. Jason, Professor, DePaul University, Director
of the Center for Community Research

4:00-4:10 PM   Q and A from Committee

4:10-4:40 PM   Sleep Disturbances in ME/CFS
Akifumi Kishi, Postdoctoral Fellow in the Division
of Pulmonary, Critical Care, and Sleep Medicine,
Department of Medicine, New York University School of
Medicine

4:40-4:50 PM   Q and A from Committee

4:50-5:20 PM   Neurocognitive Manifestations in ME/CFS
Gudrun Lange, Professor, Department of Physical
Medicine and Rehabilitation, Rutgers University-New
Jersey Medical School

5:20-5:30 PM   Q and A from Committee

5:30 PM   Adjournment of Public Session
Ellen Wright Clayton, Committee Chair

B

GRADE Grid Template

	GRADE score				
	2	1	0	-1	-2
Balance between desirable and undesirable consequences of inclusion as a core or required symptom	Desirable clearly outweigh undesirable	Desirable probably outweigh undesirable	Trade-offs equally balanced or uncertain	Undesirable probably outweigh desirable	Undesirable clearly outweigh desirable
Assessment of quality of evidence	Strong: "definitely include as required"	Weak: "probably include as required"	No specific recommendation	Weak: "probably don't include as required"	Strong: "definitely don't include as required"

For each symptom or category of symptoms below, please mark with an "X" the cell that best corresponds to your assessment of the available evidence, in terms of benefits versus disadvantages for inclusion as a core or required symptom.

Post-exertional malaise
(exacerbation of symptoms or fatigue triggered by physical or mental exertion and lasting > 24 hours after exercise)

Sleep
(unrefreshing sleep, sleep disturbance/ dysfunction)

Neurocognitive manifestations
(mental fatigue, memory impairment, concentration difficulties, confusion)

Autonomic manifestations
(orthostatic intolerance, cardiovascular irregularities, gastrointestinal impairments, genitourinary impairments)

Immune manifestations
(sore throat, tender lymph nodes)

Neuroendocrine manifestations
(loss of thermostatic stability, sweating episodes, intolerance of temperature extremes)

Pain
(headaches, muscle pain, joint pain)

Balance between desirable and undesirable effects of inclusion as a required or core symptom or symptom category
Desirable consequence: The specific symptom or symptom category is present in a majority of ME/CFS patients, and its inclusion as a required symptom could prevent incorrect diagnoses of ME/CFS in those that do not have it.
Undesirable consequence: The specific symptom or symptom category is *not* present in a majority of ME/CFS patients, and its requirement could thus exclude patients with ME/CFS from diagnosis.
The larger the difference between the desirable and undesirable effects, the more likely a strong recommendation is warranted. The narrower the gradient, the more likely a weak recommendation is warranted.
Quality of evidence: The higher the quality of evidence, the more likely a strong recommendation is warranted.

C

Disability in ME/CFS

Several ME/CFS symptoms may contribute to impairment or disability, including fatigue, cognitive dysfunction, pain, sleep disturbance, post-exertional malaise (PEM), and secondary depression or anxiety (Andersen et al., 2004; Tiersky et al., 2001).[1] This appendix presents the Social Security Administration's (SSA's) current guidelines for evaluating disability in ME/CFS patients and summarizes research to date in assessing disability and impairment in both children and adults with ME/CFS.

SSA GUIDELINES FOR EVALUATING DISABILITY

In April 2014, SSA issued updated guidelines for evaluating disability claims involving ME/CFS. Social Security Ruling (SSR 14-1p) provides guidance on how to develop evidence to establish that a person has a medically determinable impairment (MDI) of ME/CFS and explains how SSA evaluates disability claims and continuing disability reviews for ME/CFS under titles II and XVI of the Social Security Act. According to SSA, determination of an MDI includes a diagnosis of ME/CFS by a licensed physician using the Fukuda case definition, supported by specific medical evidence consisting of signs, symptoms, and laboratory findings (see Box C-1). Therefore, it is critical for health care providers to know what medical evidence is necessary and how to test for it in order for patients to receive disability status. It should be noted that the symptoms constituting this report's new diagnostic

---

[1] Personal communication; public comments submitted to the IOM Committee on the Diagnostic Criteria for Myalgic Encephalomyelitis/Chronic Fatigue Syndrome for meeting 3, 2014.

BOX C-1
Social Security Administration Evaluation of Disability

Medical Evidence

For the purposes of Social Security Disability evaluation, in addition to a diagnosis of ME/CFS that meets the Fukuda case definition, one or more of the following medical signs clinically documented over a period of at least 6 consecutive months is required to establish the existence of a medically determinable impairment (MDI) of CFS:

- palpably swollen or tender lymph nodes on physical examination;
- nonexudative pharyngitis;
- persistent, reproducible muscle tenderness on repeated examinations, including the presence of positive tender points; or
- any other medical signs that are consistent with medically accepted clinical practice and are consistent with the other evidence in the case record. For example, the Canadian Consensus Criteria (CCC) and International Consensus Criteria for ME (ME-ICC) explain that an acute infectious inflammatory event may precede the onset of CFS, and that other medical signs may be present, including
  - frequent viral infections with prolonged recovery,
  - sinusitis,
  - ataxia,
  - extreme pallor, and
  - pronounced weight change.

Laboratory Findings

Specific laboratory findings are not well established for ME/CFS. However, certain laboratory findings may support the finding of an MDI in people with ME/

---

criteria, as well as the objective tests mentioned in Chapter 7 (tilt table test, cardiopulmonary exercise test [CPET], and neuropsychological testing), are already included in the current guidelines.

ASSESSING DISABILITY

This section reviews the literature regarding the role of impairment and disability in ME/CFS patients. While it stands to reason that many of the individual symptoms of ME/CFS can cause impairment, this is not the focus of this section; it is instead discussed in various sections throughout Chapters 4, 5, and 6.

CFS even in the absence of the medical evidence listed above. It is not unusual to find standard laboratory tests in the normal range for many patients with ME/CFS, and SSA advises that such tests should not be relied upon to the exclusion of all other clinical evidence in decisions regarding the presence and severity of an MDI. The following laboratory findings establish the existence of an MDI in people with ME/CFS:

- an elevated antibody titer to Epstein-Barr virus (EBV) capsid antigen equal to or greater than 1:5,120, or early antigen equal to or greater than 1:640;
- an abnormal magnetic resonance imaging (MRI) brain scan;
- neurally mediated hypotension as shown by tilt table testing or another clinically accepted form of testing; or
- any other laboratory findings that are consistent with medically accepted clinical practice and are consistent with the other evidence in the case record (for example, an abnormal exercise stress test or abnormal sleep studies, appropriately evaluated and consistent with the other evidence in the case record).

New laboratory and clinical evidence may emerge with continued research in ME/CFS. According to SSA, these findings may be considered, in conjunction with laboratory findings discussed above, in the assessment of an MDI. Depending on the type of assessment, ongoing mental limitations or neurocognitive manifestations documented by a mental status examination or psychological testing may be considered medical signs or laboratory findings.

SOURCE: Social Security Ruling, 2014.

Challenges and Limitations

Research to date illustrates the many challenges of assessing disability in adults with ME/CFS, an illness for which cause and cure are unknown. First, the often lengthy duration of time between symptom onset and diagnosis is estimated to be at least 1 year in 67 to 77 percent of patients and at least 5 years in 29 percent of patients (CFIDS Association of America, 2014; ProHealth, 2008). Thus, many people may be disabled for years before being identified as an ME/CFS patient. Second, compared with more current case definitions (Carruthers et al., 2003, 2011), the most commonly used case definition (Fukuda et al., 1994) identifies a more broadly defined patient population in which PEM, arguably a hallmark of ME/CFS, is not required for diagnosis. Thus, evidence of disability must correspond to the unique semiology of this broadly defined patient population. Third, disability, evidenced by the persistence of illness following optimal treatment, requires consensus regarding an optimal course of treatment. A lack of consensus regarding treatment efficacy persists in the research to date and further confounds efforts to assess disability status. Fourth, studies of recovery from ME/CFS vary widely as a result of the use of different case definitions in the study samples; differing definitions of "recovery"; the lack of temporal metrics of function obtained before, during, and after treatment; and the use of patients' subjective assessment of their own progression of illness and recovery (Cairns and Hotopf, 2005). The call for objective markers of impairment that correspond to the unique symptom complex of ME/CFS patients is prudent and indicated given the lack of consensus that persists in the research literature regarding assessment of recovery.

Impact on Daily Activities, Responsibilities, and Social Interactions

Daily activities, responsibilities, and social interactions—perhaps the most important of which are adults' ability to work and children's attendance and performance in school—can be an important indicator of disability and impairment (Schweitzer et al., 1995). Patients coping with the burden of disease will often reduce certain activities such as extracurricular school activities or social gatherings in order to fulfill these essential responsibilities. Thus, it is important to exercise caution in generalizing findings on work and school to a patient's overall function.

Impairment and Employment Status

A review of studies published between 1966 and 2004 examined the extent of work-related impairment and unemployment in ME/CFS (Taylor and Kielhofner, 2005). Studies were included if work-related impairment was a primary variable and individuals met any case definition for ME/CFS. Regarding work-related impairment, unemployment rates in 13 of 15 studies varied from 35 to 69 percent. Job loss ranged from 26 to 89 percent, which was consistent with job loss among those with other chronic illnesses. Decreased work performance also was consistently reported in the literature and was attributed to impairments of short-term memory and learning, decision making, attendance, and communication skills and increased dependence on coworkers to perform work duties, among other reasons. Studies in this review were based primarily on unstandardized self-report, and some data indicated that symptom severity was associated with inability to work.

A systematic review of studies published between 1988 and 2001 examined evidence in the literature relating impairment to employment status in those diagnosed with ME/CFS (Ross et al., 2002, 2004). Evidence of impairment was found to be substantially more prevalent in ME/CFS (40 percent of 1,830 patients) than in controls (12 percent), and 54 percent of ME/CFS patients reported being unemployed, compared with 9 percent of controls.

Impairment and School Activity

For children, adolescents, and young adults who are not yet engaged in full-time occupations, physical function, impairment, and disability are more appropriately evidenced by school attendance. Additionally, assessment of social, physical, emotional, psychosocial, and cognitive domains that reflect levels and quality of overall function in this age range are warranted.

In their epidemiological study of absence due to long-term sickness in U.K. schools, Dowsett and Colby (1997) examined the results of a 5-year retrospective survey of school principals and students in six school areas. They found that 42 percent of all medically certified long-term sickness-related absence was due to ME/CFS, a figure considerably higher than those absent due to cancers (23 percent), other illnesses (13 percent), and psychiatric or psychological problems (12 percent). Crawley and colleagues (2011) performed a clinical evaluation of schoolchildren ages 11-16 years enrolled in secondary schools in the Bath region of England and who had been absent for more than 20 percent of a 6-week term (n = 461). Of this high absence group, 6 percent were identified as having ME/CFS, confirming ME/CFS as a major cause of school absence. Only 11 percent of these children had previously been diagnosed with ME/CFS, indicating under-recognition of the illness.

Bell and colleagues (2001) completed a 13-year follow-up of 35 respondents who developed an illness suggestive of ME/CFS in children and adolescents between January 1984 and December 1987 in an isolated rural community in upstate New York. All of these individuals met the Fukuda definition retrospectively. The educational impact of the illness was correlated most closely with illness outcome, with those who missed the most school (up to 2 years) reporting the poorest recovery over time. Upon follow-up, 66 percent believed that their illness had an overall social effect on their life that varied from mild to severe. In general, the social effect paralleled the perceived illness outcome. Crawley and Sterne (2009) found that reduced school attendance among children with ME/CFS was associated most strongly with poor physical function, with more than 60 percent of the 211 children with ME/CFS in their sample attending only 2 days of school or less per week. Smith and colleagues (2003) found that adolescents with ME/CFS missed 57 days of school on average over a 6-month period. Severity of fatigue was highly associated with school absence.

Health care providers should not dismiss the lack of school attendance or participation in activities in these patients as merely school phobia or having overprotective parents. Further, pediatricians should assess the risk or existence of a disability in their patients ideally at their first visit and identify those who may benefit from services under the Individuals with Disabilities Education Act (IDEA). Pediatricians should be well informed about the process for referring children and adolescents with a disabling condition to early intervention programs in the community and explain the parents' right to have their children evaluated by a multidisciplinary team from the school or a state-designated agency (American Academy of Pediatrics, 1999).

Other Indicators of Impairment

A recent Norwegian study that surveyed ME patients as defined by the International Consensus Criteria for ME (ME-ICC) (Carruthers et al., 2011) attempted to characterize the burden of disease through self-report measures in lay terms (Bringsli et al., 2014). The authors found that 75 percent of those surveyed described their impairment as being housebound most of the time (leaving home only with careful planning) if not all of the time or being fully bedridden.

The Centers for Disease Control and Prevention's (CDC's) Multi-Site Study surveyed ME/CFS patients using the Short Form 36-Item Questionnaire of the Medical Outcomes Study (MOS) (SF-36) as an indicator of function (Unger, 2013). Preliminary data from this study show that patients scored under 40 on all measures except for "role emotional" and "mental health." They scored particularly low (< 20) on "role physical" and "vitality." These findings were consistent across sites.

A comparison of quality of life (QOL) characteristics in 25 children from the United Kingdom with ME/CFS (based on the Fukuda definition) and 23 age/gender/Tanner stage-matched healthy controls found QOL in the ME/CFS children to be profoundly reduced (Kennedy et al., 2010). Only 1 of 25 children with ME/CFS attended school full time, 48 percent attended school part time, and 32 percent received home tutoring. Children with ME/CFS scored substantially lower than controls on the global health item of the Child Health Questionnaire (CHQ), as well as most other items, including physical functioning, social limitations due to emotional and health limitations, pain and discomfort, mental health, self-esteem, general health perceptions, and family activities. Most notably, a comparison of scores on nine items of the CHQ revealed that the ME/CFS children scored lower than children with type 1 diabetes and asthma as well as healthy controls.

Similarly, Rowe and colleagues (2014) compared the self-reported health-related quality of life (HRQOL) of adolescents and young adults with ME/CFS with that of healthy controls as well as published results of HRQOL in other chronic pediatric conditions. Scores on all measures of HRQOL indicated worse function among those with ME/CFS compared with controls. The mean total score on the Pediatric Quality of Life Inventory (one of the tools used to measure HRQOL) for ME/CFS was lower than published scores for children with cystic fibrosis, eosinophilic gastrointestinal disorder, epilepsy, type 1 diabetes, sickle cell disease, and renal transplants and comparable to scores for children with pediatric fibromyalgia and paraplegic cerebral palsy (Ingerski et al., 2010; Varni et al., 2007).

Duration of Disability

The length of recovery time and effectiveness of treatment for ME/CFS have important implications for defining the duration of disability.

Recovery

A recent effort to define recovery in ME/CFS employed a systematic review of 22 studies in which recovery was defined operationally by reference to one or more of these domains: (1) premorbid functioning, (2) both fatigue and function, (3) fatigue (or related symptoms) alone, (4) function alone, and/or (5) brief global assessment (Adamowicz et al., 2014). The aim was to systematically review and evaluate the different definitions of recovery proposed in the ME/CFS literature and to offer recommendations for future research.

The brief global assessment was the most common outcome measure used to define recovery, although measures of recovery varied considerably among the studies. Overall, the review revealed widely varying estimates of recovery that ranged from 0 to 66 percent in intervention studies and 2.6 to 62 percent in naturalistic studies. The review found many inconsistencies across the literature which help explain the wide range of these estimates. First, the wide range can be explained in part by whether recovery was defined by single or multiple domains. Reports of high recovery rates typically were based on single-domain definitions of recovery (e.g., fatigue or function); use of multiple criteria (fatigue scores within the normal range, normal health perceptions, no physical or social disabilities, and no negative perceptions of fatigue) within the same cohort produced rates of recovery less than half of those reported using single-domain definitions. Second, the term "recovery" often included less than full restoration of health as reported by the patients, and typically it was based on limited assessment. Thus, the authors recommend that positive changes in illness status be referred to more precisely as "clinically significant improvement" to better differentiate between "recovery" (return to premorbid functioning) and "improvement" (positive change in health but not full restoration). Third, the majority of studies relied on patient self-reports and did not utilize more objective measures of recovery, such as return to work or school- or laboratory-based assessments. Consequently, it is difficult to know whether substantial recovery occurred.

In a response to the recommendations of Adamowicz and colleagues (2014), Twisk (2014) states that subjective measures cannot dispel the debate regarding identification of full or partial recovery from ME/CFS. Instead, he recommends objective measures to characterize the clinical status and function of a patient before, during, and after treatment interventions to ascertain partial or full recovery. Further, he asserts that accurate diagnosis is crucial to establish whether a patient has recovered, and that objective assessment must address the unique symptoms in accordance with the diagnosis, whether it be ME or CFS.

The challenge of defining recovery in ME/CFS is further supported by a study of long-term health, symptom, and disability outcomes in ME/CFS patients diagnosed 25 years ago compared with healthy controls (Brown et al., 2012). Twenty of the 25 patients in the study reported no longer having a diagnosis of ME/CFS. Compared with healthy controls, those who remitted from ME/CFS showed significantly more impairment on 21 of 23 outcomes. Likewise, compared with the 5 patients who maintained a diagnosis of ME/CFS, those who remitted from ME/CFS showed no difference on 17 outcomes of impairment. The results of this study suggest that over time, most ME/CFS patients will not maintain the diagnosis, but they will not fully recover and will still be symptomatic.

A systematic review by Taylor and Kielhofner (2005) examined employment status as an indicator of recovery. The review included three longitudinal studies that found little change in employment status over time (Bombardier and Buchwald, 1995; Tiersky et al., 2001; Vercoulen et al., 1996). A 5-year follow-up study by Andersen and colleagues (2004) found that work disability of ME/CFS patients, identified in accordance with the Fukuda definition, increased from 77 to 91 percent, indicating no evidence of recovery.

Treatment

Similar to the literature on treatment in ME/CFS patients, there is little evidence on the efficacy of interventions in ME/CFS patients with respect to function and disability.

The efficacy of cognitive-behavioral therapy (CBT) in improving cognitive function in ME/CFS patients is unclear. Knoop and colleagues (2007) found a decrease in self-reported cognitive impairment following CBT, yet ME/CFS patients did not differ from a support control group on results of the subscale of alertness behavior of the Sickness Impact Profile (SIP-ab). These results do not preclude the use of CBT to mitigate cognitive impairment in ME/CFS, but they do suggest that any effects of CBT may not be measurable by a single scale such as the SIP-ab.

A systematic review showed that while a few studies found improvement in symptoms over time, no variables, including gender or length of illness, predicted improvement or positive work or functional outcomes (Ross et al., 2002). Furthermore, analysis of existing studies revealed no evidence of treatments effective at restoring the ability to work. Another systematic review found that the placebo response is lower in behavioral intervention studies than in medical intervention studies of patients with ME/CFS (Cho et al., 2005).

Consistent with the findings of the systematic review of Ross and colleagues (2002, 2004), studies reviewed by Taylor and Kielhofner (2005) provided no evidence regarding the efficacy of employment rehabilitation, such as CBT and/or graded exercise therapy. Variation in methodologies, outcome measures, subject selection criteria, and other factors precluded drawing conclusions about the efficacy of interventions designed to enable ME/CFS patients to return to work.

SUMMARY

ME/CFS clearly impairs patients' ability to function on a regular basis both cognitively and physically. This impairment often confines patients to their homes or beds and may severely restrict their ability to attend to their jobs or schoolwork, among other responsibilities and basic needs. Recovery is a highly variable and generally lengthy process with no standard course of treatment, and some patients' symptoms may persist indefinitely. Health care providers should be familiar with SSA's guidelines for evaluating disability and recognize that diagnosis alone is not sufficient for receiving a disability status.

REFERENCES

Adamowicz, J. L., I. Caikauskaite, and F. Friedberg. 2014. Defining recovery in chronic fatigue syndrome: A critical review. *Quality of Life Research* 23(9):2407-2416.

American Academy of Pediatrics. 1999. The pediatrician's role in development and implementation of an Individual Education Plan (IEP) and/or an Individual Family Service Plan (IFSP). *American Academy of Pediatrics* 104(1, Pt. 1):124-127.

Andersen, M. M., H. Permin, and F. Albrecht. 2004. Illness and disability in Danish chronic fatigue syndrome patients at diagnosis and 5-year follow-up. *Journal of Psychosomatic Research* 56(2):217-229.

Bell, D. S., K. Jordan, and M. Robinson. 2001. Thirteen-year follow-up of children and adolescents with chronic fatigue syndrome. *Pediatrics* 107(5):994-998.

Bombardier, C. H., and D. Buchwald. 1995. Outcome and prognosis of patients with chronic fatigue vs chronic fatigue syndrome. *Archives of Internal Medicine* 155(19):2105-2110.

Bringsli, G. J., A. M. Gilje, and B. K. Getz Wold. 2014. *The Norwegian ME Association National Survey: Abridged English version.* Oslo, Norway: The Norwegian ME Association.

Brown, M. M., D. S. Bell, L. A. Jason, C. Christos, and D. E. Bell. 2012. Understanding long-term outcomes of chronic fatigue syndrome. *Journal of Clinical Psychology* 68(9):1028-1035.

Cairns, R., and M. Hotopf. 2005. A systematic review describing the prognosis of chronic fatigue syndrome. *Occupational Medicine (Oxford)* 55(1):20-31.

Carruthers, B. M., A. K. Jain, K. L. De Meirleir, D. L. Peterson, N. G. Klimas, A. M. Lemer, A. C. Bested, P. Flor-Henry, P. Joshi, A. C. P. Powles, J. A. Sherkey, and M. I. van de Sande. 2003. Myalgic encephalomyelitis/chronic fatigue syndrome: Clinical working case definition, diagnostic and treatment protocols (Canadian case definition). *Journal of Chronic Fatigue Syndrome* 11(1):7-115.

Carruthers, B. M., M. I. van de Sande, K. L. De Meirleir, N. G. Klimas, G. Broderick, T. Mitchell, D. Staines, A. C. P. Powles, N. Speight, R. Vallings, L. Bateman, B. Baumgarten-Austrheim, D. S. Bell, N. Carlo-Stella, J. Chia, A. Darragh, D. Jo, D. Lewis, A. R. Light, S. Marshall-Gradisbik, I. Mena, J. A. Mikovits, K. Miwa, M. Murovska, M. L. Pall, and S. Stevens. 2011. Myalgic encephalomyelitis: International consensus criteria. *Journal of Internal Medicine* 270(4):327-338.

CFIDS (Chronic Fatigue and Immune Dysfunction Syndrome) Association of America. 2014. *ME/CFS road to diagnosis survey.* Charlotte, NC: CFIDS Association of America.

Cho, H. J., M. Hotopf, and S. Wessely. 2005. The placebo response in the treatment of chronic fatigue syndrome: A systematic review and meta-analysis. *Psychosomatic Medicine* 67(2):301-313.

Crawley, E., and J. A. Sterne. 2009. Association between school absence and physical function in paediatric chronic fatigue syndrome/myalgic encephalopathy. *Archives of Disease in Childhood* 94(10):752-756.

Crawley, E. M., A. M. Emond, and J. A. C. Sterne. 2011. Unidentified chronic fatigue syndrome/myalgic encephalomyelitis (CFS/ME) is a major cause of school absence: Surveillance outcomes from school-based clinics. *BMJ Open* 1(2).

Dowsett, E. G., and J. Colby. 1997. Long-term sickness absence due to ME/CFS in UK schools: An epidemiological study with medical and educational implications. *Journal of Chronic Fatigue Syndrome* 3(2):29-42.

Fukuda, K., S. E. Straus, I. Hickie, M. C. Sharpe, J. G. Dobbins, and A. Komaroff. 1994. The chronic fatigue syndrome: A comprehensive approach to its definition and study. *Annals of Internal Medicine* 121(12):953-959.

Ingerski, L. M., A. C. Modi, K. K. Hood, A. L. Pai, M. Zeller, C. Piazza-Waggoner, K. A. Driscoll, M. E. Rothenberg, J. Franciosi, and K. A. Hommel. 2010. Health-related quality of life across pediatric chronic conditions. *Journal of Pediatrics* 156(4):639-644.

Kennedy, G., C. Underwood, and J. J. Freda Belch. 2010. Physical and functional impact of chronic fatigue syndrome/myalgic encephalomyelitis in childhood. *Pediatrics* 125(6): e1324-e1330.

Knoop, H., J. B. Prins, M. Stulemeijer, J. W. M. van der Meer, and G. Bleijenberg. 2007. The effect of cognitive behaviour therapy for chronic fatigue syndrome on self-reported cognitive impairments and neuropsychological test performance. *Journal of Neurology, Neurosurgery & Psychiatry* 78(4):434-436.

ProHealth. 2008. *A profile of ME/CFS patients: How many years and how many doctors?* http://www.prohealth.com/library/showarticle.cfm?libid=13672 (accessed August 13, 2014).

Ross, S. D., C. Levine, N. Ganz, D. Frame, R. Estok, L. Stone, and V. Ludensky. 2002. Systematic review of the current literature related to disability and chronic fatigue syndrome. *Evidence Report/Technology Assessment (Summary)* (66):1-3.

Ross, S. D., R. P. Estok, D. Frame, L. R. Stone, V. Ludensky, and C. B. Levine. 2004. Disability and chronic fatigue syndrome: A focus on function. *Archives of Internal Medicine* 164(10):1098-1107.

Rowe, P., C. Marden, M. Flaherty, A. Johns, K. R. Fontaine, and R. Violand. 2014. Impact of adolescent chronic fatigue syndrome. Paper presented at IACFS/ME Biennial Conference, San Francisco, California.

Schweitzer, R., B. Kelly, A. Foran, D. Terry, and J. Whiting. 1995. Quality of life in chronic fatigue syndrome. *Social Science and Medicine* 41(10):1367-1372.

Smith, M. S., S. P. Martin-Herz, W. M. Womack, and J. L. Marsigan. 2003. Comparative study of anxiety, depression, somatization, functional disability, and illness attribution in adolescents with chronic fatigue or migraine. *Pediatrics* 111(4, Pt. 1):e376-e381.

Social Security Ruling. 2014. Social Security Ruling, SSR 14-1p; Titles II and XVI: Evaluating claims involving chronic fatigue syndrome (CFS). *Federal Register* 79(64):18750-18754.

Taylor, R. R., and G. W. Kielhofner. 2005. Work-related impairment and employment-focused rehabilitation options for individuals with chronic fatigue syndrome: A review. *Journal of Mental Health* 14(3):253-267.

Tiersky, L. A., J. DeLuca, N. Hill, S. K. Dhar, S. K. Johnson, G. Lange, G. Rappolt, and B. H. Natelson. 2001. Longitudinal assessment of neuropsychological functioning, psychiatric status, functional disability and employment status in chronic fatigue syndrome. *Applied Neuropsychology* 8(1):41-50.

Twisk, F. N. 2014. A definition of recovery in myalgic encephalomyelitis and chronic fatigue syndrome should be based upon objective measures. *Quality of Life Research* 23(9):2417-2418.

Unger, E. 2013. Measures of CFS in a multi-site clinical study. Paper read at FDA Scientific Drug Development Workshop, April 26, 2013, Washington, DC.

Varni, J. W., C. A. Limbers, and T. M. Burwinkle. 2007. Impaired health-related quality of life in children and adolescents with chronic conditions: A comparative analysis of 10 disease clusters and 33 disease categories/severities utilizing the PedsQL 4.0 generic core scales. *Health and Quality of Life Outcomes* 5:43.

Vercoulen, J. H. M. M., C. M. A. Swanink, J. F. M. Fennis, J. M. D. Galama, J. W. van der Meer, and G. Bleijenberg. 1996. Prognosis in chronic fatigue syndrome: A prospective study on the natural course. *Journal of Neurology, Neurosurgery & Psychiatry* 60(5):489-494.

D

Questionnaires and Tools That May Be Useful for Assessing ME/CFS Symptoms[1]

---

[1] Further evidence of utility is needed.

Symptoms/Manifestations	Tools or Questionnaires	Access Link
Fatigue	The Chalder Fatigue Scale[a]	http://www.goodmedicine.org.uk/files/assessment,%20chalder%20fatigue%20scale.pdf
	Multidimensional Fatigue Inventory[a]	http://www.cdc.gov/cfs/pdf/wichita-data-access/mfi-doc.pdf
	Fisk Fatigue Impact Scale[a]	http://www.actaneurologica.be/acta/download/2003-4/01-Kos%20et%20al.pdf
	The Krupp Fatigue Severity Scale[a]	http://www.abiebr.com/set/17-assessment-outcomes-following-acquiredtraumatic-brain-injury/177-fatigue-severity-scale-fss
	Checklist of Individual Strength[b]	http://www.ncbi.nlm.nih.gov/pmc/articles/PMC1739950/pdf/v057p00353.pdf
	DePaul Symptom Questionnaire[b,c]	http://condor.depaul.edu/ljason/cfs
	CDC Symptom Inventory for CFS[b,c]	http://www.institutferran.org/documentos/cdc_full_symptom_inventory.pdf
	NOVA form[d]	http://www.nova.edu/nim/patients/forms/fatigue-scale.pdf
Substantial decrease or impairment in function: adults	Work and Social Adjustment Scale (WSAS)[a]	serene.me.uk/tests/wsas.pdf
	Energy Index Point Score[a]	http://www.treatmentcenterforcfs.com/energy_index_score
	SF-36[b] (RAND-36 is available as a free version of SF-36)	http://www.sf-36.org/tools/pdf/SF-6v1_Standard_Sample.pdf
	The Lawton Instrumental Activities of Daily Living (IADL) Scale[d]	http://consultgerirn.org/uploads/File/trythis/try_this_23.pdf
	Katz Index of Independence in Activities of Daily Living[d]	http://clas.uiowa.edu/socialwork/files/socialwork/NursingHomeResource/documents/Katz%20ADL_LawtonIADL.pdf
	FIQR (Fibromyalgia Impact Questionnaire Revised)[d]	http://fiqrinfo.ipage.com/FIQR%20FORM.pdf
Substantial decrease or impairment in function: children	Short form of the Child Health Questionnaire[b]	http://jech.bmj.com/content/59/1/75.full.pdf+html
	Pediatrics Quality of Life Inventory (PedsQL)[d]	http://www.pedsql.org

	Functional Disability Inventory (FDI)[d]	http://www.commondataelements.ninds.nih.gov/Doc/NOC/Functional_Disability_Inventory_Parent_Form_NOC_Request.pdf
Post-exertional malaise	CDC Symptom Inventory for CFS[b,c]	http://www.institutferran.org/documentos/cdc_full_symptom_inventory.pdf
	DePaul symptom questionnaire[b,c]	http://condor.depaul.edu/jason/cfs
Sleep problems	Sleep Assessment Questionnaire[d]	http://www.completehealthsleep.com/DesktopModules/DocumentViewer/Documents%5CDocumentId5_%5CSleep%20Assessment%20Questionnaire.pdf
	Pittsburgh Sleep Quality Index (PSQI)[d]	http://consultgerirn.org/uploads/File/trythis/try_this_6_1.pdf
	PROMIS Sleep questionnaire[d]	http://www.ncbi.nlm.nih.gov/pmc/articles/PMC3261577/pdf/nihms335121.pdf
Cognitive symptoms	Wood Mental Fatigue Inventory[a]	http://www.pubfacts.com/detail/7902751/A-brief-mental-fatigue-questionnaire
	Checklist Individual Strength Questionnaire[b]	http://www.ncbi.nlm.nih.gov/pmc/articles/PMC1739950/pdf/v057p00353.pdf
	The Cognitive Failures Questionnaire[b]	http://www.yorku.ca/rokada/psyctest/cogfail.pdf
Orthostatic intolerance	Orthostatic Grading Scale[d]	http://www.thestudentroom.co.uk/attachment.php?attachmentid=139109&d=1333233284
	COMPASS 31[d]	http://www.nymc.edu/fhp/centers/syncope/COMPASS%2031.pdf

continued

Symptoms/ Manifestations	Tools or Questionnaires	Access Link
Pain	PROMIS[b]	http://www.assessmentcenter.net
	SF-36[b]	http://www.sf-36.org/tools/pdf/SF-6v1_Standard_Sample.pdf
	McGill Pain Questionnaire[d]	http://www.ama-cmeonline.com/pain_mgmt/pdf/mcgill.pdf
	Brief Pain Inventory[d]	http://www.npcrc.org/files/news/briefpain_short.pdf
	Pain diagram[d]	http://alaska.providence.org/locations/pvmc/Documents/Pain%20Diagram.pdf

[a] Questionnaires used or tested in ME/CFS patients that may be useful tools in a clinical setting.
[b] Questionnaires used or tested in ME/CFS patients that may be difficult to apply in a clinical setting.
[c] Questionnaires that evaluate the full range of ME/CFS symptomatology (fatigue, decrease in function, post-exertional malaise [PEM], sleep problems, cognitive symptoms, pain).
[d] Questionnaires not formally tested in ME/CFS patients that may be useful tools in a clinical setting.

E

Biographical Sketches of Committee Members, Consultants, and Staff

COMMITTEE MEMBERS

Ellen Wright Clayton, M.D., J.D. (*Chair*) is an internationally respected leader in the field of law and genetics who holds appointments in both the law and medical schools at Vanderbilt University, where she also co-founded the Center for Biomedical Ethics and Society. She has published 2 books and more than 100 scholarly articles and chapters in medical journals, interdisciplinary journals, and law journals on the intersection of law, medicine, and public health. In addition, she has collaborated with faculty and students throughout Vanderbilt and in many institutions around the country and the world on interdisciplinary research projects and has helped to develop policy statements for numerous national and international organizations. An active participant in policy debates, she has advised the National Institutes of Health (NIH) as well as other federal and international bodies on an array of topics ranging from children's health to the ethical conduct of research involving human subjects. Professor Clayton has worked on a number of projects for the Institute of Medicine (IOM), five of which she has chaired or co-chaired, and she is currently a member of the IOM Council. She is an elected fellow of the American Academy for the Advancement of Science.

Margarita Alegría, Ph.D., is the director of the Center for Multicultural Mental Health Research at Cambridge Health Alliance and a professor in the Department of Psychiatry at Harvard Medical School. Dr. Alegría has an extensive publishing history, with more than 200 titles that include journal articles, book chapters, editorials, and research training manuals focused on services research, conceptual and methodological issues with minority populations, ways to bring the community's perspective into the design and implementation of health services, and disparities in service delivery. She is also on the editorial board of *Health Services Research* and served as the guest editor of the June 2012 supplemental issue. In addition to her partnerships and collaborations, research work, and publishing, Dr. Alegría has continued her commitment to mentoring and training. She has mentored more than 50 pre- and postdoctoral faculty members, trainees, and junior investigators whose interests are in disparities and other emerging concerns in the mental health field, such as immigration, acculturation, and the role of culture and context in both illness and treatment. She has received several Robert Wood Johnson Foundation grants, which have greatly enabled her mentoring work to continue. She has been recognized for her mentoring leadership with the 2011 Excellence in Hispanic Mental Health Research Advocacy and Leadership award by the National Resource Center for Hispanic Mental Health and the 2011 Excellence in Mentorship award by the National Hispanic Science Network. Dr. Alegría has been honored nationally with the 2003 Mental Health Section Award of the American Public Health Association, the 2006 Greenwood Award for Research Excellence from the Research Centers in Minority Institutions Program Directors Association, and the 2008 American Psychological Association's Presidential Recognition Award. She received international recognition when she was appointed as a member of the IOM in 2011.

Lucinda Bateman, M.S., M.D., is an internal medicine doctor at the Fatigue Consultation Clinic in Salt Lake City, Utah. She completed medical school at the Johns Hopkins School of Medicine and internal medicine residency at the University of Utah and was certified by the American Board of Internal Medicine. She practiced general internal medicine until 2000, when she changed her focus to the diagnosis and management of chronic fatigue, chronic fatigue syndrome (CFS), and fibromyalgia syndrome (FMS). Dr. Bateman's goal in establishing her Fatigue Consultation Clinic and the nonprofit OFFER (Organization for Fatigue & Fibromyalgia Education & Research) was to encourage a thoughtful evaluation process, better sharing of information, and more research efforts aimed at understanding the cause(s) and treatment of CFS and FMS. In addition to being co-founder, executive director, and board chair of the Utah-based nonprofit OFFER, she has been on the boards of the CFIDS Association of America and the International Association for Chronic Fatigue Syndrome/Myalgic Encephalomyelitis (IACFS/ME), and was board chair of Easter Seals of Utah.

Lily Chu, M.D., M.S., is a board member of IACFS/ME and Stanford University's ME/CFS Initiative. She has a background in internal/geriatric medicine and public health. She graduated from the University of Washington with a B.S. (molecular and cellular biology) and an M.D.; trained in internal medicine at the University of Rochester (New York) and in geriatric medicine at the University of California, Los Angeles (UCLA); and obtained an M.S. in health services research, also while at UCLA. Dr. Chu has experience working in academic, small private, the Veterans Health Administration, and large integrated multispecialty health care systems. She is interested in all aspects of ME/CFS, ranging from pathophysiology, diagnosis, and treatment to epidemiology, health care provider education, and access to quality medical care. Dr. Chu also has personal experience with ME/CFS.

Charles S. Cleeland, Ph.D., is a McCullough professor of cancer research and chair, Department of Symptom Research, at the University of Texas MD Anderson Cancer Center. He is a leader in the area of cancer symptom epidemiology, assessment, and treatment. He has directed epidemiological studies of pain and other symptoms in patients with cancer; studies of the mechanisms of pain and other symptoms; studies using positron emission tomography (PET) and functional magnetic resonance imaging (fMRI) to examine the effects of pain on cortical activity; and clinical trials aimed at reducing the risk of inadequate symptom control, including in underserved populations. Dr. Cleeland is a member and past president of the board of directors of the U.S. Cancer Pain Relief Committee. He is also past president of the American Pain Society. His research is widely published. He has published numerous studies on the prevalence and severity of cancer symptoms, on U.S. and international symptom management practice patterns, and on potential biological mechanisms underlying the symptoms produced by cancer and its treatment.

Ronald W. Davis, Ph.D., is a professor of biochemistry and genetics at the Stanford University School of Medicine in Stanford, California. He is a world leader in the development of biotechnology, especially the development of recombinant DNA and genomic methodologies and their application to biological systems. At Stanford University, where he is director of the Stanford Genome Technology Center, Dr. Davis focuses on the interface of nano-fabricated solid state devices and biological systems. He and his research team also develop novel technologies for the genetic, genomic, and molecular analysis of a wide range of model organisms as well as humans. The team's focus on practical application of these technologies is setting the standard for clinical genomics.

Betty Diamond, M.D., is chief of the Autoimmune Disease Center at the Feinstein Institute for Medical Research. She graduated with a B.A. from Harvard University and an M.D. from Harvard Medical School. She performed a residency in internal medicine at New York-Presbyterian/ Columbia University Medical Center and received postdoctoral training in immunology at the Albert Einstein College of Medicine. Dr. Diamond has headed the rheumatology divisions at the Albert Einstein School of Medicine and at Columbia University Medical Center. She also directed the Medical Scientist Training Program at the Albert Einstein School of Medicine for many years. She is currently head of the Center for Auto-immune and Musculoskeletal Diseases at the Feinstein Institute for Medical Research and director of the Ph.D. and M.D./Ph.D. programs at the Hofstra North Shore–LIJ School of Medicine. A former president of the American Association of Immunology, Dr. Diamond has also served on the board of directors of the American College of Rheumatology and the Scientific Council of the National Institute of Arthritis and Musculoskeletal and Skin Diseases. She is a fellow of the American Association for the Advancement of Science and a member of the IOM.

Theodore G. Ganiats, M.D., is a professor in the Department of Family Medicine and Community Health at the University of Miami Miller School of Medicine. Dr. Ganiats attended the University of California, San Diego, School of Medicine, where he completed both his medical degree and his family medicine residency. He is a member of many professional associa-tions, including the Society for Medical Decision Making, Academy Health, the American Public Health Association, and the International Society for Quality of Life Research. Dr. Ganiats's research interests are in out-comes research, focusing on quality-of-life assessment and cost-effectiveness analysis. He has delivered more than 100 lectures throughout the United States and Europe. In addition, he was a member or chair of more than 50 national guideline and quality/performance panels spanning multiple disciplines. He has published more than 100 manuscripts in peer-reviewed journals, such as *Diabetes Care*, *Medical Care*, and the *American Journal of Preventive Medicine*. Dr. Ganiats is currently on the editorial boards of the *Journal of Family Practice* and *Family Practice News* and is a member of the IOM.

Betsy Keller, Ph.D., is a professor in the Department of Exercise & Sport Sciences at Ithaca College in New York. She received her Ph.D. in exercise science from the University of Massachusetts Amherst. Her research has focused on physical inactivity and obesity in children, wellness in older adults, occupational physiology, and ME/CFS. For the past 10 years she has tested persons ill with ME/CFS for purposes of research and/or to provide an objective assessment of functional capacity and ability to perform and recover following physical work. Recently, she collaborated on an NIH R21 grant to study the effects of physical activity in ME/CFS on parameters of physiological and immune function. Dr. Keller has given many scientific, invited, and lay presentations on physical inactivity and obesity; the effects of ME/CFS on physiological and physical function; and the role of physical activity in health, wellness, physical function, and injury prevention. She is a fellow of the American College of Sports Medicine (ACSM), past member of the Board of Trustees of ACSM, and past president and former department chair of the Mid-Atlantic Regional Chapter of ACSM.

Nancy Klimas, M.D., is chair of clinical immunology at Nova Southeastern University (NSU). She is one of the world's leading researchers and clinicians in ME/CFS and recently joined the faculty of NSU's College of Osteopathic Medicine. An expert in immune disorders, Dr. Klimas retired from the University of Miami as professor emeritus to establish the NSU College of Osteopathic Medicine's Institute for Neuro-Immune Medicine, which is conducting cutting-edge research and treats patients suffering from ME/CFS and Gulf War illness, as well as other immunologic disorders. Dr. Klimas is director of research for the clinical AIDS/HIV and Gulf War illness research programs at the Miami Veterans Affairs Medical Center. She is immediate past president of the IACFS/ME, an organization of researchers and clinicians dedicated to furthering knowledge of this disabling illness. She continues to work nationally and internationally to bring a better understanding of ME/CFS to clinicians and policy makers.

A. Martin Lerner, M.D., M.A.C.P., is a professor of infectious diseases at Oakland University William Beaumont School of Medicine. He is certified by the American Board of Internal Medicine. He was resident in internal medicine, Washington University in St. Louis, 1954-1955, and U.S. Public Health Service assistant surgeon, Laboratory of Infectious Diseases, NIH, 1955-1957. He was awarded a 1-year fellowship in molecular biology under the direction of Dr. James Darnell at the Massachusetts Institute of Technology, 1962-1963. Dr. Lerner was Commonwealth of Massachusetts fellow in infectious diseases, Dr. Maxwell Finland sponsor, Harvard Medical School, 1958-1963. He was chief of the Division of Infectious Diseases and professor of internal medicine at Wayne State University School of Medicine from 1963 to 1982. He established a clinical virology laboratory and trained 33 physicians in the subspecialty of infectious diseases at Wayne State University from 1963 to 1982. Dr. Lerner was an elected member of the American Society for Clinical Investigation, American Association of Physicians. He was also a member of the committee that prepared the National Boards in Medical Examiners, US; a member of the training grant committee, National Institute of Allergy and Infectious Diseases, NIH; and governor for the Michigan American College of Physicians, 1991-1994. Dr. Lerner is honorary master of the American College of Physicians. The Dr. A. Martin Lerner CFS Foundation was formed to ensure that his past 25 years of CFS-specific work would be recognized and communicated to CFS sufferers and physicians worldwide. The foundation, established in early 2007, conducted a major study that documented Dr. Lerner's successful antiviral subset treatment. The foundation officially closed in July 2011 after achieving its projected objectives. Dr. Lerner's work in CFS continues.

Cynthia Mulrow, M.D., M.Sc., is senior deputy editor of *Annals of Internal Medicine* and adjunct professor of medicine at the University of Texas Health Science Center at San Antonio. She has been program director of the Robert Wood Johnson Foundation Generalist Physician Faculty Scholars Program and director of the San Antonio Cochrane Collaboration Center and the San Antonio Evidence-based Practice Center. Dr. Mulrow was elected to the American Society of Clinical Investigation in 1997; served as a member of the U.S. Preventive Services Task Force, 1998-2002; was honored as a master of the American College of Physicians in 2005; and was elected to the IOM in 2008. Her academic work focuses on systematic reviews, practice guidelines, research methodology, and chronic medical conditions. She contributes to several groups that set standards for reporting research: PRISMA (systematic reviews and meta-analyses), STROBE (observational studies), and CONSORT (clinical trials).

Benjamin H. Natelson, M.D., received his bachelor's and medical degrees at the University of Pennsylvania in Philadelphia and then did his neurology residency at the Albert Einstein College of Medicine in New York City. He then completed two postdoctoral fellowships: one in behavioral neurosciences at the Cornell University Medical Center in White Plains, New York, and one in physiologic psychology at the Walter Reed Army Institute of Research in Washington, DC. He then moved to the New Jersey Medical School in Newark and the Veterans Affairs Medical Center in East Orange. He rose through the ranks, attaining the position of professor of neurosciences in 1981, and leaving in 2008 as an emeritus professor. Dr. Natelson had continual funding from the Department of Veterans Affairs through 1999 for his experimental work on stress and chronobiology. With the award of a federally funded research center to explore the causes of CFS in 1991, he shifted his research to studies of people with CFS and more recently has extended those studies to include people with fibromyalgia. Dr. Natelson served as president of the Pavlovian Society, the Academy of Behavioral Medicine Research, and the IACFS/ME. He has had more than 250 papers published in peer-reviewed journals and has authored 3 books for lay audiences. In 2008, Dr. Natelson moved his activities to the Department of Pain Medicine and Palliative Care at Mount Sinai Beth Israel in Manhattan, where he directs the Pain & Fatigue Study Center. In that capacity, he is also a professor of neurology at the Icahn School of Medicine at Mount Sinai.

Peter Rowe, M.D., has directed the Chronic Fatigue Clinic at the Johns Hopkins Children's Center since 1996 and is the inaugural recipient of the Sunshine Natural Wellbeing Foundation Chair in Chronic Fatigue and Related Disorders. He graduated from McMaster University Medical School, Hamilton, Ontario, Canada, in 1981. From 1981 to 1987, he was a resident, general academic pediatrics research fellow, and chief resident in pediatrics at Johns Hopkins Hospital. Between 1987 and 1991, he was a staff member at the Children's Hospital of Eastern Ontario, Ottawa, and an assistant professor of epidemiology and community medicine and of pediatrics. Dr. Rowe returned to Johns Hopkins University in 1991. His work focuses on conditions characterized by chronic fatigue, particularly the relationship between CFS and treatable orthostatic intolerance syndromes, as well as the association between Ehlers-Danlos syndrome and CFS. His work has been funded by NIH, the Department of Defense, and the CFIDS Association of America, as well as by private donations.

Michael Shelanski, M.D., Ph.D., serves as chairman of the department of pathology and cell biology at Columbia University, co-director of the Taub Institute, and director of the Medical Scientist Training Program. He is a member of the American Society for Cell Biology, the American Society for Investigative Pathology, the Association of American Physicians, and the IOM. Dr. Shelanski's laboratory has been responsible for the identification and purification of several of the major cytoskeletal proteins and has served as a training ground for a number of outstanding scholars of the neurode-generations. The laboratory is using a combination of cell biological and molecular biological approaches to unravel the pathways of "cell suicide" or apoptosis in Alzheimer's disease and other neurodegenerations, to understand the alterations in gene expression that occur in these diseases, and to dissect the regulation of synaptic responses in these diseases.

CONSULTANTS

Rona Briere has worked as an independent writer/editor for the National Academies and numerous governmental and private organizations since 1980. During that time, she also has taught courses in report writing and editing at the National Academies and elsewhere. She is the author of the texts *Writing to Inform and Persuade* and *Writing with Clarity and Precision*. Ms. Briere received her undergraduate degree from Syracuse University and her graduate degrees from Johns Hopkins University.

René Gonin, Ph.D., is a senior biostatistician, academician, and medical researcher with 35 years of experience. He has directed or conducted methodological statistical and medical research, primarily in the areas of hematology and oncology (including surgical and radiation oncology). He has also conducted collaborative research in dermatology, infectious diseases (including HIV), nephrology, radiology, gastroenterology, ophthalmology, and nursing (behavioral and cancer control). At Westat Inc., he was principal investigator for the National Institute of Neurological Disorders and Stroke (NINDS) Pilot Therapeutics Network Clinical Operations Center (NPTUNE COC). This network is undertaking early phase I, I/II, and II trials in neuromuscular diseases. Dr. Gonin collaborated on analyses for the Disability Evaluation Study, sponsored by the Social Security Administration, particularly in developing a measure of Social Security Disability using Rasch partial credit models. Before joining Westat in 1997, Dr. Gonin served as director of biostatistics at the Indiana University (IU) Cancer Center and as associate professor of medicine at the IU School of Medicine. Between 1989 and 1993, he served concurrently as assistant professor in the Department of Biostatistics at the Harvard School of Public Health and at the Dana-Farber Cancer Institute. During his tenure, he was a collaborating statistician in the Eastern Cooperative Oncology Group, with overall responsibilities for cancer control and health practices. At Dana-Farber, he had several responsibilities, including oversight of the bone marrow transplant program (allogeneic and autologous). Dr. Gonin has extensive experience in the design and analysis of phase I through III clinical trials and in behavior and health practices studies, and has more than 100 publications to his name. He also has many years of experience in the field of nonlinear optimization and numerical analysis.

Troy Petenbrink is a seasoned marketing communications specialist at Caduceus Marketing. His more than 20 years of experience combines in-house, agency, and consulting roles, whereby he has developed strong brand-building and results-driven skills. He has helped shape issues ranging from increasing awareness of HIV, by creating National HIV Testing Day, to fighting underage drinking, by preserving the voluntary ban on alcohol commercials on network television. His clients have included the National Library of Medicine, the American Society for Parenteral and Enteral Nutrition, the National Certification Commission for Acupuncture and Oriental Medicine, and the Global Virus Network.

IOM STAFF

Sulvia Doja, M.S.H.C.P.M., is a senior program assistant in the Board on the Health of Select Populations at the IOM. She began working as a senior program assistant for the present study in May 2014. She earned her M.S. degree in health care policy and management from Carnegie Mellon University's H. John Heinz III College and her undergraduate degree in biology with a minor in chemistry from Chatham College. Before coming to the IOM, Ms. Doja researched the effect of national health care reform on American Indian and Alaska Native populations and pioneered a social media marketing outlet designed to increase customer visibility and enhance communication with those populations.

Frederick (Rick) Erdtmann, M.D., M.P.H., is the director of the Board on the Health of Select Populations at the Institute of Medicine (IOM). Prior to joining the IOM he was a career military physician in the U.S. Army. While in the military he served as chief of several large departments of preventive medicine at U.S. installations at home and overseas. He also was commander of the military community hospital at Fort Carson, Colorado, and later served as hospital commander for the Walter Reed Army Medical Center. He had several assignments at the Army Surgeon General's Office working on military health care policies. He received his undergraduate degree from Bucknell University and an M.P.H. degree from the University of California, Berkeley. He is a graduate of the Temple University Medical School and is board certified in the specialty of preventive medicine.

Kate Meck, M.P.H., is an associate program officer in the Board on the Health of Select Populations at the IOM. Prior to joining the Board on the Health of Select Populations, Ms. Meck spent 5 years with the IOM's Board on Global Health, where she is wrapping up a workshop report on large-scale program evaluation methods and a report on preventing a tobacco epidemic in Africa. She previously worked on an IOM study that produced an evaluation of the President's Emergency Plan for AIDS Relief and with the Committee on the U.S. Commitment to Global Health. Ms. Meck received her B.A. in international relations from American University and her M.P.H. in global health program design, monitoring, and evaluation from the George Washington University School of Public Health and Health Services.

Adriana Moya is a senior program assistant in the Board on the Health of Select Populations at the IOM. Prior to joining the IOM, Ms. Moya spent a summer during her undergraduate career at the Fred Hutchinson Cancer

Research Center (FHCRC) in Seattle, Washington. As a research intern at FHCRC, she worked on the Thompson studies, focusing on the prevention of cancer disparities among minorities in Washington State's Yakima Valley. She received her B.A. in political science with a minor in public health from the George Washington University Columbian College of Arts and Science.

Carmen C. Mundaca-Shah, M.D., Dr.P.H., is a senior program officer with the IOM's Board on the Health of Select Populations. Prior to directing the present study, she served as a postdoctoral fellow with the IOM's Board on Global Health on the *Outcome and Impact Evaluation of Global HIV/AIDS Programs Implemented Under the Lantos-Hyde Act of 2008.* Prior to joining the IOM, Dr. Mundaca-Shah was employed as head of the Surveillance Center of the Emerging Infections Program in the U.S. Naval Medical Research Unit 6 in Lima, Peru. In that role, she led the successful implementation of a technology-based disease surveillance system (Alerta) at sites across the nation and initiated the broad adoption of Alerta in five other countries in South America. Alerta is a partnership involving the Peruvian Navy and the U.S. Navy. Dr. Mundaca-Shah also led the collaborative syndromic surveillance pilot implementation in the Peruvian Ministry of Health. She was part of the Early Warning Outbreak Recognition System (EWORS) Working Group and participated in several studies, including a field visit to evaluate the performance of the system in Lao People's Democratic Republic. She obtained her M.D. from San Marcos University, Lima, Peru, and her M.P.H. and Dr.P.H. degrees from the Uniformed Services University of the Health Sciences, Bethesda, Maryland. Her dissertation work focused on developing a framework that will serve as a guideline for the implementation of disease surveillance systems in developing countries. Dr. Mundaca-Shah completed a certificate in emerging infectious disease epidemiology at the University of Iowa.

Jonathan Schmelzer, M.P.H., is a research associate at the IOM. He has worked at the IOM since January 2010, providing administrative and research support on several studies addressing environmental exposures, health outcomes, program evaluation, and treatment guidelines. Mr. Schmelzer holds a B.A. in political science from Miami University and an M.P.H. in epidemiology from George Washington University.